Migration and Health

Migration and Health

EDITED BY SANDRO GALEA,
CATHERINE K. ETTMAN,
AND MUHAMMAD H. ZAMAN

THE UNIVERSITY OF CHICAGO PRESS   CHICAGO AND LONDON

The University of Chicago Press, Chicago 60637
The University of Chicago Press, Ltd., London
© 2022 by The University of Chicago
Published 2022
Printed in the United States of America

31 30 29 28 27 26 25 24 23 22   1 2 3 4 5

ISBN-13: 978-0-226-82248-8 (cloth)
ISBN-13: 978-0-226-82250-1 (paper)
ISBN-13: 978-0-226-82249-5 (e-book)
DOI: https://doi.org/10.7208/chicago/9780226822495.001.0001

Library of Congress Cataloging-in-Publication Data

Names: Galea, Sandro, editor. | Ettman, Catherine K., editor. | Zaman, Muhammad H.
    (Muhammad Hamid), editor.
Title: Migration and health / edited by Sandro Galea, Catherine K. Ettman, and
    Muhammad H. Zaman.
Description: Chicago ; London : The University of Chicago Press, 2022. |
    Includes bibliographical references and index.
Identifiers: LCCN 2022015149 | ISBN 9780226822488 (cloth) | ISBN 9780226822501
    (paperback) | ISBN 9780226822495 (e-book)
Subjects: LCSH: Emigration and immigration—Health aspects. | Immigrants—
    Health and hygiene. | Immigrants—Medical care.
Classification: LCC RA408.M5 M524 2022 | DDC 362.1086/912—dc23/eng/20220502
LC record available at https://lccn.loc.gov/2022015149

♾ This paper meets the requirements of ANSI/NISO z39.48-1992 (Permanence of Paper).

Contents

PART I

Why Migration and Health?

CHAPTER ONE

An Introduction to Migration and Health

Sandro Galea, Catherine K. Ettman, and Muhammad H. Zaman

1.0 Introduction

Population migration — the movement of people across and within borders — has long been, remains today, and will likely continue to be one of the central demographic shifts shaping the world around us. It is therefore unsurprising that population migration is also associated with the health of populations. The world's history — and its health — is shaped and colored by stories of migration patterns, the policies and political events that drive these movements, and narratives of individual migrants. Petroglyphs in Azerbaijan, more than ten thousand years old, depict humans migrating.[1] Europeans' migration to the Americas resulted in widespread infectious disease outbreaks, affecting the health of millions of native Americans and also changing the history of the world as the Americas emerged as an important center of geopolitical power. Marie Curie migrated from her native Poland to Paris, where she carried out groundbreaking science, doing work that was instrumental to establishing radiology and becoming the first person in history to receive two Nobel Prizes. These are just some examples of the formidable influence of migration on human advancement.

2.0 The Global Demographics of Migration

Migration, therefore, is an indelible part of human history. It is increasingly so today. Together with population aging and urbanization, the movement of people within countries and across international borders is rapidly coming to define the mid-twenty-first century. A brief summary of the current demographics of migration illustrates the scope of the impact migration has on the world.[2] It is estimated that there are 272 million international migrants today, about 3.5 percent of the world's population. This is an increase from the 258 million international migrants in 2017, which itself was a 50 percent increase since 2000. If international migrants made up one country today, they would be the fifth largest country in the world after China, India, the United States, and Indonesia.

The countries that are the largest recipients of migrants overall are the United States, followed by Saudi Arabia, Germany, and the Russian Federation. One hundred forty-one million—more than half—of all international migrants live in Europe or North America. In North America, more than 40 percent of population growth is accounted for by positive net migration. India, Mexico, and China are the countries with the largest number of migrants living abroad. Internal migration represents an even larger flow of populations globally, with about 750 million persons being internal migrants. Taking internal and external migration together, about one in seven people globally are migrants. A number of cities now house more people from other countries than those who are native to the country itself, and it has become unsurprising to find foods from all corners of the world readily available in global cities.

Out of the 272 million international migrants globally in 2019, 74 percent were between the ages of twenty and sixty-four (i.e., working age adults who contribute substantially to the economies of their country of origin and their host country). Global remittances sent by migrants back to their country of origin topped 689 billion US dollars in 2018, with the top three remittance recipients being India, China, and Mexico. The United States is the leading remittance-sending country, consistent with its status as the country receiving the most migrants, followed by the United Arab Emirates and Saudi Arabia. There is substantial variability in migration patterns from region to region. Most international migrants born in Asia, Africa, and Europe stay within their regions of birth, while the majority of migrants from Latin America, the Caribbean, and North America live outside their regions of birth. The number of refugee and asylum seekers is estimated at around 14 percent of the total number of migrants. The Syrian Arab Republic was the origin—and Turkey the recipient—of most refugees globally. Canada is the country that hosts the most permanently resettled refugees.

Such large population demographic shifts might be reasonably expected to affect many aspects of populations, including how cities are organized and evolve, who lives in rural areas, the foods we eat, the people in our neighborhood, and our social networks. These shifts also have been responsible for some of the most heated political rhetoric of the past decade, as nativist political leaders all over the world have used an "othering" of migrants to drive narrow political agendas, resulting in seismic political shifts ranging from the United Kingdom to China. Several chapters in this book present data about the impact of migration on demographic shifts and how those demographic shifts are shaping the world around us.

3.0 Key Definitions in Migration

Chapters of this book make use of definitions relevant to migration that are particular to their area of inquiry and reflect the substantial variability in the realities of migration within and across regions. However, we recognize, as have others, that some of these definitions may present challenges in measurement and comparability across contexts.[3] Therefore, we offer a brief synthesis of the most relevant definitions around migration. At the most fundamental level, *migration* refers to the movement of people, individually or in groups, as well as persons moving within or between countries. The International Organization for Migration defines a *migrant* as anyone who has moved either across borders or to a state outside the person's habitual residence.[4] Migration can be voluntary or involuntary, transient or permanent. Short-term migration is generally considered to be three to twelve months, while more than twelve months is considered to be long-term. People may pass through several countries and stay for varying periods of time in several states before eventually reaching a place where they live for an extended period. In the past two decades, circular migration has also become more common, with migrants moving temporarily for economic opportunities and returning to their home countries.

Migration can happen for any range of reasons, such as economic or environmental, and can be initiated by the migrants themselves or by official efforts to expel them from their home country. Forced migration is generally considered to be migration that is propelled by an external compelling reason, such as violence or disasters. Voluntary migration is, in contrast, considered to be migration initiated at the person's choice. The boundaries demarcating these definitions are clearly not rigid and have evolved over the years. While a person who is migrating to improve economic context may not be forced to migrate, it is entirely plausible that that person felt little choice but to migrate to improve their or their children's opportunity set. A forced migrant may also become an economic migrant during the course of his or her lifetime or even in the course of the journey. In addition, formal definitions distinguish between internal migration (movement within a country) and external migration (movement across countries). Persons who are migrating across nation states owing to fear of persecution for reasons of race, religion, nationality, or membership in a particular group are called refugees. Persons who are awaiting decisions on their refugee status are called asylum seekers. We refer the reader who is interested to some very good work that includes more comprehensive definitions of different types of migrants,[5] as well as official United Nations reports on the topic.[6]

4.0 This Book's Approach

There is a growing body of scholarship in the field of migration and health, and more scholars are dedicating themselves to the field. This is all heartening and, to our minds, commensurate with the importance of this area of inquiry. Therefore, this book, grounded in the scholarship that has come before us, aims to be a comprehensive text that interrogates the complex relationship between migration and health, bringing to bear insights from across disciplines to do so. This book is predicated on the idea that understanding how migration affects health requires a comprehensive grappling with the processes that explain migration and a rigorous analysis of the consequences of migration for the health of populations.

Three observations may be helpfully grounding to readers of this book.

First, migration matters, and it matters to the health of populations. How migration intersects with and affects the health of populations is complex and is not readily reduced to simple summaries. This book is premised on the importance of the role migration plays in shaping health and also of the complexity of the relationship between migration and health.

It is important to note that the relation between migration and health cannot readily be reduced to simple risk factor and health outcome dichotomies. Migration is, in and of itself, not harmful to health, in much the same way that, for example, urbanization is not as a single entity harmful to health. Rather, there are features of migration that influence health—some positively, some negatively. What is of interest is not the reductive simplification of a linear, predictable relationship between migration and health, but rather a full understanding of the features and processes of migration that matter for the health of populations. One of the challenges with these ideas in a book such as this one is that the chapters are written by experts in one aspect of migration and health and the focus is often on why that aspect challenges the health of migrant populations. This may leave the reader with the impression that migration is a net negative, which is not the case. If it were, it is unlikely that migration would have long been such an important—and growing—force in the world. Migration in the net exists because migrants move to better and healthier lives. However, an exploration of migration and health casts a spotlight on the aspects of migration that negatively affect health with the goal of identifying those elements so that we can intervene and do better. Insofar as this book helps hold a magnifying glass to those processes, it is doing its job to help motivate action on improving the health of migrants.

Second, those affected by migration include both the receiving (host) populations and migrants themselves. That association, however, is not straightforward. There is the health of the migrants themselves. The health of migrants is a product of the migrants' baseline health—generally better than that of the population where the migrants came from—of the migration experience, and of the social, economic, mental, and physical conditions that the migrants encounter in their destination. There is also the health of the migrants' descendent groups. As populations assimilate in new environments, health behaviors and exposures change, often resulting in subsequent generations being less healthy than the migrants themselves. There are important issues in health access, nutrition, disease exposure, and health policies at the intersection of migrant and host populations that have short- and long-term impacts on the community as a whole. Communities are shaped and reshaped by waves of migration, changing local social and economic environments in a way that influences the health of all within these populations.

Third, this book builds on existing scholarship and expertise, aiming to be a synthesis of what we know and how we think and to push the field forward. Although we tried to address the dominant challenges in the field, the book is limited in areas where the field is limited. For one, the book, by design and intention, does not focus on either internal or global migration, as it considers the migratory journey—be it domestic or international—to be just one part of the set of forces shaping how migration affects health. That design tilts the chapters of the book to focus more on international migration than on intranational. This reflects the preponderance of academic work, and that is in turn driven by the much more readily apparent international migrant populations, rather than internal migrant populations. In a similar vein, the scholarship documented here represents more perspectives of migration from low- and middle-income countries to high- or higher-income countries than of migration among low- and middle-income countries. This reflects the state of the scholarship, but we note it here as a call for future action and as a marker for readers who are using this work to ground their learning in the field. And, finally, reflecting the state of the field, different chapters in the book sometimes bring different conceptual lenses and approaches to their subject matter. While this is a common challenge with edited volumes like this one, it is particularly true for a field that is as much in its infancy as is migration and health. This book aims to weave together data from different disciplines to create a framework for understanding the relationship between migration and health that can serve us well as we move to the middle of the twenty-first century, where migration is increasingly shaping where and how we live. Although we have worked with the chapter authors on harmonizing key aspects of each contribution to the broader agenda of this volume, we opted to allow for heterogeneity of perspective where there was such, leaving that to reflect genuine differences between authors, and respecting readers' discernment to develop their own narrative, informed by the state of the field.

This book is divided into six parts. First, we present a comprehensive framework from which the reader can understand the issue of migration and population health. Second, we discuss the mechanisms that intersect with migration to shape population health. Third, we discuss particular topics that intersect with migration and health—the domains in which migration's health impacts manifest. This part will discuss, for example, nutrition, aging, maternal and reproductive health, mental health, access to health care, and the health of children. The fourth part brings a methodologic lens to the topic, bringing together authors who approach the issue from different disciplinary perspectives, including, for example, anthropology, sociology, economics, engineering, and epidemiology. The fifth part includes case studies, focusing on countries and regions like Nepal, the United States, China, and the Persian Gulf, where migration has been increasingly shaping the political, social, and economic milieu over the past decade. We end with a part about the future of migration and health, focusing on how we can best educate the next generation of scholars in the area, articulating areas where the field can productively grow, and answering questions that need to be answered to the end of improving the health of populations.

It is our hope that this book represents a comprehensive text that synthesizes the state of the science surrounding human migration and health. To us, the study of migration and population health represents an exciting evolution in an interdisciplinary field. As more scholarship emerges in the area, the opportunity for transdisciplinary synthesis increases, paving the way for a whole new scholarship that helps us better understand the particular challenges and opportunities presented by migration and health as it adopts methods and approaches from long-established disciplines. The synthesis, therefore, aims to do more than summarize; it aims to clarify what we know and what we do not know to the end of informing what we do today and what we shall do in the coming decade. We are publishing this book at a time when we think we are at an inflection point in the field of migration and health. This book aims to be part of the movement toward making that inflection steeper and to help point it in the right direction and will hopefully aid the teachers, scientists, and programs in the field that will emerge. We look forward to reading and learning from the scholarship that shall emerge as other authors and thinkers build on this work to advance our understanding of migration and the health of populations.

CHAPTER TWO

Understanding Migration and Health

Social-Ecological and Lifecourse Perspectives

Catherine K. Ettman, Muhammad H. Zaman, and Sandro Galea

1.0 Introduction

The first chapter of this book framed how migration has been a major driver in population movement and that trends past, present, and future indicate that migration is, and will remain, an important driver of the health of populations in coming decades. Migration, whether forced due to conflict or climate change or driven by economic incentives, shapes health in a number of ways. This chapter aims to provide three frameworks that can be useful in organizing our thinking about migration and health in particular: the social-ecological model, the lifecourse perspective, and the migration process itself. The chapter will discuss how these three frameworks may be used to understand the relation between migration and health, anchored in mental health as one example of a health indicator influenced by migration. We first introduce the three frameworks, and then we expand with specific examples using each framework. We conclude by summarizing the goals of the book and how these concepts will be addressed throughout the volume.

2.0 Three Frameworks

2.1 The Social-ecological Model

Health is the product of a set of influences, at multiple levels, ranging from the personal to the societal, that intersect, modify each other in a mutually codependent manner, and produce health.[1] The social-ecological model summarizes how multiple levels of context produce health in persons. Personal—and population—health is a product of social relationships, living conditions, neighborhood conditions, institutions, and social and economic policies that govern the places where populations live.[2] This is true of all people and particularly of people who migrate. Figure 2.1 shows how the health of people who migrate is a function of multiple levels of context across multiple levels. The health of persons who migrate is in part a product of the social, environmental, and political institutions and public resources available in their country of birth, current country of residence, and any countries where they may have lived over the lifecourse. In this way, personal relationships, physical living conditions, neighborhoods, institutions, and national policies influence the health of migrants.

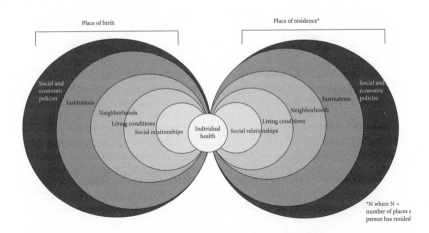

FIGURE 2.1. Social-ecological framework for understanding health, in the context of migration

Source: Modified from Kaplan, George A., "What's Wrong with Social Epidemiology, and How Can We Make It Better?" *Epidemiologic Reviews* 26, no. 1 (2004): 124–35, https://doi.org/10.1093/epirev/mxh010.

2.2 The Lifecourse Perspective

Exposure to contexts—and their influence on health—varies throughout the lifecourse. Birth and death bookend health throughout the lifecourse. Exposures in utero and during critical development periods in childhood and adolescence influence later health outcomes. The experience of migration can expose persons to contexts that improve or harm health, and *when* that exposure happens also influences the importance of each factor. The lifecourse approach allows us to visualize how experiences mount over time to accumulate in health.[3] Figure 2.2 describes health as a function of life stage across five periods: prenatal, infancy and childhood, adolescence, adult life, and older age. Although the demarcation between each stage is ultimately arbitrary, conceptually each stage presents unique opportunities and challenges for health for all people. A lifecourse framework can help situate how experiences that are unique to persons who migrate can affect their health in different ways at different periods in their lives. Figure 2.2 highlights health risks at every developmental stage and how exposure to them can cause good or poor health. It also shows that health is cumulative over the course of a person's life. The migration process can influence health in different ways, depending on when in life and how a person migrates.

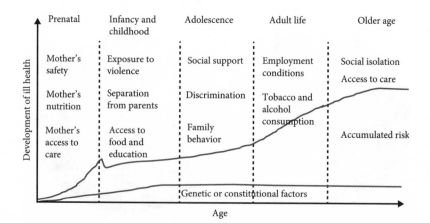

FIGURE 2.2. Health across the lifecourse, in the context of migration

Source: Adapted from Uauy, Ricardo, and Noel Solomons, "Diet, Nutrition, and the Life-Course Approach to Cancer Prevention," *Journal of Nutrition* 135, no. 12 (2005): 2934S–45S, https://doi.org/10.1093/jn/135.12.2934S.

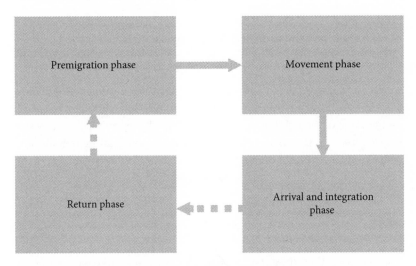

FIGURE 2.3. The determinants of health through the migration process

Sources: Modified from Vearey, Hui, Wickramage, Migration and Health: Current Issues, Governance, and Knowledge Gaps, *World Migration Report* (2020): 209–28. Figure 1. The Determinants of Migrant Health throughout the Migration Cycle, adapted from Gushulak, Weekers, and MacPherson, 2009; IOM, 2008, https://publications.iom.int/books /world-migration-report-2020.

2.3 The Migration Process

Migration itself is a complex and multipart process. The migration process framework shows simplified stages, within which exposures can influence health. Figure 2.3 shows one possible three-step process of migration with a potential fourth step: premigration, movement, arrival and integration, and return. Health may intersect with each phase, and understanding what exposures occur and when they happen in the course of the migration process can help to organize our understanding of how these factors shape health.[4] This framework is a generalized one, and variations exist based on context. There are many other context-specific scenarios, but this framework aims to present a more generalized approach to considering the various stages of migration and health.

3.0 Applications of the Frameworks

Here we use the example of mental health to show how these three frameworks can be applied in organizing how migration affects health. Mental health is sensitive to physical, economic, and social contexts, and may present sooner than physical health disparities;[5] additionally, mental health is inseparable from physical health, with mental illness associated with additional comorbidities.[6] Thus, the mental health effects of migration may serve as an effective illustrative example of the application of these frameworks on understanding migration and health. The examples cited below are used for illustrative purposes; chapter 10 will delve into greater depth on the topic of mental illness, substance use, and migration. The processes in the three frameworks featured—the social-ecological model, the life-course perspective, and the migration process—serve as organizing metaphors, helping us better understand what are ultimately complex and dynamic relations that produce health.[7]

3.1 Social-ecological Model

The social-ecological model can help organize our thinking around the relation between migration, context, and health. The social-ecological model reflects the multiple contexts within which people live and within which health is ultimately realized. Experiences in social relationships, living conditions, neighborhoods, institutions, and social and economic policies shape personal and population health,[8] and in particular the health of migrant populations.[9]

Starting at the personal level, personal characteristics, including genetic traits and dispositions, influence health. It is not at all clear if migrants overall have better or worse mental health than nonmigrants. A "healthy migrant" effect has been noted, where persons who are able to migrate have better health than their native-born counterparts, potentially representing a health selection bias in those who are able to migrate.[10] Although some studies show a physical health[11,12,13] and a mental health advantage,[14] there is substantial heterogeneity of findings across subpopulations.[15] For example, immigrant mothers in Canada exhibit worse mental health than their native-born counterparts.[16] Fundamentally, it is competing forces over the social-ecological model that influence the production of mental health in migrant populations.[17,18,19] Chapter 4 will expand on the health of persons before migration and the "healthy migrant" effect, adding to our understanding of personal constitutional factors and individual risk factors before, during, and after migration.

At the social relationship level, family and interpersonal relationships can serve to protect against or exacerbate poor mental health of persons who migrate. For married female immigrants, spousal alcohol consumption, intimate partner violence, marital distress, and family-related stressors such as intergenerational cultural conflict are associated with poor mental health.[20,21,22] Numerous studies document the effect of parental mental health on children[23] and of the separation of families, such as the ill effects of parental migration on children "left behind."[24] The experience of parenthood and family dynamic is shaped by the heterogeneous experiences of migration, leading to improved or deteriorated health outcomes.[25] Positive factors such as family efficacy,[26] ethno-cultural identity, and broader social support can serve as a protective factor against ill health.[27,28,29]

Living conditions shape many measures of health.[30] For migrant populations in particular, their living conditions may be a function of their resources and the terms of their migration. Housing instability and substandard living conditions have been well documented among migrant farm workers,[31,32,33] temporary foreign workers,[34] and general migrant populations.[35] Substandard housing may include crowding, mold, mildew, structural deficiencies, and pesticides, which in turn can cause poor mental and physical health.[36,37,38] Access to living conditions is in no small part a function of economic status, with low economic resources leading to poor or unsafe housing conditions among migrant populations.[39,40]

At the neighborhood level, environmental factors shape the context in which migrant populations live. Neighborhood characteristics such as violence, walkability, access to healthy foods, and green space have been associated with health outcomes among refugee and migrant populations.[41,42] Living in disadvantaged neighborhoods has been shown to be associated with withdrawal, somatic complaints, and depressive/anxious behaviors in first- and second-generation immigrant adolescent Latinx populations in the United States.[43] Similar associations have been observed for other health conditions. For example, refugees assigned to live in more disadvantaged neighborhoods in Denmark were found to have increased risk for hypertension, diabetes, and myocardial infarction several decades later than their counterparts placed in wealthier neighborhoods.[44] In this way, exploring characteristics of neighborhoods that migrants have lived in, both before and after migration, can help in our understanding of mental and physical health among populations who migrate. Chapter 12 will assess nutrition, exploring in part how access to healthy foods, as a function of neighborhood resources, leads to improved health. Chapter 17 will expand on violence and health, touching on exposures to violence at different stages of migration.

Interactions with public, private, and civic institutions can harm or promote migrant health. Interactions that shape health may occur in workplace, medical, and religious and cultural institutions, as examples. Migrant employees may face greater discrimination or risk of injury at the workplace than nonmigrant employees, as has been documented in nurses,[45] farm workers,[46] and other workers.[47] Interactions with medical institutions have been well established as unequal between immigrant and nonimmigrant populations for a number of reasons.[48,49] International migrant children use health-care services such as general, primary, and dental care less than native-born children, with the exception of hospital and emergency services.[50] For mental health care use in particular, lack of insurance, high costs, and language barriers have been reported as key obstacles to access among immigrant populations.[51] Interactions with other organizations, such as religious and cultural institutions, can facilitate social support, which in turn protects against poor mental health. For example, older Latinx women in the United States who attended regular church services reported lower levels of depression before and after a spouse's death than their counterparts who did not regularly attend.[52] Chapter 3 discusses global drivers that shape health, which often overlap with institutional engagement. Chapter 6 explores migration and access to health care in particular. Chapter 20 expands on interactions between migrants and systems more broadly. Engaging institutions may be influenced by the macro level of the social-ecological model, in which national policies shape contexts in which migrants live.

The macro-determinants of health include the social and economic policies that shape migrant experiences at all other levels. Examples of policies that may particularly affect migrant populations are those around immigration, health-care coverage, access to a social safety net, and discrimination. Broadly, recognition of legal status of migrant populations allows for access to a whole suite of public resources that improve mental and physical health. Restrictive policies for migrant entry and legalization are associated with poor health in migrant populations in high-income countries.[53] Countries with robust social safety-net programs may more readily provide access to health care, housing, and food, translating to better health for all residents and particularly for the health of its migrant populations.[54,55] Access to health care in particular also varies by country. The United States does not provide health care as a human right, and policies such as expansion of the definition of public charge to include Medicaid use may also stifle the use of health care for persons who migrate. Immigrants in the United States who use social services for twelve months within a thirty-six-month period including food assistance, housing assistance, or Medicaid can be denied visa extension or entry to the United States due to their potential "charge" to the public.[56] Fear of using public assistance for determinants of health such as housing or nutritional services may lead to widened health gaps between migrant populations and nonmigrant populations. However, even in countries that provide universal health-care coverage, such as Canada, barriers to care still exist for immigrant populations. Barriers to accessing care include language barriers, cultural barriers, and barriers in navigating services.[57] Finally, policies that discriminate against ethnic minorities or that remove protections from discrimination are associated with worse mental health outcomes. In 2017, the United States limited immigration for persons from a set of countries that have majority Muslim populations. Those policies, coupled with an increase in Islamophobia and discriminatory acts, were associated with an increase in poor mental health.[58] Discrimination has been well documented to lead to poor mental health in migrant and non-majority populations in general[59] and Latinx,[60] Arab American,[61] Asian,[62] and refugee populations in particular.[63] Laws, policies, and practices at the broader national and societal level can promote health or worsen health. Chapter 8 will explore global governance and the health of migrants. Chapter 28 will explore the relation between law, migration, and health in the US context. Chapter 21 will discuss the concepts of ethics and justice surrounding migrant health and will touch on the macro-social and economic policies shaping the health of populations who migrate.

The social-ecological model serves as one framework to organize the connection between the multiple, complex causes of health and the migrant experience. It should be noted that persons who migrate live under multiple contexts; many of the studies mentioned in this chapter refer to immigrant populations, citing the associations between context and health after persons have migrated. Additionally, migration can also be seen as a continuous process or one that does not end. A person's health will be the function of his or her cumulative life experiences; thus, their contexts before, during, and after migration matter, as well as their age and life phase when the exposures occur.

3.2 Lifecourse Framework

A second framework that may be useful for considering the health of persons who migrate is the lifecourse framework. Figure 2.2 shows health across the lifecourse, in the context of migration. Health happens over the lifecourse, with exposures before birth influencing outcomes and with health slowly deteriorating over a life until eventual death. As such, experiences at different developmental moments affect health differently. For example, maternal violence or exposure to violence in the surrounding environment during pregnancy is linked to developmental difficulties in children.[64] Adversity in childhood[65] and adolescence[66] has been linked to negative health outcomes including obesity, asthma, and recurrent infections requiring hospitalization.[67] A robust literature exists on the health and behavior of children who migrate in particular, although this work is limited by a reliance on parental or adult accounts of children's experiences.[68] Risky behavior during adulthood, such as consumption of alcohol and tobacco and physical inactivity, leads to ill health. Finally, in older age, factors such as social isolation can lead to poor mental health outcomes.[69]

Health benefits and risk accumulate over time and are a function of when in his or her lifetime a person migrates. Differences in psychological distress may be explained by exposures over the lifecourse.[70] For example, exposure to reduced social cohesion, lower socioeconomic status, and discrimination account for a large portion of differences in health between native-born and non-native-born persons. In Sweden, poorer self-rated health was associated with later age of migration and fewer than fifteen years of residence in the country.[71] In the United States, Australia, and Canada, the health outcomes of immigrants converge with those of native-born residents after residency in the host population for ten to twenty years.[72] While people who migrate to these countries may be healthier to begin with, those benefits appear to fade through aging and assimilation.[73] Exposure to different experiences and environments at different points in time will translate to different health outcomes. In this way, persons who migrate will have unique health outcomes depending on the intersection of their experiences in place and time over the course of their lives. Thus, age and experiences through the lifecourse matter for all persons and particularly for persons who migrate, and the lifecourse approach offers another tool to organize our understanding of migration and health. Chapter 16 explores the health of children in particular, and chapter 15 explores the health of older people. Health risks vary depending on life stage during migration,[74] leading to the third framework to consider.

3.3. Migration Process

A third framework that may be helpful for considering migration and health is the migration process framework. Figure 2.3 shows the distinctive stages of migration: premigration, movement, arrival and integration, and potential return. The experience of migration at any of these phases may shape health. Premigration experiences have been found to shape mental health in youth.[75] Having a high socioeconomic status premigration may not necessarily protect refugees from the ill effects of migration during or after the first few years of integration.[76] The movement phase can expose people to stressors that in turn affect mental health.[77] For example, exposure to violence during migration leads to poor mental health.[78,79] Similarly, experiences during arrival and integration can affect both physical and mental health outcomes.[80] Exposures during the first year of arrival also contribute to youth mental health[81] and adult health. Persons who experience downward social mobility upon migration are more likely to report poor mental health than persons who experience upward or unchanged mobility.[82] Persons who migrate may face different risks of infectious disease across each stage of migration.[83] Additionally, for some communities, the process of migration may not end, and these populations may continue to move and may remain displaced for long periods. It is important to note that while migration can be a stressful exposure, not all persons who migrate go through the same process and, therefore, their health outcomes may vary as a result.[84] The migration process framework, however, may serve as an additional mechanism for organizing and understanding the connection between migration and health. Chapter 5 explores more fully health and the process of migration. Chapter 14 expands on forced migration, and Chapter 17 discusses the impact of violence through all migration phases on health.

4.0 Conclusion

Ample evidence shows that migration is a factor in population health. Additionally, health is a function of context, and context matters across the lifecourse. Differential experiences across contexts have led researchers to identify immigration itself as a social determinant of health.[85,86]

This chapter presented three frameworks to guide our thinking on migration and being a migrant: the social-ecological model, health across the lifecourse, and the migration process. In sum, these three frameworks can help focus research and action that address how health is influenced by context, which affects health throughout the lifecourse and through stages of migration. These are but three frameworks to use; there are countless others, many of which will be discussed throughout this volume. We offer these three at the outset, presenting them as overall frames within which subsequent chapter-specific discussions can be situated.

CHAPTER THREE

The Global Drivers of Migration

Francesco Castelli

1.0 Introduction

Migration is an extremely complex phenomenon that leads individuals, families, entire communities, or even mass populations to move definitively from their usual place of residency.

During the last fifty years, the absolute number of international migrants has more than tripled, from 84 million in 1970 to nearly 272 million in 2019.[1] However, the proportion of international migrants over the total world's population has only risen from 2.3 percent to 3.5 percent over the period, and especially so during the last thirty years, when the proportion rose from 2.9 percent in 1990 to 3.5 percent in 2019 (table 3.1). Of note, contrary to public perception, international migrants from the South are equally relocated in both Southern and Northern countries. In 2018, the number of asylum seekers and refugees was estimated to be twenty-six million globally.[2] Apart from international migrants, as many as 740 million individuals are estimated to have moved internally away from their usual place of residency to other areas in the same country.

The rising absolute flow of migrants in the last two decades has sometimes prompted a negative reaction from the host communities in the Western industrialized world, fueled by prejudices regarding safety and health issues.[3] Although the health profile of migrants may vary according to their geographical provenance, the infectious risk to the host communities has been proven negligible from a public health perspective.[4]

According to the various factors that drive migrations and that often act in combination, attempts have been made to classify the heterogeneous

TABLE 3.1 **International migrants by calendar year, 1970–2019**

Year	Absolute number	Percentage of the total world population
1970	84,460,125	2.3%
1975	90,368,010	2.2%
1980	101,983,149	2.3%
1985	113,206,691	2.3%
1990	153,011,473	2.9%
1995	161,316,895	2.8%
2000	173,588,441	2.8%
2005	191,615,574	2.9%
2010	220,781,909	3.2%
2015	248,861,296	3.4%
2019	271,642,105	3.5%

Note: International Organization for Migration (IOM), "World Migration Report 2020," accessed October 10, 2020, https://publications.iom.int /system/files/pdf/wmr_2020.pdf.

population of migrants, summarized in chapter 1.[5] However, it should be noted that the motivations forcing people to permanently leave their country of origin may even change during the migration process as the situation changes and evolves, as was the case for Afghan children arriving in Belgium.[6] Further, most economic and sociopolitical drivers are strictly interconnected, as sometimes even push and pull factors are and often hardly separable from one another, making mutually exclusive classifications most probably overly simplistic.

The literature exploring the causes of migration flows is often divergent and contradictory, largely because the perspective of the authors differs from methodological (quantitative *versus* qualitative studies) and geopolitical or socioeconomic standpoints.[7] Given the complexity of the matter, a multidisciplinary effort is needed to appreciate the evolving nature of the causes of such a relevant phenomenon that has a profound social and economic impact on both origin and hosting societies.

The classic *push and pull* framework trying to describe and classify the global drivers of migration was initially proposed by Everett S. Lee in 1966.[8] Briefly, the *push and pull* theory tried to identify those negative elements that may affect satisfactory life in the country of origin (e.g., conflicts, dictatorships, discrimination, unemployment, low wages, etc.) leading to the migratory project (*push factors*), and those attracting factors (*pull factors*) that conversely are regarded as positive elements to ameliorate the life of the individual and of their family (e.g., welfare, job opportunities, peace, presence of co-ethnic communities, etc.). Lee also addressed the issue of *intervening obstacles* that may prevent migration despite the presence of effective push and pull factors. The *push and pull* conceptual frame has the advantage of linearity and simplicity. However, it fails to explain why, for example, people living in the same area and suffering from the same negative conditions may make different choices with regards to migration or why the same area may be at the same time a place of emigration and immigration.[9] Other elements to be taken into consideration include individual characteristics and aspirations within a broader evolving socioeconomic perspective. To overcome the limit of the somehow static *push and pull* theory while maintaining its linearity and clarity, some authors have proposed a revised version called *push and pull plus*.[10] The push and pull plus framework tries to assess the impact of structural (pushing and pulling) macro-factors on the individual characteristics of the subject (micro-level) or their social network (meso-level), leading to the final decision to migrate or not to migrate.[11]

2.0 Drivers of Migration

The following is a brief description of the evidence supporting the roles of the main structural *macro* (pushing and pulling) and the *meso and micro* factors—most often acting in combination—in determining the final individual decision to move.

2.1 Pushing Macro-factors

Pushing macro-factors are those factors producing dangerous or unpleasant living conditions in one specific area that act as expelling forces and are not under the control of the individual or the community.

2.1.1 DEMOGRAPHIC INCREASE, URBANIZATION, AND POPULATION DENSITY. The world population has sharply increased in the last two centuries, from the estimated 1 billion individuals living in the year 1800 to the nearly 7.8 billion reported by the United Nations Department of Economic and Social Affairs (UNDESA) in the year 2020. However, the increase in population has not been even in the different parts of the world. Between 1950 and 2020, the African population increased from 227 million to 1.340 billion (+490%) and the Asian population from 1.404 billion to 4.641 billion

(+230%). In the same period, Europe has grown from 549 million to 747 million (+36%) and North America from 172 million to 368 million (+113%), a much lower increase as a result of different fertility rates in Africa (4.4 live births/woman in the period 2015–2020), Asia (2.15), Europe (1.61), and North America (1.75).[12] According to UNDESA forecasts, given the existing conditions, the world total population will approach eleven billion in the year 2100, with Africa and Asia totaling nine billion individuals and Europe experiencing a shrinking of its population to 629 million. The net result will be a progressive demographic decline characterized by an aging population in today's Western industrialized countries, compared to a much younger working-age population living in resource-limited countries in the Global South. This demographic unbalance is coupled with the progressive urbanization rate taking place in Africa (from 14.3% in 1950 to 43.5% in 2020) and Asia (from 17.5% to 51.1%), exposing younger generations to an increasingly densely populated urban environment with a strikingly uneven wealth distribution.

2.1.2 INADEQUATE HUMAN AND ECONOMIC DEVELOPMENT, THE INVERSE U CURVE.   The United Nations Development Programme (UNDP) created the Human Development Index (HDI) in 1990 to rank the state of development of any individual country. The HDI is a complex indicator assessing the three key dimensions of development: healthy life, knowledge, and standard of living, respectively measured by life expectancy at birth, years of schooling for adults aged twenty-five or more, and gross national income per capita. The top twenty HDI ranked countries in 2019 are European (13), North American (2), and Australasian (3), while as many as eighteen out of the bottom ranked twenty countries belong to the African continent, with gross national income per capita ranging from US$68,059 to US$912.[13] Although the African continent has witnessed remarkable economic growth in the last decades, the distribution of wealth in African resource-poor countries has not been even, leaving a large majority of the workforce in the poorly profitable informal sector without social security coverage. Interestingly enough, the educational gap between the countries with a very high human development index (12 years of schooling, on average) and developing countries (7.4 years of schooling) is not as dramatic as the economic gap, as a probable result of the ongoing efforts put in place to reach the Millennium Development Goals and the Sustainable Development Goals.[14] Evidence points to the fact that initial economic development in a given low-income country is not immediately followed by a fall in the emigration rates, but rather by an increase. Only when development has reached a certain level does emigration tend to lower, a pattern referred to as the inverse U curve theory.[15]

2.1.3 DISEASE PREVALENCE AND HEALTH SYSTEMS. In 1978, the World Health Organization launched the Health for All goal, based on the implementation of the Primary Health Care (PHC) strategy and on the strengthening of the health systems in resource-poor countries, to be reached by the year 2000.[16] Many economic and political factors have prevented the full implementation of the PHC, leading to large health sector privatization and out-of-pocket expenses and leaving many poor people entrapped in poverty with little access to health-care services.[17] The Millennium Development Goals, launched in the year 2000 and targeted to 2015, have contributed significantly to ameliorating the living conditions of resource-poor settings, but the infant mortality rate in low-income regions in 2015 was still 47 per 1,000 live births (compared to 6/1,000 in developed regions) and the maternal mortality rate was 230/100,000 live births (compared to 16/100,000).[18] The Covid-19 pandemic is expected to set back all the Sustainable Development Goals indicators to a large extent, making living conditions in resource-poor settings worse.[19] However, little is known about the role of disease prevalence and access to care on migration flows.

2.1.4 CLIMATE CHANGES, FOOD, AND WATER SECURITY. Little doubt exists that the planet has undergone a warming process largely due to the emission in the atmosphere of greenhouse gases (in particular carbon dioxide, methane, and nitrous oxide) of an anthropogenic nature.[20] Most greenhouse gases enter into the atmosphere by affluent countries (estimated 97%),[21] but the most negative consequences even in terms of mortality are suffered by resource-poor countries.[22] The warming of the planet has many negative environmental consequences possibly influencing the final decision to migrate. First, it may cause dryness and drought in large areas, making the soil unsuitable for cultivation and breeding and eventually leading to severe food insecurity. Such conditions may affect vast areas in sub-Saharan Africa (for example, those surrounding Lake Chad) and other arid zones in Asia and Latin America. Further, extreme weather events may have a direct impact on health conditions of the populations. Second, it may facilitate the incidence and prevalence of communicable (vector borne and waterborne) and noncommunicable (mental, cardiovascular, allergic, etc.) conditions to an extent that living conditions become unbearable.[23] Third, melting glaciers can produce floods and even raise the sea level, forcing people living in the

coastal areas to move internally. An example of such a situation is the expected migration from the coastal areas of Bangladesh as a consequence of
the melting of the large Himalaya glaciers.[24] People may consider escaping a
hostile environment in search of better living conditions for themselves and
their families (environmental migrants), although migration itself may conversely affect health in a vicious circle.[25] According to the UCL-Lancet Commission on Migration and Health, climate changes are a major trigger for
human mobility, possibly forcing as many as 200 million people to move from
their place of residency by the year 2050,[26] even if factor-specific forecasts
are difficult to perform, as many confounding social, economic, and political
variables are likely to act in combination to drive environment-related migration. Further, the evidence that many individuals continue residing in hostile environments, possibly due to the lack of resources to move, makes the
specific role of climate change in exclusively driving migration uncertain.[27]

2.1.5 LAND GRABBING.   The intensive exploitation of rural areas in low-
income countries, usually by international enterprises or even foreign
governments, is referred to as *land grabbing*. Large areas are exploited
to cultivate mainly biofuels or food crops or even to build large tourist
resorts, with little (if any) economic benefit to the native communities and
a negative impact on land impoverishment, agricultural biodiversity, and
the local economy, adding to the consequences of climate changes.[28] Poor
rural villagers, often devoid of land property documents, are obliged to
leave their native areas with little compensation to move elsewhere in the
country.[29] They often reach the degraded peripheries of the main cities, a
setting that is largely hostile and different from the one their families have
been living in for centuries, with physical and psychological detriments for
them and their children.

2.1.6 WARS, AUTHORITARIAN REGIMES, INSECURITY, AND DISCRIMINATION.
According to the Uppsala Conflict Data Programme (UCDP) of the University of Uppsala, a major observatory of organized violence operating
for over forty years, the number of wars or conflict outbreaks is on the
rise.[30] In this time period, the number of non-state violent conflicts (n = 67)
has surpassed the number of officially declared state violent conflicts
(n = 54), making the recognition of asylum seekers difficult to ascertain under different national regulations. These bloody conflicts are happening
in virtually all continents, offending civilians and denying civil and social
rights to populations who are eventually forced to leave by dictatorships.
The long-lasting wars in Syria and Afghanistan are forcing millions of

individuals to leave their country of citizenship. Other conflicts taking place in the Horn of Africa (Eritrea, Somalia), Northern Africa (Libya), West Africa (Mali, Nigeria), and Latin America (Venezuela) are somehow undeclared but equally socially disrupting, denying basic human rights and access to quality education and a dignified life, especially for the fragile female population.[31] It is to be noted that many people escaping conflicts and wars are relocated within national borders (as is the case for Yemen), thus they are not numbered in the international migrants count and instead are considered internal refugees.

3.0 Pull Macro-factors

3.1 Job Opportunities

The main pull factor for economic migrants is the prospect of labor in receiving countries, where there are low-skill job opportunities and higher salaries that may be partially returned to the origin families (remittances). This is not new; for example, Italian workers were incentivized by the Italian government to migrate from Southern Europe to the Central and Northern European Countries after the Second World War as a means to obtain return remittances and to prevent high internal unemployment.[32] Migrants are often available to perform unattractive duties (such as agricultural or low-level services) that the nationals of destination countries are not willing to do anymore, mainly due to improved lifestyles and the aging of the population.

This may be viewed as a "risk stratification" strategy that makes migration a component of the economic perspective of the origin communities.[33] This remains true as long as the migrants reference group is the primary origin reference group, but it may change over time with better integration in the new society.

Of course, the economic attractiveness of a specific country or continent may vary over time and cycles are to be expected, as evidenced by the decreasing pulling economic strength of Southern Europe after the economic crisis that started in 2008.[34]

3.2 Welfare Magnet

A precarious welfare state (lack of quality free education and accessible health systems) in the country of origin is an obvious push factor. However, it has been suggested that better service provisions may also be a push factor, as they provide people with a higher level of awareness and resources to migrate long distances.[35] On the other hand, the existence of a generous welfare state in the destination country is an attractive pull factor (the "magnet" hypothesis) that may discourage migrants from returning to their homeland. The cuts in welfare benefits offered in the destination country, a policy that is sometimes implemented to decrease the attractiveness for migrants, bear negative consequences for health and integration.[36]

4.0 Meso-factors

4.1 Community and Ethnic Networks

The presence of ethnic networks of successfully migrated nationals in the destination country appears to be an evident factor attracting migrants, due to expectations of economic and societal support. Ethnic and family networks also drive migrants to specific regions and countries, perpetuating cluster migration. Advanced communication technologies, favoring awareness of better living conditions elsewhere and linking potential migrants with their ethnic communities abroad, act as a boosting factor for leaving the country of origin. However, the relative weight of such factors is still under debate.[37]

4.2 Social Investment and Support, Remittances

As already noted, migration can also be viewed as a "risk stratification" strategy by communities or families in developing countries in transition. The amount of remittances from international migrants (US$ 689 billion in 2018) is much higher than the amount (US$ 152.8 billion in 2019) granted by the Official Development Assistance (ODA) Programme provided by the Organization for Economic Co-operation and Development (OECD) countries.[38]

5.0 Micro-factors

5.1 Education

Most reports indicate that the level of education of international migrants is appreciable[39] and is usually higher than the level of education that of their age-matched peers left behind in their country of origin and sometimes in the destination country.[40] International economic and forced migrants are most often individuals with some skills and economic resources who are searching for a better future. When family members have already successfully migrated in the past, the ethnic or familiar network is an additional driver of migration.[41] Persons with higher skills may better pursue their aspirations, providing additional explanations of the apparent paradox existing between transitional development and migration.[42] As conceptualized by the inverse U curve theory, the initial stages of educational development that are not accompanied by concrete job possibilities may paradoxically create the conditions for migration.[43]

These people may well constitute an economic gain for the host communities. However, at the same time, it is a loss of skilled and qualified human resources for the country of origin. This phenomenon is called brain drain and is considered to be one of the main barriers to the autonomous development of resource-limited countries, although it may provide huge economic return as remittances, as already discussed.

5.2 Religion

Many mass migrations in history have been driven by religious intolerance and persecution. Followers of many religions (the monotheistic Muslims, Jews, Christians, and others) have been forced to leave their land in search of a place where their faith could be freely practiced. The interconnections between religion and migrations are tight. The presence of religious communities plays a role in the choice of the destination country and may influence the resilience of the migrant in his/her new environment.[44]

5.3 Sexual Identity

Although difficult to quantify, there is little doubt that restrictive policies of various countries on sexual identity and LGBTQI+ individuals (lesbian, gay, bisexual, transgender, queer, and intersex or questioning people) play a role as a micro-factor of migration.[45] People persecuted because of their sexual orientation may be more likely to migrate to find better living conditions and social integration.

6.0 Conclusions

The above factors—and many others, such as marital status and family obligations, food/water and energy security, and the cost of moving—are often deeply interconnected and act together to inform the final decision of an individual to migrate, alone or with his/her family. Macro-, meso-, or micro-factors may prevail in the single individual. The ethnic network, particularly in times of global communication, is of utmost importance, as are family supports, educational levels, and personal aspirations.[46]

The perceived initial main motivation may also change during the migration itinerary and even after settlement in the receiving country according to the dynamic of the prevailing pushing or pulling factor.

Far from being overwhelming, the present flow of international migrants is increasing slowly compared to the total world population, growing from 2.9 percent in 1990 to 3.5 percent in 2019. Given the degradation of living conditions in many parts of the world, the question *Why do so few people migrate?* has also been raised.[47]

Given the complex interconnection of many different factors (social, environmental, economic, political, individual, etc.) eventually driving individual or mass population movements, a collaborative multidisciplinary effort is needed to better assess the deep roots of migration and propose solutions to the benefit of the people on the move and of both the sending and receiving countries.

PART I I

How Migration Affects
Population Health

CHAPTER FOUR

Health of People Before Migration, the "Healthy Migrant"

Yudit Namer and Oliver Razum

1.0 Introduction

The term *migration* describes a process encompassing not only the actual act of moving and the time in the new host country, but also the period before migration, or premigration, during which experiences accumulate leading to the decision or the forced choice to move to a new place. These experiences may range from economic uncertainty and lack of opportunities to political unsettlement and war. The decision or the forced choice to migrate is not taken lightly and implies a certain strength and resilience to construct a new life someplace else.

In this chapter, we focus on the state of health of people before migration. In doing so, we briefly describe the phenomenon called the *healthy migrant effect* and discuss the factors that create seemingly healthy migrants, drive migration to begin with, and influence the physical and mental health of migrants.

2.0 The Paradox of Healthy Migrants

Migrants fare better in terms of health when compared to the host population, a finding which has baffled scientists since it emerged. A mortality advantage was first documented in the United States in relation to migrants from Latin America in the 1970s[1,2] and was thus christened as "the Hispanic Paradox."[3] In Britain, scientists found that Vietnamese refugees or "boat people" showed lower overall mortality, as well as lower mortality from ischemic heart disease, non-cerebrovascular circulatory disease, and certain types of cancer compared to the population of England and Wales.[4] The healthy migrant effect was considered a paradox: the overall health status of the migrant population was closer to that of the majority host population and not the minority host population with whom many social disadvantages were shared.[5]

Researchers have replicated a healthy migrant effect mostly with first-generation migrants or people who migrated themselves. A Mediterranean paradox, whereby people who migrated from Mediterranean countries to Northwest Europe had lower mortality than the host population, was subsequently described.[6] For example, a mortality advantage was documented for migrant men from Morocco in France, compared to the majority population in France and the general population in Morocco.[7] Similarly, migrants from Turkey had significantly lower mortality than the majority population in Germany and in the capital of Turkey, an effect that persisted into the second generation.[8] A mental health advantage was also documented in international migrants in Germany compared to internal migrants.[9] These findings implied that the migrants were healthier than not only the populations they migrated to, but also the populations they left behind.

There is by now solid evidence for the healthy migrant effect. A more nuanced lifecourse approach to our understanding of migration shows that health is not fixed but is a process and that the health of migrants evolves over time, particularly as migrants adapt to their host country. The classic Irish brothers study documented that Irish American men had a higher mortality risk from arteriosclerotic heart disease than their brothers living in Ireland.[10] Another classic epidemiological study, the Ni-Hon-San study, showed that men from Japan had the lowest risk for coronary heart disease in Japan, higher risk in Hawaii, and the highest risk in mainland United States.[11] This meant that in the context of coronary heart disease, past exposures in the countries of origin were relevant to migrant health, health risks changed during the process of migration, and social processes, such as adopting the lifestyle of the host country, should be taken into account when assessing risk.[12] Subsequent studies were able to show that such an adoption often meant a convergence to the mean health of the majority population in terms of health risks, such as increased body mass index in migrant children in the second generation[13] and increased smoking frequency in second-generation migrant women.[14]

Following the findings that the health of migrant populations may eventually converge to the mean of the host population, some alternative (complementary)[15] explanations attempted to contextualize the healthy migrant effect. These explanations include:

1) A *selection bias*,[16] which suggests that the healthy members of populations choose, are physically and mentally able to, and are invited or permitted by states to migrate and corresponds to the *healthy worker effect*,[17] which involves the selection of healthy people in the workforce;

2) *Ethnic enclave hypothesis* or *barrio advantage*,[18] which proposes that residential stability, a cohesive environment, and support networks that come with segregated neighborhoods overcome the socioeconomic disadvantages of being members of a minority community;

3) The *time travel metaphor*,[19] which argues that migrants profit from not yet adopting the industrialized societies' dietary practices and deskbound lifestyles but immediately benefiting from industrialized health technologies and lower incidence of communicable diseases;

4) The *salmon effect*,[20] which claims that migrants may choose to return to their country of origin when they age or become seriously ill, to be cared for by family members or their communities;

5) An *unhealthy remigration hypothesis*,[21] a variant of the salmon effect, which postulates that the healthy migrants remain in the countries to which they migrated, but the unhealthy migrants return to their country of origin; and

6) Forms of *data artifact*,[22] such as misreport or misclassification of age, nationality and/or ethnicity, and the overlook of return migrants (e.g., salmon effect), multiple reentries, or cumulative migration experiences in population registries or census data.

It should be noted that much of the research on the healthy migrant effect is rooted in the dominant paradigms within public health. Some epidemiological inquiries into migrant health pay attention only to migrant-specific diseases and reduce explanations to cultural factors and migrants' health behaviors. Other inquiries neglect the temporality and liminality of migration and lack focus on intersectionality, heterogeneity, social, and environmental factors. Although interdisciplinary and mixed-methods inquiries are on the rise in the field of migrant health, much of the epidemiological inquiries do not adequately engage with broader social sciences. In other words, research on the healthy migrant effect is not always situated within the macro societal dynamics and does not always reflect the complex nature of migration.[23,24]

To summarize, despite certain limitations inherent in studies on migrant health, migrants are seemingly healthier members of the populations of their countries of origin who are able to or selected to migrate (see our previous work for a more detailed discussion)[25], warranting a discussion of health before migration.

3.0 Health Before Migration

Migrants, due to their act of moving when their compatriots stayed (in the context of non-forced migration), are considered to be outliers.[26] The issue of health before migration is thus closely related to the questions of who immigrates and why. There have been many attempts to answer these questions in various migration contexts.[27] Due to the nature of migration, it is not always possible to empirically observe migration before it happens. For example, in the context of free mobility and open borders, such as within the European Union, it is difficult to establish the reason citizens move from one country to another unless explicit data are collected.[28]

Most studies therefore (as summarized above) compare the health of migrants to that of the population of their countries of origin in the absence of premigration data. Some studies, however, were able to follow cohorts before migration, mostly in the context of internal migration; some visa lottery-based studies measured health before or immediately after migration, and others have examined the intention to migrate in order to describe certain psychological factors contributing to migration. We now discuss such findings in terms of physical and mental health.

3.1 Physical Health

The Migration and Health in Malawi cohort study follows the internal migration activity of people identified through a larger panel and is one of few cohort studies investigating the premigration period.[29] So far, they reported that participants are physically healthier before migration from rural settings than nonmigrants who stayed in rural areas, an effect that disappears for women when controlled for age but remains in place for men. In addition, healthier men and women migrated to urban areas, regardless of HIV status, which is a factor for migration selection in Malawi. Healthier men were also more likely to be permanent migrants than return migrants.[30] These relationships exist only for adults in Malawi, however, as children who migrate have premigration health similar to that of children who do not.[31]

Similar findings have been reported in internal migration contexts: in Indonesia, internal migrants were found to be healthier than nonmigrants and also than household members who stayed.[32] In China, those who internally migrated far away were healthier, but the unhealthy among the migrated returned home or closer to home,[33] as explained by the *unhealthy remigration hypothesis*. In Thailand, on the other hand, no physical health advantage in rural to urban internal migrants was observed in a multivariate framework, suggesting that the observed better health was explained by socioeconomic factors.[34]

Visa-based studies offer a unique opportunity to examine migrant health in international migration. Visa lotteries create a natural experiment in that lottery winners are not self-selected into migration, although lottery participants are. Other visa-based studies define a premigration period following the granting of the visa, prior to the move, with often sufficient time to conduct health-based measurements. One example is the New Immigrant Survey (NIS), a representative cohort of contemporary migrants who have just been granted permanent residency to the United States with work, family reunion, refugee, or diversity lottery visas or whose residency status has just changed.[35] One study found a positive health selection at the point of obtaining permanent residence, with women, refugees, and migrants from Mexico showing a lower level of selection than their counterparts.[36] More specifically, migrants who won the diversity lottery had the highest selection for health,[37] and refugees exhibited a health disadvantage compared to nonrefugee migrants.[38] The Health of Philippine Emigrants Study (HoPES), another visa-based cohort study, recruited migrants from the Philippines to the United States in a mandatory predeparture seminar following the granting of the visa.[39] Overall, migrants reported better self-rated health yet higher systolic blood pressure premigration than nonmigrant counterparts in the Philippines.[40] When visa type was considered, marriage (or fiancé) visas accounted for the health selection compared to employment and family reunification visas.[41] Those who were considered "pre-acculturated" in terms of more frequent contact with family or friends in the United States and more preparation to migrate had higher body mass index and larger waist circumference than nonmigrant counterparts in the Philippines, suggesting pre-acculturation to be a health risk factor. For the nonmigrant counterparts, however, increased communication with friends and family indicated a lower body mass index and smaller waist circumference, highlighting the complexity of selection into migration.[42]

An analysis of the Finnish cohort participants who migrated to Sweden and their twins who remained in Finland revealed that higher rates of smoking and alcohol consumption preceded and predicted migration in the future.[43] The Mexican Migration Project, a life history study investigating international migration from Mexico to the neighboring United States, found that perceived excellent early life health (at age fourteen) predicted both documented and undocumented migration.[44] Migrants were also found to be taller than nonmigrants, although this is a post-migration measurement. An interesting finding from the study reveals the complex nature of migration decisions: in moderately dry regions of Mexico, a positive health selectivity is documented during higher rainfall but not during scarce rainfall.[45] A limitation of this project is that questions on health are asked retrospectively.

3.2 Mental Health

Findings related to mental health are sparser than those to physical health in investigations of premigration health. The Malawi cohort study was not able to find a healthy migrant effect for mental health.[46] The aforementioned Thailand study, on the other hand, showed that internal rural to urban migrants had worse mental health before than after migration, which perhaps explained the motivation to move.[47] In the NIS, newly migrated women were more likely than men to experience sadness or depressive feelings due to visa stress, even when they had a family member who was a citizen of the United States (which was a protective factor for men).[48] For refugees in the NIS sample, harm experienced prior to migration was related to depression.[49] On the contrary, the HoPES found that migrants predeparture reported less depression than their nonmigrant counterparts in the Philippines.[50]

In the absence of mental health data, personality psychology may shed light on who migrates. Personality psychology studies showed, for example, that the personality traits of "openness to experience" (i.e., being imaginative, creative, and intellectually curious and favoring variety) and "extraversion" (i.e., seeking human interaction, taking pleasure in and being energized by social activities) were associated with the intention to migrate. Specifically, openness to experience influenced the intention to migrate in a complementary manner to education (i.e., greatest intention in people with both high level of education and openness to experience). In contrast, extraversion did so in a compensatory manner (i.e., the gap in education drops with increase in extraversion).[51] The Finnish twin study also found extraversion and "neuroticism" (i.e., being anxious, irritable, and prone to stress) to be related to an increased likelihood to migrate, in addition to life dissatisfaction, to which migration seems to be a response. The personality traits may also explain risky health behaviors such as alcohol intake and smoking.[52]

3.3 Type of Migration

The discussion so far mostly relates to migration situations other than forced migration. Studies available, as reported above (e.g., NIS), suggest that the healthy migrant effect does not necessarily apply to forced migrants. Extremely distressing interrelated experiences—famine, natural disasters, war, and political persecution, for example—that lead to displacement and/or fleeing are themselves health-related exposures. This means that their effects are difficult to disentangle from that of migrating. Although the Vietnamese refugees or "boat people" reported above showed lower overall mortality, this could be partly explained by a survival bias at the onset of the journey or at sea. Indeed, a significant number of people did not survive the journey.[53] The urgency and the destruction of infrastructure often inherent in forced migration further reduce the availability of meaningful data to draw conclusions regarding people's health before migration. Based on this discussion, we suggest adapting the migrant health research agenda to such issues.

4.0 A New Research Agenda

In this chapter, we summarized existing research on the health of migrants, mostly in non-forced migration contexts. The evidence points toward a healthy migrant effect that is transitory, shows gender differences, and may not extend to mental health. There is an opportunity for a mental health advantage, especially when premigration conditions are poor, but this requires equitable conditions in the host county. However, due to the low number of studies that were able to measure health before migration, these findings are not yet conclusive. We thus recommend a research agenda that considers migration within a lifecourse, thereby including the period before migration.[54]

First, we echo the call of Maria Roura for a "trans-disciplinary research agenda" in migration and health that includes a critical inquiry into dominant paradigms in public health, an examination of how research on migrant health contributes to discriminatory discourses, an intersectional perspective, longitudinal research designs, and qualitative, participatory, co-creative inquiries into health and migration phenomena.[55]

Second, more cohort studies that follow different migration routes (e.g., work resettlement, visa lottery, humanitarian resettlement) and focus on mental health in addition to physical health would help unveil migration as a complex determinant of health. An ideal cohort, although requiring considerable resources, could be achieved by enrolling potential participants in cohort studies before they migrate and following them up in their journey abroad and their possible return and/or by establishing a health record linkage across countries that allow for tracking people's lifecourse as they move between (hopefully) post-migration societies.[56]

Third, premigration accounts already exist in different forms, such as archives, documentaries, blog posts, and social media groups. Narrative inquiries into existing stories, in collaboration with the owners of these stories, could generate rich and profound knowledge to complement the knowledge garnered by epidemiological studies.

CHAPTER FIVE

Health and the Process of Migration

Santino Severoni, Richard Alderslade, and Palmira Immordino

1.0 Introduction

Population movement is one of the defining phenomena of our time. In today's world, marked by economic inequalities, easily transmissible information, and ease of travel, more people are moving in search of better living conditions for themselves and their families.[1] Our political and social structures often struggle to rise to the challenge of responding to displacement and migration of populations in a humane and positive way. Yet the relationship between displacement, migration, and development, including health, has become more prominent recently in global and regional policy agendas,[2] and it has emerged as a theme of common interest for all countries.

Migration has many positive societal effects, including economic, employment, and development benefits for host countries.[3] Refugees and migrants bring new ideas, innovations, and entrepreneurial commitment to the societies they have entered and replenish the labor supply.[4]

In addition, refugees and migrants sustain families and communities in their countries of origin by providing a flow of remittances. For example, the World Bank estimates that the officially recorded flow of remittances to low-income countries was US$429 billion in 2016. Global remittances, which include flows to high-income countries, were US$575 billion in 2016.[5]

Most recently, migrant workers have made great contributions to keeping societies' essential services and health systems functioning during the Covid-19 crisis and will undoubtedly continue to do so during the period of social and economic recovery.[6]

Yet despite these positives, we have seen a rejection of migrants in many countries worldwide, fueling populist and nationalist reactions.[7] These global political forces, the migration process itself, the impact of the social determinants of health, and the risks and exposures in the origin, transit, and destination environments interact with biological and social factors to create health challenges for refugees, migrants, and host populations.

Improving the health and well-being of refugee, migrant, and host communities contributes to reducing anti-migrant sentiment, discrimination, antisocial behaviors, and possible violence, which have profound implications for refugees' social welfare and health-care entitlements as they migrate to and settle in new host communities.[8] This chapter will consider these issues from the perspective of health and health services.

First, a word on definitions. What are refugees and migrants? This chapter uses the term *refugees and migrants* to refer to refugees and all groups of migrants, unless one specific subgroup is intended. The term *refugee* is defined precisely in the 1951 United Nations High Commissioner for Refugees Convention Relating to the Status of Refugees and the 1967 Protocol thereto.[9] The International Organization for Migration indicates that *migrant* is an umbrella term, not defined in international law.[10] It reflects the common lay understanding of a person who moves away from his or her place of usual residence, whether within a country or across an international border, temporarily or permanently, and for a variety of reasons.[11,12]

Refugees and migrants remain distinct groups governed by separate legal frameworks. Only refugees are entitled to specific international protections, as defined by international refugee law.

Today, approximately one in seven of the world's population is a migrant, some one billion people.[13] Based on official government data, some 763 million are internal migrants, with an estimate of 150 million in China alone. The number of international migrants at mid-2019 is estimated to be around 272 million persons, defined for statistical purposes as persons who changed their country of residence, including refugees and asylum seekers.[14]

Many are forced to move because of wars, complex emergencies, or natural disasters. At the end of 2020 the United Nations High Commission on Refugees (UNHCR) estimated that more than 82.4 million were forcibly displaced, of which 42% were children.[15] Among them were nearly 20.7 million refugees under UNHCR's mandate and 5.7 million under UNWRA's mandate. Forty-eight million were internally displaced. In addition, there are also millions of stateless people globally, who have been denied a nationality and access to basic rights such as education, health care, employment, and freedom of movement.

Work is a major reason that people migrate internationally, and migrant workers constitute a large majority of the world's international migrants, with most living in high-income countries. Food security is also one of the key drivers of migration, even as migration itself affects food security and nutrition.[16]

2.0 Migration, Displacement, and Its Impact on Health and the Health Sector

The public health challenges affecting migrants are influenced by various factors and may be specific to each phase of the migration and displacement cycle (i.e., predeparture, departure, travel, destination, and possible return).[17] Most available evidence suggests that a combination of multiple factors, including displacement and migration, influences the health status of refugees and migrants, with some studies identifying lower socioeconomic status and social exclusion as the reasons for disparities seen between migrant and nonmigrant populations.[18]

While most refugees and migrants are healthy young working age adults, many are not. Migrant populations may include elderly and disabled persons, as well as minors, often unaccompanied, who can be particularly vulnerable to the health effects of migration.[19] Children may be accompanied by persons other than their parents or guardians, who may not be able, or suitable, to assume responsibility for their care. The identification and registration of these children can be difficult.[20]

Women, including pregnant women, make up about half of migrant populations and are often disproportionately represented in vulnerable groups, such as victims of sexual and gender-based violence, human trafficking, and sexual exploitation. For female refugees and migrants, most research indicates a trend toward poorer maternal and newborn health outcomes in migrants.[21]

Many refugees and migrants may have been exposed to hazards and stress, including excessive heat or cold, wet weather, poor sanitation, and lack of access to healthy food and a safe water supply, as well as distress, torture, and violence.[22] Access to preventive and curative services before arrival in the host country may have been difficult or absent.

Migrants may come from countries where communicable diseases are endemic or may be at risk of developing communicable diseases, such as HIV, infection, tuberculosis, malaria, and hepatitis, as well as food- and waterborne diseases during their journey, or due to poor conditions when they arrive. Access to immunization and continuity of care is more difficult to ensure when people are on the move.

Gender is one of the key determinants of health and has important implications for health policy and for equitable health care for all. Women and girls are often disproportionately disadvantaged, often losing access to critical quality sexual and reproductive health services. Maternal and perinatal outcomes may be diminished.[23] Also, the migration process may lead to the disruption of infant and young child feeding practices and care.

Displacement and migration can also increase vulnerabilities to non-communicable diseases through interruptions in management or loss of medication or equipment during travel or through legal status issues. For example, refugees and migrants in Europe have a higher incidence of and mortality rate for diabetes than the host population,[24] with higher rates in women depending on the country of origin. Although generally a higher risk of ischemic heart disease and stroke is seen among refugee and migrant populations, there is no clear pattern for cardiovascular diseases, and prevalence may be linked as much to socioeconomic factors as to migration-specific factors.[25,26] While refugees and migrants have a lower risk for all neoplasms except cervical cancer, they are more likely to be diagnosed at a later stage in their disease than the host population in Europe.[27]

The prevalence of disorders in refugees and migrants shows considerable variation depending on the population studied and the methodology of assessment.[28] Mental health outcomes are particularly at risk, as they are affected by social isolation, barriers to access, discrimination, poor living conditions, and irregular utilization of health care.[29] Migrant situations may contribute to social exclusion, depression, and early onset cardiovascular disease.[30] Often there may be no specialist mental health services available for refugee and migrant populations.

Many migrants, particularly those in low- or semiskilled labor, work in dirty, dangerous, and demanding low-paid jobs, sometimes with illegal contracts. They may work for longer hours and in worse conditions than host populations, resulting in worse work-related health outcomes.[31] This is especially the case for female migrants in irregular situations and precarious employment in the informal economy.[32]

For migrants in detention, the potential for harm to physical and mental health increases with increasing length of detention.[33] Fear of jeopardizing an asylum application and social taboos can inhibit the disclosure of psychological symptoms. Structural features, such as insecure asylum status, financial difficulties, and discrimination may affect children and unaccompanied refugee minors.

3.0 Health and Health Policy Issues

Refugees and migrants have the fundamental human right, as do all human beings, to the enjoyment of the highest attainable standard of health, without distinction of race, religion, political belief, economic, or social condition.[34] Fulfilling this right requires nondiscriminatory, comprehensive laws, policies, and practices including health and social protection.

At the national level, the entitlement and access to health services for the various refugee and migrant groups are determined by national contexts, priorities, and legal frameworks. While not all countries are party to the 1951 Convention Relating to the Status of Refugees, those countries that have agreed to accord to refugees lawfully staying in their territory, the same access to health care and treatment as accorded to their host country nationals.

However, despite these rights-based perspectives and extant international conventions and resolutions, in practice refugee and migrant health policies are strongly influenced by non-health agendas. Many present laws and policies that prevent refugees and migrants from accessing health and social services are in contrast with governments' international legal obligations.[35] As a result, many refugees and migrants lack access to health services, prevention and promotion measures, and financial protection based on their health and migration status.

Responding to the needs of refugees and migrants provides a powerful impetus for the strengthening of health system capacities in countries. The current infrastructure and arrangements for the funding of health care for the general population will significantly affect the ability of a country to provide health care for refugees and migrants. In countries where health infrastructure is underdeveloped or where refugees are not legally recognized, access to care is inevitably poor.

Countries need in the first instance to systematically assess whether their health system and public health interventions are meeting the needs of refugees and migrants as part of their processes of health policy development to achieve universal health coverage.[36]

The utilization of health services by refugees and migrants is affected by the organization of the health system and whether payments are required for access. Adverse social and economic determinants of health affecting refugees and migrants may also contribute to worse health outcomes.[37] For refugees and migrants who spend more than a brief time in resettlement, care for chronic as well as acute health needs may be required.

There are a variety of other inhibitory barriers,[38] such as a lack of information about entitlements, high costs, language and cultural differences, discrimination, administrative hurdles, the inability to affiliate with local health financing schemes, and adverse living conditions (e.g., living in camps), that make seeking care difficult, and there is a lack of recognition of professional qualifications.

An inability to affiliate with local health financing schemes is often seen. Here social insurance-based systems may be particularly problematic for asylum seekers and refugees, since registration is usually more complex than in tax-funded systems.[39] The aim should be to provide culturally and linguistically informed care. Achieving this goal requires culturally supportive staff and training for clinical, support, and administrative personnel. Wherever possible, refugee and migrants with health-related professional backgrounds should be incorporated into the health workforce.[40]

Humanitarian situations may create specific needs.[41] In urgent situations, parallel health systems may be established to serve refugee and migrant populations, though wherever possible, parallel health systems should be avoided. In wars or complex emergencies, health workers may be killed, injured, too distressed to work, displaced, or exposed to physical assault, threats, and sexual violence, or they may have fled. Health infrastructure may be disrupted or destroyed, including through deliberate assault.

Refugees and migrants often settle in large cities, where they have better job prospects, existing social connections, and opportunities for money transfer. The responsibilities facing these cities and municipalities include housing, training, and integrating individuals from different cultures, with different education levels.

It is imperative to promote an intersectoral approach in dealing with the complex and multifaceted social and health dynamics and needs of refugees and migrants. This needs coordination between national and local authorities, civil society, nongovernmental organizations (NGOs), and charity and religious organizations to optimize the use of resources and promote structural interventions. Important also will be the development and opening of alternative, protected, legal migration routes, allowing for refugee- and migrant-sensitive health services en route.[42]

4.0 Health Information, Surveillance, Risk Communication, and Advocacy

Robust evidence and good surveillance systems are required to develop informed policies, enhance service delivery, and support the work of health and non-health workers in multiple areas.[43] Unfortunately, refugee and migrant specific data is sparse, with limited specific evidence available on the health status of refugees and migrants. Few country health information systems disaggregate data in a way that permits analysis of the main health issues.

This lack of records and data, also disaggregated by ethnicity, gender, and age, hinders efforts to fully understand the extent of the health challenges and to develop evidence-informed health policies and public health interventions. Yet accurate advocacy, communication, and public information on refugee and migrant health are of paramount importance to reduce discrimination and stigmatization, eliminate barriers to health care, and offer the requisite conditions for mobile populations to enjoy a healthy life.

5.0 Barriers of Communication, Language, and Culture

While a common language is crucial, culturally competent services should offer more than just minimal communication. Ideally, a health care professional should be able to explain to a refugee or migrant the host country's system of health care as well as understand the political situation of the migrant's country of origin and the specific diseases common in the countries of origin.[44] Also important are legal knowledge, the impact of migration on health, and the capacity to ask questions sensitively about traumatic events.

6.0 Global Policy Responses and the Role of the World Health Organization

How can the world best respond to the challenges of refugee and migrant health? The Global Compact on Refugees[45] and the Global Compact for Safe, Orderly and Regular Migration (GCM)[46] set out specific global expectations and commitments. The adoption of the GCM was followed by the establishment of the United Nations Network on Migration[47] to ensure effective, timely, and coordinated system-wide support to member states.

Within the United Nations system, the World Health Organization (WHO) has a constitutional function to act as the "directing and coordinating body on international health work"[48] and has a primary organizational and technical commitment to promoting and achieving health for all and universal health coverage (UHC) within the context of the United Nations Agenda 2030 and the Sustainable Development Goals (SDGs).

The WHO and its governing World Health Assembly (WHA) have considered refugee and migration health on several occasions. In May 2017, the World Health Assembly adopted WHA 70.15 "Promoting the Health of Refugees and Migrants."[49] This referred to the WHO Executive Board Framework of priorities and guiding principles,[50] also adopted in 2017, as a means to increase advocacy for the health of refugees and migrants, as well as leadership and support to countries to develop capacities and best practices.

In May 2019, the World Health Assembly adopted the WHO Global Action Plan (GPA), "Promoting the Health of Refugees and Migrants" (2019-2023),[51] which had been developed in close collaboration with the International Organization for Migration, UNHCR, and other international organizations and stakeholders.

The key priority objectives of the WHO GPA are:

1) Promote the health of refugees and migrants through a mix of short-term and long-term public health interventions.
2) Promote continuity and quality of essential health care while developing, reinforcing, and implementing occupational health and safety measures.
3) Advocate the mainstreaming of refugee and migrant health into global, regional, and country agendas and the promotion of refugee-sensitive and

migrant-sensitive health policies and legal and social protection; the health and well-being of refugee and migrant women, children, and adolescents; gender equality and empowerment of refugee and migrant women and girls; and partnerships and intersectoral, intercountry, and interagency coordination and collaboration mechanisms.

4) Enhance capacity to tackle the social determinants of health and to accelerate progress toward achieving the Sustainable Development Goals, including universal health coverage.

5) Strengthen health monitoring and health information systems.

6) Support measures to improve evidence-based health communication and to counter misperceptions about migrant and refugee health.

To support this work at the global level, WHO has now established the Health and Migration Program (PHM), which will explore the potential of migration as a development strategy and the ways in which integration of refugees and migrants into health policies and services in the destination country can contribute to the health and well-being of the whole population on the basis of universal health coverage.

A priority for WHO will be to assist and coordinate the development of evidence-informed global norms and standards on health and migration. WHO will work with member states, IOM, UNHCR, and other UN and international organizations to promote technical assistance; improved information systems, communication, and knowledge sharing; and coherent country policy development. It will promote intercountry dialogue and interregional collaboration, as well as provide specialized technical assistance, response, and capacity-building support to countries, WHO technical departments, and regional and country offices and partners in addressing the public health challenges associated with human mobility.

Support will also be given to countries to expand systems of access to health services, for example by encouraging country initiatives to expand financing through cross-border agreements on remittances and portable social entitlements. Intercountry, interregional, and global collaboration for continuity of care and coherent and integrated actions will also be promoted.

A further priority will be supporting the establishment of reliable cross-border health information systems, fully respecting the rights of refugees and migrants to privacy and confidentiality. WHO will also promote a research agenda aimed at generating evidence- based information to support decision-making and global guidance for new tools and strategies on health and migration.

A core function will be providing support to countries implementing core capacities for national and international application of the *International Health Regulations (2005)*.[52]

7.0 How Will This Make a Difference?
What Would Success Look Like?

We can imagine what success would look like from several perspectives, based on the provisions and recommendations of the WHO Global Action Plan for promoting the health of refugees and migrants.[53]

At the national level, countries will have introduced national standards and policies on the protection of refugees and migrants based on the human right to health, both in national law and in practice, and with adequate resources.

This would require coherence among the policies of various sectors, other than health, that may affect the ability of refugees and migrants to access health services (e.g., ministries of finance, interior, and foreign affairs). Such effective policy development would be based on prior assessments of whether the health system is meeting the needs of refugees and migrants.

Such policies would deal specifically with the needs of some particularly vulnerable population groups and should address, inter alia:

1) The immediate health risks resulting from inadequate migration policies (e.g., working conditions, accommodation, camps, access to health care, prevention, sexual and reproductive health [SRH] services, etc.).
2) The needs of women, children, and vulnerable populations on the move, in order to protect them from exploitation, abuse, and discrimination.
3) The needs of those affected by gender-based challenges, exclusionary processes, stigma, and discrimination.
4) The special needs for support and developmental interventions required by children on the move, and most particularly unaccompanied children.

Achieving accountability for delivering on these objectives will be supported by country-by-country progress reports produced on the health status of refugees and migrants.

Public health systems and capacities will be strengthened across the board to address the health needs of refugees and migrants and of receiving populations. Strengthened epidemiological surveillance capacities will produce migrant-sensitive data. Adequate immunization programs will be established for refugees and migrants. Core capacities will provide for national and international implementation of the *International Health Regulations (2005)*. The health needs of refugees and migrants will be met within the national strategy for the prevention and control of noncommunicable diseases.

Health systems will provide at least minimum capacities to respond to the health needs of refugees and migrants, while also enhancing continuity and quality of care. Health services will be delivered to refugees and migrants in a gender-sensitive and culturally and linguistically appropriate way while enforcing laws and regulations that prohibit discrimination. Any screening and mandatory examinations will be migrant sensitive and implemented based on risk-specific evidence and best available advice.

Culturally appropriate provisions will be supported wherever possible by the inclusion of diaspora health workers included in the design, implementation, and evaluation of migrant-sensitive health services and educational programs. Migration health will be included in the graduate, postgraduate, and continuous professional training of all health personnel. Information systems will be strengthened to collect data on refugees and migrants through innovative approaches including surveys and qualitative methods. Awareness will be raised about data collection methods and uses and data sharing related to refugees and migrants among governments, civil society, and international organizations. The responsibility to guarantee privacy and confidentiality will be upheld, and the use of data to limit access to services avoided. Through explanation, refugees and migrants will be helped to understand why nondiscriminatory health-related data is being collected and how this can benefit them.

The health opportunities and risks faced by refugees and migrants within countries will be assessed according to the social, economic, and environmental determinants of health. The relevant sectors that have policy responsibility in these areas will be systematically involved in dialogue and joint action, and appropriate multisectoral interventions will be implemented using the whole of government and the whole of society and health in all approaches, which will involve all stakeholders.

Mechanisms will be identified for extending social protection for health and, where necessary, increasing social security coverage for refugees and migrants. Advocacy and public education efforts will be implemented to build support for responding to the health needs of refugees and migrants and to promote wide participation among the public, government, and other stakeholders.

CHAPTER SIX

Migration and Access to Health Care

Barriers and Solutions

Marie Norredam and Allan Krasnik

1.0 Introduction

Formal and informal health care constitute an essential element of all societies and have an important impact on the life and welfare of the population. The access to care for different groups of the population is a major and often controversial issue in health policy and service development. It is determined by several interacting factors, including legal frameworks and structural or organizational characteristics, as well as individual factors. Migrants' access to health care may be challenged in their country of origin due to insufficient provision (availability), poverty, and conflict and during their migration trajectory in transit countries due to many challenges, such as the lack of available care, limited resources, and insufficient data transfer. This chapter focuses on issues of special importance for the access to health care for immigrants in their destination country after arrival. These include legal restrictions that are mainly related to the formal status of the immigrants after arrival as well as structural and individual factors that may impact all immigrant groups in different ways. First, we will present a conceptual framework explicating migrants' access to health care. Next, we will describe the different factors or barriers affecting access, well knowing that they may differ between and within destination countries depending on legal, structural, economic, and sociocultural features of the health service provision for the general population as well as for the migrants. It is important to keep in mind that determinants of access to the respective health services should be seen and taken into account within the corresponding national context. A systematic review of the international evidence on access to health care from 2015 clearly demonstrated that barriers for migrants range from *entitlement* in nonuniversal health systems to *accessibility* in universal ones.[1] Lastly, we will present some general ways forward for promoting access to health care for immigrants in practice and policies.

2.0 Conceptual Framework and Human Rights

Migrants' right to access care is often argued within a rights framework. The right to health was first articulated in the 1946 Constitution of the World Health Organization (WHO). According to WHO, the right to the enjoyment of the highest attainable standard of physical and mental health is a fundamental part of our human rights.[2] The right to health may sound like an intangible concept, but in principle it implies that all individuals should have the possibility to realize their full health potential and that none should be disadvantaged from doing this. The right to health care has also been recognized and developed within the framework of human rights in the 1948 Universal Declaration of Human Rights, which states, "Everyone has the right to a standard of living adequate for the health and well-being of himself and of his family including food, clothing, housing and medical care and necessary social services."[3] Thereby, health care is seen as a basic right equal to other basic living conditions. Article 12 of the 1966 International Covenant on Economic, Social and Cultural Rights (CESCR) further recognizes "the right to the enjoyment of the highest attainable standard of physical and mental health" and notes that states should ensure the "creation of conditions which would assure access to all medical services and medical attention in the event of sickness."[4] The human rights framework has received increasing attention in relation to access to care for vulnerable migrant groups such as undocumented migrants, asylum seekers, unaccompanied minors, and labor migrants and emphasizes the importance of seeing these rights in the light of universal entitlements for all human beings, rather than just a right for citizens. The right to health is thereby closely related to the concept of equity in health care, implying that resource allocation and access should be determined by health needs irrespective of factors such as socioeconomic status, ethnicity, or migration history.[5] Equity in health concerns fairness and implies that sometimes you have to treat people differently (i.e., targeted interventions) to obtain it.

3.0 Barriers to Access to Care

3.1 Legal Restrictions to Care

Legal barriers to health-care provisions differ between migrant groups, depending on their legal status as well as the individual country context. In most countries, asylum seekers and undocumented migrants experience some extent of restrictions on their access to health care. Asylum seekers are legally residing in the country of destination while applying for asylum but do not yet have a residence permission. In many countries, they are only entitled to emergency care and to some extent to primary care services, but generally they do not have access to care at the same level as locally born persons. Such restrictions also often exist for asylum-seeking children. A recent study showed that twelve out of thirty European countries had limited entitlements to health care for asylum-seeking children. Germany stood out as the country in Europe with the most restrictive policy for migrant children. In Australia, entitlements were restricted for asylum-seeking children in detention and for undocumented migrants.[6]

Undocumented migrants are residing without legal residence permission in the receiving country and are therefore most often only entitled to emergency care or no care at all. Even when care is accessible, undocumented migrants may refrain from seeking care due to fear of deportation. Further, when care is received, it is often inadequate or insufficient, and many undocumented migrants are unfamiliar with their entitlements.[7] As a result, undocumented migrants may seek alternative health-care strategies provided by nongovernmental organizations as well as by doctors via telephone or mail in their country of origin.[8]

3.2 Structural Barriers to Care

Structural barriers are related to the organization of health-care services and may include general user payments, especially in systems that are private or insurance based, but also as co-payments in many tax-financed health systems. This may particularly affect immigrants, as they often experience lower socioeconomic status in the immigration country compared to those locally born. This is particularly clear in the case of high-income destination countries with large socioeconomic disparities between the majority population and many migrant groups arriving from low-income countries. Additionally, user fees may be introduced as part of integration policies, as in the Netherlands and Denmark, where user fees for interpreter services in health care have been introduced.[9] This policy is based on the argument that user fees for interpretation services will motivate immigrants to learn the language of the immigration country and thus improve integration. Structural barriers may also exist if there is no provision of interpreter services or interpreter services are of low quality. For the provision of the best possible interpreter services, interpreters have to be easily available and educated about health care, which includes knowledge on anatomical and medical terms and about ethical concepts (e.g., informed consent and confidentiality).[10] Structural barriers to migrants' access to care are often also an effect of lack of diversity competences among health-care professionals (see below).

Structural racism or discrimination in health care refers to a pattern of institutional, historical, cultural, and interpersonal practices within the system. These patterns and practices in turn reinforce discriminatory beliefs, values, and distribution of resources. The result of structural racism is that one racial or ethnic group is in a better position to succeed and at the same time disadvantages other groups in a consistent and constant manner so that disparities develop between the groups over a period of time.[11] This may lead to the development of health-care policies and institutions that are adapted to the needs and expectations of the majority population and neglect those of immigrants, who often belong to ethnic minority groups (institutional discrimination). Attempts to bridge the gap have been developed in the form of intercultural mediators. A WHO Health Evidence Network synthesis report has found that intercultural mediators are highly effective in bridging linguistic and cultural gaps and therefore promoting comprehensive health-care provision for immigrants.[12] However, the report also shows that the impact of intercultural mediators is hindered by a lack of professionalization, insufficient training, and the non-systematic and inconsistent implementation of intercultural mediation programs.

3.3 Individual Barriers

Barriers on an individual level include language problems, sociocultural norms regarding expectations to medical care and health-care providers, poor education, marginalization, transnational livings, and "newness."

Language is essential for diagnosis and treatment. Refugees with post-traumatic stress disorder (PTSD) may experience problems with language learning due to difficulties with concentration and memory. Further, some migrants may be illiterate, having never learned to read and/or write in their native tongue. These groups are naturally challenged in accessing written and oral information from health-care providers. Moreover, a larger group of migrants may have learned to speak the language of the immigration country to some degree but still be unable to understand medical terms regarding anatomy, specific procedures, confidentiality, medical side effects, and the organization of services. In all these cases, there is a need for qualified, easily available interpreters to avoid misunderstanding, noncompliance, and medical errors. In contrast, the use of a professional interpreter's service is associated with better quality of care and has been shown to reduce inequalities.[13] Language is part of communication in prevention, diagnosis, and treatment, and health information has to be translated for newcomers and for immigrants with longer-lasting language difficulties. But the information also requires cultural validation in order to ensure that immigrant patients with different backgrounds will have access to and benefit from different explanations and interventions.

Furthermore, education level, health literacy, and marginalization may affect immigrants' access to care, leaving some immigrants less exposed and less likely to seek advice in regard to health information and services. Cultural framing in regard to health includes different perceptions of health beliefs and practices and may thereby also affect communication and expectations about health care. Some migrants may be used to a more paternalistic system in their country of origin, resulting in dissatisfaction and frustration with providers and systems in the immigration country that are less so. This may provide a barrier to seeking care and create risks of delay in cases of need. A recent literature review regarding mental-health services utilization among migrants in Europe suggested inadequate access due to major barriers such as language, help-seeking behaviors, lack of awareness, stigma, and negative attitudes toward and by providers.[14]

Finally, "newness" may hamper access to services. Newly arrived immigrants' need to learn about the health-care system of the immigration country before they are able to navigate between services. However, different groups of immigrants are introduced differently to the available services, if at all. Refugees are sometimes part of resettlement programs that provide some kind of introduction about the structure of the health-care system. In comparison, families reunified with immigrants and labor migrants often depend on their relatives or others with more experience for an introduction to health services and advice regarding how best to access the health service when needed.

There is increasing evidence on the effect of less optimal access to care among immigrants leading to delayed diagnostic procedures and thereby more serious disease outcomes. An example of this is the late diagnosis of cancer, implying a more advanced disease stage at the time of diagnosis, as a result of patient delay in seeking health care when early symptoms appeared.[15] A special concern is access to population-based preventive health programs. These may include preventive health examinations among children, vaccination programs, and breast cancer screenings, all with defined target groups by age or gender but clearly showing lower participation rates among some immigrant groups than in the native-born population,[16] with potential serious long-term effects on future health and survival.

4.0 Promoting Immigrants' Access to Health Care

To promote health equity for immigrants, it is crucial to focus on multiple dimensions, including the right to access care, the organization of services, diversity sensitivity education, data collection, and health-care policies. Many countries have signed international declarations regarding the universal right to health care, but it is essential that these intentions are also reflected in national laws. Universal access is far from reality globally—in many countries even for the native-born population, not least in low-income countries in regions of conflicts and wars that receive the majority of the global refugees. However, immigrants are often given even less entitlements, resulting in formal inequities and potential serious health consequences. A special concern is the lack of formal access for asylum seekers, undocumented migrants, and children. For these groups, the provision of care by NGOs is often essential in order to ensure basic services reflecting the needs of the particularly vulnerable groups of refugees.[17]

Beyond the legal frameworks, it is important that immigrants' access to health care is included as a topic of its own in local, regional, and national policies and guidelines. This is necessary to be able to address the specific needs and barriers that immigrant groups may have. Only a few countries have developed national immigrant health policies indicating defined objectives and measures for better access. In order to overcome structural barriers, it is crucial to examine and improve the way health-care services are organized in light of the general increasing diversity of the population in many countries. For example, do we increase equity by providing separate services like special clinics for refugee health and torture survivors[18] or should we rather provide mainstream services to be more inclusive and able to accommodate the needs of all immigrant groups?[19] The answer depends on the particular population composition and the health system of the country. An argument for separate immigrant-focused services is that they render more empowerment and focus on different groups, ensuring special expertise on immigrant health issues and easier communication. But an argument against is that they marginalize immigrants and reduce their integration and the general professional insights and competences regarding the health and welfare of migrants.

Even with some services developed specifically for immigrants, there is still a need for diversity sensitivity or cultural competence to be enhanced in the meeting between health-care professionals and patients, both in general primary and secondary services. Medical professionals sometimes stereotype groups of immigrant patients, which may lead to errors or problematic communication and thereby to less access to qualified care. Consequently, education in diversity sensitivity and cultural competence is crucial, as part of both pre- and postgraduate training. Both concepts refer to the promotion of three general ideas among health-care providers and institutions: (1) knowledge on immigrant's health issues and risk factors hereof; (2) the ability to reflect on the identity of one's own and that of others; and (3) language and communication.[20] It is about how professionals and institutions create stereotypes and unintentional assumptions, which may contribute to health disparities by impacting medical decision-making and interpersonal communication. Instead, health-care professionals need to train their awareness and critical reflexivity about the role of culture, identity, stigma, power, and privilege in the patient.[21]

Finally, to be able to promote migrants' access to care in immigration countries and during migration, data collection is crucial for all groups of immigrants—both about the individual immigrant to ensure quality and continuity of care and on the group level to produce evidence on met and unmet needs and barriers and promoters for health-care access within special groups. Also, data collection on similar immigrant groups across countries is important for better understanding the different societal factors and structural differences in the organization of services that may influence access to care.[22]

Improving health equity for immigrants involves some direct costs—
for instance, for establishing reception programs offering information and
examinations or providing full health-care entitlements for newcomers
soon after their arrival. However, there is good evidence that these investments do pay off by better health-seeking behaviors among new immigrants[23] and early access to medical interventions leading to less costly
services in the long run.[24]

In addition, it is very likely that efforts to reduce barriers for health
care for immigrants will also benefit other vulnerable groups in society.
Easy access based on diversity competence among health professionals,
better communication between patients and professionals, and support in
navigating complex care organizations is not only crucial for immigrants,
but also for many other disadvantaged population groups. An inclusive
system for immigrants may therefore very well prove inclusive for all and
thereby support a further process toward meeting the United Nations
Sustainable Development Goals for more global equity in health.

Topics in Migration and Health

CHAPTER SEVEN

Climate Change, Migration, and Population Health

James M. Shultz and Andreas Rechkemmer

"Mobility has emerged as the 'human face of climate change.'"—François Gemenne, 2011a

1.0 Introduction

Climate change influences and interacts with social, political, economic, environmental, and demographic factors and circumstances in communities worldwide, threatening population health and survival and sometimes setting populations on the move. Human mobility takes many forms. Rapid-onset, climate-driven extreme weather events are associated with traumatic exposures to disaster hazards and "distress displacement" lasting months or years for those who sustain severe damage or loss during impact. Pervasive, slower-onset, climate-induced processes lead to soil erosion, land degradation, water scarcity, food insecurity, and loss of life- and livelihood-sustaining territory. These processes drive larger population flows internally and sometimes lead to sustained migration across borders or even continents over more extended time frames. Climate-induced displacement and migration may be internal (within country) or external (cross-border), voluntary or forced, and proactive—often adaptive—or reactive. At the most fundamental level, climate migration may be possible for populations at risk or under threat, or it may not be possible, trapping some of the most vulnerable populations in precarious immobility. This chapter shall discuss the intersection of climate change, population health, and population mobility, introducing each component of this trifecta in sequence.

2.0 Climate Change

Climate change refers to "a change of climate that is attributed directly or indirectly to human activity that alters the composition of the global atmosphere and that is in addition to natural climate variability observed over comparable time periods" (UNFCCC 2011). The Intergovernmental Panel on Climate Change (IPCC) has concluded that human (anthropogenic) influences on the climate system are clear and produce cascading impacts on human and natural systems (IPCC 2014). Indeed, human actions have ushered in the Anthropocene, our contemporary geological epoch where humans have become a major force of nature, dominating the Earth system and influencing climate and population health globally (Crutzen 2006; Laurance 2019).

The burning of fossil fuels is the primary source of heat-trapping greenhouse gases (GHGs), particularly carbon dioxide and methane, released into the atmosphere. One hundred fossil fuel producers have accounted for 71 percent of global GHG emissions (CDP 2017). In addition, nitrous oxide from the use of fertilizers and "fugitive methane" from mining and hydraulic fracturing ("fracking") are now major GHG sources as well (IPCC 2019). GHGs cause the Earth to retain more heat energy than it is releasing, leading to a warming planet.

Recent worldwide temperature anomalies are unprecedented over a period of at least two thousand years. Seven consecutive years, 2015 through 2021, have been the hottest on record (Neukom et al. 2019; WMO 2020). Indeed, two years, 2016 and 2020, have been the warmest ever; NASA declared a tie (NASA 2021), while NOAA estimated that 2016 was fractionally warmer by hundredths of a degree (NOAA 2021).

The warming of Earth by 1.5 degrees Celsius this century is already irreversible. A fraught global struggle is underway to contain the temperature rise during the twenty-first century below a critical tipping point of 2.0 degrees Celsius above preindustrial levels (UNFCCC 2015), but obstacles include a global neoliberal economic regime and profit-driven human actions that relentlessly feed GHGs into the atmosphere.

Climate change is hastening environmental degradation and worsening natural hazards. The World Bank Group's monumental analysis, *Groundswell: Preparing for Internal Climate Migration*, examined the nexus of climate change, migration, and development with a primary focus devoted to internal, rather than cross-border, migration. *Groundswell* coauthors asserted that climate change will pose one of the paramount threats to the health and survival of people and ecosystems by midcentury (Kurmari Rigaud et al. 2018; IPCC 2014). These alarming trends prompted 11,263 scientists from 153 countries to publish a position paper, "World Scientists Warning of a Climate Emergency" (Ripple et al. 2020). These scientists document how the climate crisis has arrived full force, as originally predicted forty years ago, and is accelerating based on the review of a suite of measures that collectively portray Earth's vital signs. Authors propose interventions in six realms: (1) energy conservation practices that prioritize replacing fossil fuels with low-carbon renewables; (2) reduction of short-lived climate pollutants (methane, black carbon, hydrofluorocarbons) to decrease warming trends; (3) protection and restoration of Earth's ecosystems; (4) worldwide changeover to a plant-based diet; (5) economic transition away from the excessive consumption wealthy lifestyle toward a carbon-free existence; and (6) limitation of population growth.

3.0 Climate Change and Population Health

Alterations in the climate system affect population health through multiple mechanisms. The US Global Change Research Program coordinated the enterprise and consolidated the wisdom of hundreds of researchers representing dozens of agencies to produce a comprehensive work outlining the human health impacts of climate change (USGCRP 2016). Researchers identified major "climate drivers"—essentially hazards on a macro scale— including increased temperatures, enhanced precipitation, extreme weather events, and sea level rise, and causally connected these climate drivers to a panoply of health outcomes. Then they connected the dots, scrutinizing the extant scientific literature to specify the "exposure pathways" linking climate change to health consequences. Climate-associated health concerns include temperature-related illness and heat-related mortality, respiratory ailments and allergies associated with pollution and poor air quality, water shortages and waterborne diseases, food insecurity related to droughts and crop failures, intensification of extreme weather events leading to widespread destruction, expansion of the geographic range of vector-borne diseases, and debilitating mental health consequences (USGCRP 2016). For each health outcome, experts presented key findings and rated the strength of the scientific evidence supporting their assertions (table 7.1). USGCRP findings corroborate those of other global, regional, and national assessments

TABLE 7.1 **Climate-related exposures, health outcomes, and evidence-based findings linking climate change to health**

Climate-related exposures	Health outcomes	Key evidence-based findings linking climate change to health effects
Extreme heat	Temperature-related illness and death	Future increases in temperature-related deaths Small differences from seasonal average temperatures result in illness and death Changing (diminished) tolerance to extreme heat Populations at greater risk: children, older adults and frail elderly, persons who work outdoors, persons with chronic diseases
Outdoor air quality impacts	Premature death, acute and chronic cardiovascular and respiratory illnesses	Exacerbated ozone health impacts Increased health impacts from wildfires Worsened allergy and asthma conditions
Climate-driven extreme events	Injuries, drowning, mental health consequences, gastrointestinal and other illnesses related to post-disaster exposures	Increased exposure to extreme events Disruption of essential infrastructure Vulnerability to coastal flooding
Expansion of vector range and emergence of new pathogens	Vector-borne diseases	Changing distributions of vectors and vector-borne diseases Earlier tick activity and northward range expansion Changing mosquito-borne disease dynamics Emergence of new vector-borne pathogens
Rising sea temperatures, precipitation changes	Waterborne diseases	Seasonal and geographic changes in waterborne illness risk Runoff from extreme precipitation increases exposure risk Water infrastructure failure
Rising temperatures/humidity favoring pathogens; increasing carbon dioxide	Foodborne infections and diseases	Increased risk of foodborne illness Chemical contaminants in the food chain Rising carbon dioxide lowers nutritional value of food Extreme weather limits access to safe foods
Increased temperature and precipitation, climate-driven extreme events, sea level rise	Detrimental impacts on mental health and well-being	Exposure to disasters results in mental health consequences Specific groups of people are at higher risk Climate change threats result in mental health consequences and social impacts Extreme heat increases risks for people with mental illness
All climate-related exposures discussed	Populations of concern are at disproportionate risk for climate impacts: communities of color, low income, immigrants, limited English proficiency groups, indigenous peoples, pregnant women and infants, older adults, occupational groups, persons with disabilities, persons with chronic medical conditions	Vulnerability varies over time and is place-specific Health impacts vary with age and life stage Social determinants of health interact with climate factors to affect health risks Mapping tools and vulnerability indices identify climate health risks

Source: Key findings in the table adapted from US Global Change Research Program, 2016, *The Impacts of Climate Change on Human Health in the United States: A Scientific Assessment*, edited by Allison Crimmins, John Balbus, Janet L. Gamble, Charles B. Beard, Jesse E. Bell, Daniel Dodgen, Rebecca J. Eisen, Neal Fann, Michelle D. Hawkins, Stephanie C. Herring, Lesley Jantarasami, David M. Mills, Shubhayu Saha, Marcus C. Sarofim, Juli Trtanj, and Lewis Ziska. Washington, DC: USGCRP. http://dx.doi.org/10.7930/J0R49NQX.

and special reports that have explicated the linkages between climate change and human health (McMichael et al. 2006; IPCC 2014; WHO 2018; Watts et al. 2019; UNFCCC 2020).

4.0 Climate Change and Mobility

One primary ramification of climate change that contributes uniquely to population health risks is the focus of this volume: setting people on the move. The Foresight Project, sponsored by the UK Government Office for Science, brought together an independent panel of experts to explore how human population movements worldwide would be influenced by global environmental changes through the year 2060 (Foresight 2011). The team developed an elegant framework for conceptualizing mobility and migration in terms of five interrelated categories of drivers: social, political, environmental, economic, and demographic (SPEED) (Foresight 2011). As conceptualized, climate-induced human mobility, migration, and displacement are propelled by the dynamic interplay among these socio-ecological drivers.

Climate change influences the movement and distribution of individuals, families, communities, and populations through such push factors as progressive temperature elevations triggering reoccurring heat waves and wildfires across broad swaths of a warming planet; droughts, aridity, and ecosystem degradation rendering areas unlivable; sea level rise and reoccurring floods submerging once inhabitable communities; and worsening impacts from extreme weather events.

In any year, an ever-changing mix of climate-related events may trigger human mobility. Severe loss and damage from geographically circumscribed, rapid-onset climate disasters—such as floods and storm surges, tropical cyclones, or wildfires—create short-term, short-distance population displacement. Following recovery and reconstruction—often guided by the premise of building back better—many disaster survivors are able to return to their communities and homesites. The term *distress displacement* is used to define these episodes of climate mobility and migration that, while extremely disruptive, may be temporary.

Meanwhile, far more ominous undercurrents are unfolding quickly on a warming and crowded planet that portend long-term or even irreversible migratory upheaval for ever-larger numbers of world citizens. Insidious but relentless, slower-motion processes measured over decadal time frames—including land degradation and droughts, vegetation cover changes, decreased crop yield, ocean acidification and coral bleaching, rising seas, and coastal inundation—progressively usurp habitats and render territories inhospitable. People must vacate lands that can no longer support life and livelihoods.

5.0 Climate Change, Population Health, and Population Mobility

As is generally the case with highly complex systems, there is no clear through-line linking climate change, population health, and population mobility (Schütte et al., 2018). Rather, all three elements are multicausal and mutually influential. Stefanie Schütte and colleagues offer an explanatory framework illustrated by a triangular configuration connecting the three. This conceptualization shows how climate change can directly impact health (independent of migration), particularly as a consequence of heat waves, extreme weather events, and threats to food security. Furthermore, climate change can directly affect migration (independent of health effects), particularly as an outcome of sea level rise, land degradation, food and water scarcity, and again, extreme weather events. That leaves the third side of the triangle, representing the bidirectional influences of health and migration acting upon each other. The commentary also describes the potential for migration to be an adaptive response to climate change that may potentially enhance the health of those migrants who are able to move to safer locales that are more conducive to sustenance. This is a simple concept: favorable environments attract people who are on the move. An influential study from Australia came to a similar conclusion (McMichael et al. 2006). While McMichael and colleagues clearly emphasize that most climate migration results in adverse health consequences, they also present this counterpoint: when mobility is employed as a purposeful adaptation strategy, health risks may diminish and health gains may be observed (McMichael et al. 2006).

6.0 Terminology in Search of Consensus

Currently, there is no unified terminology to describe climate-induced migration and the populations affected. Therefore, terms like *migration*, *displacement*, and *mobility* are used imprecisely and often interchangeably. The continuing saga to develop consensus terminology has spanned decades and has been described as "complex and contentious" (Zickgraf 2020). In the 1990s, the terms *environmental refugees* and *climate refugees* were popularized, and the reception to these terms was instantly polarized. There was strong pushback from forced migration experts for whom *refugee* is a legal term, generally reserved for persons who cross international borders to seek safety in another nation (most climate migrants remain within their countries of birth). However, the news media liked the use of the word *refugee* in this context, picking up on the crisis themes and portraying a future of mass migrations comprised of the world's most deprived peoples flooding northward from the Global South (Zickgraf 2020). While having no resemblance to reality, such misrepresentations provoked fear-related and xenophobic reactions toward migrants, adding to their health risks along the journey and during adjustment to destination communities (Zickgraf, 2020).

Migration and health experts now do not generally use the refugee label in this context, frequently substituting the term *migrant*. In 2007, the International Organization for Migration introduced this definition: "Environmental migrants are persons or groups of persons who, predominantly for reasons of sudden or progressive change in the environment that adversely affect their lives or living conditions, are obliged to leave their habitual homes, or choose to do so, either temporarily or permanently, and who move either within their country or abroad" (IOM 2007, 2009).

More recently, the World Bank Group's landmark *Groundswell* analysis took a deep dive into systematically parsing terms (Kumari Rigaud et al. 2018). In what sounds tautological, "climate migrants are people who move because of climate change-induced migration." In turn, climate change–induced migration (climate migration for short) refers to "migration that can be attributed largely to the slow-onset impacts of climate change on livelihoods owing to shifts in water availability and crop productivity, or to factors such as sea level rise or storm surge" (Kumari Rigaud et al. 2018).

Springboarding from the Foresight Project, the World Bank Group's *Groundswell* team presents *environmental mobility* as the overarching term for people on the move. Mobility is partitioned into multiple subcategories, including migration, displacement, and planned relocation. Mobility is contrasted with the worst-case scenario of *immobility*, a term that aptly describes the fate of populations dwelling in zones of risk who cannot leave and remain trapped. We illustrate these terms in a schematic fashion (table 7.2).

TABLE 7.2 **Terminology for climate-based migration**

Environmental Mobility

Time frame	Internal (within country)	External (across borders)
Sudden onset	Climate-driven disaster "distress" displacement	Climate-driven disaster "distress" displacement
Shorter term	Environmental hazard-driven displacement	Environmental hazard-driven displacement
Longer term	Environmental migration due to progressive risks	Environmental migration due to progressive risks
Longer term	Planned relocation	Planned relocation

Environmental Immobility

7.0 Numbers in Search of Validation

There has also been considerable controversy surrounding estimates of numbers of persons on the move because of climate change (Gemenne 2011b; Ionesco et al. 2017; Zickgraf 2020). A widely circulated projection of two hundred million global climate migrants by the year 2050 (Myers 1997, 1993, 2002) has been subscribed to by the media throughout the 2000s and still appears in some stories but lacks scientific underpinning (Gemenne 2011b; Zickgraf 2020). Fortunately, the impossibility of producing robust evidence-based estimates of total global climate migrants for some future decade has given way to scenario modeling that yields sensible predictions for geographically defined subpopulations based on clearly specified — and modifiable — assumptions.

The World Bank Group's *Groundswell* project is the most trusted example to date. *Groundswell* investigators focused their sophisticated analyses on slow-onset impacts of climate change in three regions: sub-Saharan Africa, South Asia, and Latin America. Collectively, these regions account for 55 percent of global citizens living in low- and middle-income countries. Absent any action on climate and development, these researchers estimate that more than 117 million people (95% confidence range: 92–143 million) will need to vacate their climate-vulnerable communities and migrate within their countries by the year 2050. The investigators model actions and interventions that can avert or substantially mitigate these dire scenarios.

8.0 Dynamics of Climate-Driven Population Mobility

Four major takeaways were summarized at the conclusion of the *Groundswell* report that help to frame the challenges and the opportunities inherent in the evolving climate migration saga.

First, if no action is taken on climate change and human development, internal climate migration is expected to increase dramatically by 2050—and not stop. In fact, thereafter, climate migration is likely to escalate even more explosively, as critical tipping points are surpassed. Moreover, the sobering mean estimates of 117 million climate migrants by 2050—across just three regions (71 million in Ethiopia and surrounding sub-Saharan Africa, 36 million in Bangladesh and Southeast Asia, and 10 million in Latin America), with the most severe impacts on the poorest citizens in the poorest nations—is not the totality of the story. These focused estimates do not account for sizable numbers of other communities at risk throughout the entire planet. Estimates are restricted to slow-onset events and do not include the approximately twenty million persons who are displaced annually, although usually temporarily, by rapid-onset, climate-driven extreme events.

Second, the nature of climate migration is much more nuanced than summary numbers are able to convey. Most climate migration takes place internally, within countries. Climate migrants do not just leave an unviable locale (out-migration), they also arrive at a destination (in-migration) that, ideally, will be more hospitable, life-sustaining, and livelihood-sustaining. Within each nation experiencing climate-related internal population movements, there will be identifiable hot spots for both climate-induced out-migration (sending communities) and in-migration (receiving communities). The health and welfare of both must be considered.

Third, migration can be an adaptation strategy if mobility is managed in a planful manner. The population health attributes of the sending and receiving communities must be considered in addition to supporting relocation through sound development policies. Climate migrants are both pushed to out-migrate from communities that climate change has degraded ecologically, thereby posing threats to life and health, and pulled to in-migrate into communities that offer healthier environments with opportunities to pursue livelihoods and raise families safely. Part of the draw of in-migration hot spots is that these communities are less vulnerable to climate change impacts—a fundamental and defining requirement—and more likely to produce and promote health through occupational and educational options for advancement and accessible health-care systems. Purposeful migration should be structured in a manner that enhances the resilience of the climate migrants themselves and their target communities.

Fourth, the predicted rise in internal climate migrants over the next three decades is not inevitable. Mitigation and prevention strategies implemented now in three major areas can redirect the future course of climate migration. The three strategies are: (1) aggressively cap GHG emissions in accordance with the Paris Agreement goal of keeping global warming below the 2 degree Celsius threshold throughout the twenty-first century; (2) prioritize climate migration in national and international disaster risk reduction planning (e.g., Sendai Framework for Disaster Risk Reduction) and development strategies (e.g., Sustainable Development Goals—SDGs—specifically targeting migration) to insightfully manage population movements and enhance resilience; and (3) invest in globally networked research and surveillance of climate migration to be able to monitor mobility patterns and intervene to protect population health and livelihoods.

The *Groundswell* team modeled three scenarios for the three regions they studied. The pessimistic baseline of high emissions and unequal development produced a mean estimate of 117 million (95% confidence interval: 92–143 million) climate migrants by 2050. The more inclusive development scenario, where emissions remained high but equitable development policies were enacted, reduced the number of climate migrants to 85 million (range: 65–105 million). The climate-friendly scenario, with low emissions but continued unequal development, lowered climate migrants even more, to 51 million (range: 31–71 million). Although not estimated, by extension the most ideal option would strive to achieve lower emissions and equitable development concurrently, perhaps generating an even lower estimate for internal climate migrants by 2050.

While some climate migration is deemed inevitable, the numbers of migrants and the extremity of population health impacts can be substantially reduced. Clearly, setting these interventions in motion now will set fewer people in motion in the future.

9.0 Case Examples of Climate Migration

In addition to quantifying future foreseeable mass movements involving large-scale, slower-onset, internal climate migration, discrete climate migration events have occurred, are in process, or are imminent. We provide several case examples from the across the landscape of climate migration.

Climate-driven displacement of indigenous communities in the Arctic and Himalayas. Climate change impacts on the Arctic cryosphere are affecting life and livelihoods for fifty thousand to one hundred thousand Saami (Laplanders) in Arctic Scandinavia (primarily northern Norway). The Saami were the first humans to settle in these Arctic Circle latitudes as the glaciers were receding following the last ice age. The Saami are nomadic indigenous peoples best known for reindeer herding, and more recently, their lifestyles have attracted tourism to the area. Rising temperatures, accompanied by loss of sea ice and diminished snowpack, are affecting the seasonality, geographical distribution, and quantity of natural vegetation on which reindeer rely for their food source. Given the long tenure of the Saami, these abrupt shocks to Arctic ecosystems jeopardize their way of life that still revolves around reindeer husbandry.

Indeed, harms to the cryosphere have already resulted in planned relocations. Severe shoreline erosion led to the US government–supported relocation of the Iñupiat indigenous community from their traditional homelands in Shismaref, Alaska. Meanwhile, in Nepal, residents of three villages in the high Himalayas must move to lower altitudes because planetary warming has dramatically reduced soil moisture and decreased snow cover, leading the freshwater springs, upon which they have relied for centuries for irrigation, to dry up. They currently face severe food insecurity.

Climate impacts in the South Pacific and Southeast Asia. The Republic of Kiribati is an independent central Pacific nation comprised of thirty-two coral atolls and one island. Sea level rise poses an existential threat for 120,000 I-Kirabati citizens as their islands progressively submerge. The government has implemented a Migration with Dignity climate adaptation policy to increase educational attainment and provide job skills training for I-Kirabati to make them competitive for labor migration (temporary or permanent resettlement) to New Zealand and other nearby nations with strong job markets. Furthermore, given Kiribati's lack of terrain above sea level, the government purchased land on Fiji's second largest island, Vanua Levu, for food security and economic development.

On a similar theme, population relocation is planned due to sea level rise and coastal erosion for the residents of Taro, a provincial capital in the Solomon Islands. As a third regional example, Vietnam is transitioning rural populations living in the Mekong Delta—coastal areas prone to flooding and vulnerable to climate-driven super-typhoon strikes—to industrialized urban centers with strong employment opportunities, including Ho Chi Minh City.

Double displacement. As this volume makes abundantly clear, human migration is multicausal. Colombia, South America, is noteworthy for having the Western Hemisphere's largest population of internally displaced persons (IDPs) due to the fifty-two-year armed insurgency. In 2010 and 2011, Colombia was the scene of a prolonged climate disaster; inundating rains caused flooding across twenty-four of Colombia's thirty-two departments over a period of ten months. Flooding resulted in "distress" disaster dis-placement of 2.2 million Colombian citizens. Many whose homes were most vulnerable to severe flooding were IDP survivors of the armed conflict—persons who had already migrated to escape guerrilla and para-military occupation in their communities of origin. The floodwaters dis-placed them from homesites where they had settled following conflict dis-placement; they were, in essence, doubly displaced.

Double environmental injustice: Caribbean island populations and climate-driven Atlantic hurricanes. Climate change is modifying the haz-ard properties of Atlantic hurricanes, making these storms stronger, wet-ter, and slower-moving after making landfall. Island-based populations that contribute nil to GHG emissions are nevertheless the most vulnerable populations for impacts from these climate-driven storms. Island-based populations cannot evacuate from an oncoming hurricane. There is no *in-land* on an island. By default, islanders are directly exposed to traumatizing hurricane winds, rains, and storm surges. In 2017, Hurricane Maria bisected Puerto Rico, taking out electrical power for the entire island population. Only a fraction of the populace was able to move off-island in the months following impact. Most were left to swelter for months in heat and humid-ity without power. Health-care systems were hobbled. As a consequence, over a period of five months, an estimated three thousand persons died from preventable causes related to austere conditions and lack of health services. Maria's assault on Puerto Rico represents a prime example of immobility, where most storm-affected citizens had no option to migrate.

In 2019, Hurricane Dorian slammed into the Abacos islands, the stron-gest hurricane in Bahamas history. The eye passed directly over Marsh Harbour, the capital of the Abacos; survivors whose homes had been rav-aged by the front eyewall scrambled to seek safer shelter as the eye passed overhead. Destruction was so devastating that the majority of the Marsh Harbour population, particularly the children, migrated to other islands during reconstruction, in many cases splitting families apart. Just months later, in the midst of this distress displacement, the Covid-19 pandemic arrived, borders closed, and both interisland and international travel sum-marily ceased. Recovery was put on hold while family separation persisted.

10.0 Concluding Comments

Mobility has emerged as the "human face of climate change," according to François Gemenne (2011a). Climate-induced population mobility is a complex phenomenon ranging from distress displacement, to forced migration, to planful and preemptive relocation in order to maintain or diversify livelihoods and improve economic and lifestyle prospects for families and communities. Population health impacts are many and varied, given the extraordinary variability of climate change presentations.

What is clear is that human actions throughout the ongoing Anthropocene era, representing a fraction of an eyeblink in planetary time, have placed Earth's populations and ecosystems in a precarious struggle for survival—the ultimate threat to population health. However, where we live, in human time, there are still opportunities to change course. This includes both mitigating climate threats that trigger environmental mobility and migrating adaptively when necessary.

References

CDP. 2017. "The Carbon Majors Database: CDP Carbon Majors Report 2017." July 10. https://6fefcbb86e61af1b2fc4-c70d8ead6ced550b4d987d7c03fcdd1d.ssl .cf3.rackcdn.com/cms/reports/documents/000/002/327/original/Carbon-Majors -Report-2017.pdf?1501833772.

Crutzen P. J. 2006. "The 'Anthropocene.'" In *Earth System Science in the Anthropocene*, edited by E. Ehlers and T. Krafft. Springer, Berlin, Heidelberg. https://doi .org/10.1007/3-540-26590-2_3.

Foresight. 2011. *Migration and Global Environmental Change. Future Challenges and Opportunities. Final Project Report.* London: Government Office for Science.

Gemenne, François. 2011a. "How They Became the Human Face of Climate Change: The Emergence of 'Climate Refugees' in the Public Debate, and the Policy Responses It Triggered." In *Migration and Climate Change*, edited by Etienne Piquet, Antoine Pécoud, and Paul de Guchteneire, 225–59. Cambridge: Cambridge University Press.

Gemenne, François. 2011b. "Why the Numbers Don't Add Up: A Review of Estimates and Predictions of People Displaced by Environmental Changes." *Global Environmental Change* 21, no. 1(December): S41–S49. https://doi.org/10.1016/j .gloenvcha.2011.09.005.

Gemenne, François, and Julia Blocher. 2017. "How Can Migration Serve Adaptation to Climate Change? Challenges to Fleshing out a Policy Ideal." *The Geographical Journal* 183, no. 4 (December): 336–47. https://doi.org/10.1111/geoj.12205.

Ionesco, Dina, Daria Mokhnacheva, and François Gemenne. 2017. *The Atlas of Environmental Migration*. London: Routledge/Earthscan. https://environmen talmigration.iom.int/atlas-environmental-migration.

Intergovernmental Panel on Climate Change (IPCC). 2014. *Climate Change 2014: Impacts, Adaptation, and Vulnerability. Part A: Global and Sectoral Aspects.*

Contribution of Working Group II to the Fifth Assessment Report of the Intergovernmental Panel on Climate Change. Edited by Christopher B. Field, Vicente R. Barros, David Jon Dokken, Katharine J, Mach, Michael D. Mastrandrea, T. Eren Bilir, Monalisa Chatterjee, Kristie L. Ebi, Yuka Otsuki Estrada, Robert C. Genova, Betelhem Girma, Eric S. Kissel, Andrew N. Levy, Sandy MacCracken, Patricia R. Mastrandrea, and Leslie L. White. Cambridge: Cambridge University Press. https://www.ipcc.ch/report/ar5/.

International Organization for Migration. 2007. *Discussion Note MC/INF/288: Migration and the Environment.* November 1. Geneva: IOM. https://www.iom.int/jahia/webdav/shared/shared/mainsite/about_iom/en/council/94/MC_INF_288.pdf.

International Organization for Migration. 2009. *Migration, Environment, Climate Change: Assessing the Evidence.* Edited by Frank Laczko and Christine Aghazarm. Geneva: IOM. https://environmentalmigration.iom.int/migration-environment-and-climate-change-assessing-evidence.

IPCC. 2019. "2019 Refinement to the 2006 IPCC Guidelines for National Greenhouse Gas Inventories." Adopted/accepted on May 12, 2019 (Decision IPCC-XLIX-9). https://www.ipcc.ch/report/2019-refinement-to-the-2006-ipcc-guidelines-for-national-greenhouse-gas-inventories/.

Kumari Rigaud, Kanta, Alex de Sherbinin, Bryan Jones, Jonas Bergmann, Viviane Clement, Kayly Ober, Jacob Schewe, Susana Adamo, Brent McCusker, Silke Heuser, and Amelia Midgley. 2018. *Groundswell: Preparing for Internal Climate Migration.* Washington, DC: The World Bank.

Laurance, William F. 2019. The Anthropocene. *Current Biology* 29 (October 7): R953–54.

McMichael, Anthony J., Rosalie E. Woodruff, and Simon Hales. 2006. "Climate Change and Human Health: Present and Future Risks." *Lancet* 367, no. 9513 (March): 859–69.

Myers, Norman. 1993. "Environmental Refugees in a Globally Warmed World." *BioScience* 43, no.11 (November): 752–61.

Myers, Norman. 1997. "Environmental Refugees." *Population and Environment* 19, no. 2: 167–82.

Myers, Norman. 2002. "Environmental Refugees: A Growing Phenomenon of the 21st Century." *Philosophical Transactions of the Royal Society B* 357, no. 1420 (April): 609–13.

NASA. 2021. "2020 Tied for Warmest Year on Record, NASA Analysis Shows." January 14. https://www.nasa.gov/press-release/2020-tied-for-warmest-year-on-record-nasa-analysis-shows.

Neukom, Raphael, Nathan Steiger, Juan José Gómez-Navarro, Jianghao Wang, and Johannes P. Werner. 2019. "No Evidence for Globally Coherent Warm and Cold Periods Over the Preindustrial Common Era." *Nature* 571 (July): 550–54. https://doi.org/10.1038/s41586-019-1401-2.

NOAA. 2021. "2020 was Earth's Second Hottest Year, Just Behind 2016." January 14. https://www.noaa.gov/news/2020-was-earth-s-2nd-hottest-year-just-behind -2016.

Ripple, William J., Christopher Wolf, Thomas M. Newsome, Phoebe Barnard, William R. Moomaw, and 11,258 signatories from 153 countries. 2020. "World Scientists' Warning of a Climate Emergency." *Bioscience* 70, no. 1 (January): 8–12.

Schütte, Stefanie, François Gemenne, Muhammad Zuman, Antoine Flahault, and Anneliese Depoux. 2018. "Connecting Planetary Health, Climate Change, and Migration." *Lancet Planetary Health* 2, no. 2 (February): e58–e59. https://doi.org /10.1016/S2542-5196(18)30004-4.

UNFCCC. 2015. "Paris Agreement." https://unfccc.int/sites/default/files/english_paris _agreement.pdf.

UNFCCC. 2020. "COP 26 Presidency's Report on Climate Change and Health." https://www.who.int/publications/i/item/cop26-case-studies-climate-and-health.

United Nations Framework Convention on Climate Change (UNFCCC). 2011. "Fact Sheet: Climate Change Science—The Status of Climate Change Science Today." https://unfccc.int/files/press/backgrounders/application/pdf/press _factsh_science.pdf.

US Global Change Research Program. 2016. *The Impacts of Climate Change on Human Health in the United States: A Scientific Assessment.* Edited by Allison Crimmins, John Balbus, Janet L. Gamble, Charles B. Beard, Jesse E. Bell, Daniel Dodgen, Rebecca J. Eisen, Neal Fann, Michelle D. Hawkins, Stephanie C. Herring, Lesley Jantarasami, David M. Mills, Shubhayu Saha, Marcus C. Sarofim, Juli Trtanj, and Lewis Ziska. Washington, DC: USGCRP. http://dx.doi .org/10.7930/J0R49NQX.

Watts, N., M. Amann, N. Arnell, S. Ayeb-Karlsson, K. Belesova, M. Boykoff, P. Byass et al. 2019. "The 2019 Report of The Lancet Countdown on Health and Climate Change: Ensuring That the Health of a Child Born Today Is Not Defined by a Changing Climate," *Lancet* 394 (10211): 1836–78. DOI: 10.1016/S0140-6736(19) 32596-6. PMID: 31733928.

WHO. 2018. "Climate Change and Health Fact Sheet." https://www.who.int/news-room /fact-sheets/detail/climate-change-and-health.

World Meteorological Organization (WMO). 2020. "State of the Global Climate 2020: Provisional Report." December 2. https://reliefweb.int/report/world/wmo-provi sional-report-state-global-climate-2020.

Zickgraf, Caroline. 2020. "Climate Change and Migration: Myths and Realities." *Green European Journal* (January). https://www.greeneuropeanjournal.eu/climate -change-and-migration-myths-and-realities/.

CHAPTER EIGHT

Global Governance and the Health of Migrants

Agis D. Tsouros

1.0 Introduction

The global governance of migration has been the subject of concern and criticism for many years, especially because of its fragmented global architecture (institutional gaps) and substantial normative and policy gaps. However, following a landmark Summit at the United Nations (UN) in 2016,[1] the global governance of migration landscape changed significantly, principally through the adoption in 2018 of two global compacts, one for migration and the other for refugees. These developments occurred against a backdrop of rising international migration at unprecedented levels, mainly displacements of millions of people due to conflict. There has also been growing recognition of the impacts of environmental and climate change on human mobility.[2]

Global migration involves a wide range of actors; it is complex, and it is interconnected with the governance of several other transnational issues, including trade, security, finance, and the environment. Human rights have been the most significant constant in all efforts to develop legal and policy frameworks to manage migration and address the needs of migrants and refugees. A major issue of concern has been the growing numbers of migrants around the world who are vulnerable, exploited, and insufficiently protected by either states or international institutions.

The health of migrants and refugees and its determinants gained increasing prominence and understanding in these new migration-specific frameworks as well as in a number of global and regional health strategies.

The Sustainable Development Goals (UN 2030 Agenda), with multiple references to migration, have been a key driving force of commitment and legitimacy for developments in this domain since their adoption in 2015.

This chapter will bring into a unifying context the key components of the global governance of migration with relevant health priorities and considerations identified in global instruments, strategies, and action plans.

2.0 The Complex and Fast-Changing Landscape of Global Migration Governance

Migration governance is about the combined frameworks of legal norms, laws and regulations, policies, traditions, and organizational structures (subnational, national, regional, and international) and the relevant processes that shape and regulate states' approaches with regard to migration in all its forms, addressing rights and responsibilities and promoting international cooperation.[3,4,5] In contrast with many other cross-border issues of our time, such as trade, finance, or the environment, international migration lacked a coherent institutional framework at the global level. International law recognizes a significant role for unilateral state action in regulating migration, but their authority is restricted through multilateral treaties, bilateral agreements, and customary international law.[6] The legal and normative framework affecting international migrants cannot be found in a single document but is derived from customary law, a variety of binding global and regional instruments, nonbinding agreements, and policy understandings reached by states at the global and regional level. The strongest and oldest legal and institutional frameworks related to refugees, with a widely ratified UN convention and a clear lead agency, is the UN High Commissioner for Refugees (UNHCR).[7]

Given that human rights are based on a person's status as a human being and not because of citizenship, the vast majority of human rights are guaranteed to migrants and citizens alike. Asylum seekers and torture victims have the right to seek protection on the basis of human rights treaties and customary law. In the case of smuggling, which is a key means of irregular migration, while smugglers can be subject to prosecution, smuggled migrants are not.[8] In contrast to movements associated with persecution, torture, trafficking, and smuggling, there is less convergence and cooperation at the global level on laws and norms for migrant workers.

There are a number of international laws—most notably the International Convention on the Protection of the Rights of All Migrant Workers and Members of Their Families (ICRMW)[9]—that have not been widely ratified.[10]

The global governance of migration has evolved very significantly since 2016, but the key new elements of its enhanced architecture have not yet been fully activated or shown that they make a difference.[11] In other words, these new instruments and frameworks have been poorly implemented and have not yet changed reality on the ground.

The most notable developments are the United Nations 2016 New York Declaration for Refugees and Migrants; the International Organization for Migration (IOM) formally joining the UN family in 2016; the Global Compact for Safe, Orderly and Regular Migration in 2018; the Global Compact on Refugees in 2018; and the formation of the United Nations Network on Migration in 2018.

The United Nations 2016 Summit[12] represents the most high-profile plenary meeting to take place on human movements at the UN General Assembly following long efforts to build confidence in multilateral approaches. The New York Declaration set out the intention of states to develop a global compact on migration and a global compact on refugees. The two global compacts were adopted in 2018 and are rooted in the 2030 Agenda[13] and the Addis Ababa Action Agenda,[14] both agreed on in 2015.

3.0 Global Compact on Refugees

The Global Compact on Refugees[15] (GCR) was drafted by the UNHCR and focuses on international cooperation at large. The GCR is a framework for more predictable and equitable responsibility sharing, recognizing that a sustainable solution to refugee situations cannot be achieved without international cooperation. Its four objectives are to (1) ease pressure on host countries; (2) enhance refugee self-reliance; (3) expand access to third-country solutions; and (4) support conditions in countries of origin for return in safety and dignity. An integral part of the GCR is the Comprehensive Refugee Response Framework (CRRF).[16] The GCR includes a program of action that builds on the CRRF. A Global Refugee Forum is to be convened every four years and has its follow-up, review, and implementation mechanisms.

4.0 Global Compact for Safe, Orderly and Regular Migration

The Global Compact for Safe, Orderly and Regular Migration[17] (GCM) represents a 360-degree vision of international migration addressing risks and challenges for individuals and communities in countries of origin, transit, and destination.[18] It sets twenty-three objectives (table 8.1) to better manage migration at the local, national, regional, and global levels. Each objective has several associated actions from which countries will

TABLE 8.1 **Global compact for migration's twenty-three objectives for safe, orderly, and regular migration**

1. Collect and utilize accurate and disaggregated data as a basis for evidence-based policies.
2. Minimize the adverse drivers and structural factors that compel people to leave their country of origin.
3. Provide accurate and timely information at all stages of migration.
4. Ensure that all migrants have proof of legal identity and adequate documentation.
5. Enhance availability and flexibility of pathways for regular migration.
6. Facilitate fair and ethical recruitment, and safeguard conditions that ensure decent work.
7. Address and reduce vulnerabilities in migration.
8. Save lives and establish coordinated international efforts on missing migrants.
9. Strengthen the transnational response to the smuggling of migrants.
10. Prevent, combat, and eradicate trafficking in persons in the context of international migration.
11. Manage borders in an integrated, secure, and coordinated manner.
12. Strengthen certainty and predictability in migration procedures for appropriate screening, assessment, and referral.
13. Use migration detention only as a measure of last resort and work towards alternatives.
14. Enhance consular protection, assistance and cooperation throughout the migration cycle.
15. Provide access to basic services for migrants.
16. Empower migrants and societies to realize full inclusion and social cohesion.
17. Eliminate all forms of discrimination and promote evidence-based public discourse to shape perceptions of migration.
18. Invest in skills development and facilitate mutual recognition of skills, qualifications, and competences.
19. Create conditions for migrants and diasporas to fully contribute to sustainable development in all countries.
20. Promote faster, safer, and cheaper transfer of remittances, and foster financial inclusion of migrants.
21. Cooperate in facilitating safe and dignified return and readmission, as well as sustainable reintegration.
22. Establish mechanisms for the portability of social security entitlements and earned benefits.
23. Strengthen international cooperation and global partnerships for safe, orderly, and regular migration.

Source: International Organization for Migration, "Global Compact for Migration," March 6, 2017, https://www.iom.int/global-compact-migration.

draw in order to realize their commitment to the stated goal. A key element of the GCM deals with implementation, which is the responsibility of countries. Although it is not legally binding, the GCM represents a cooperative framework of 164 member states.

Progress on implementation of the GCM's objectives will be examined every four years in the General Assembly, starting in 2022, in an International Migration Review Forum.

The adoption of the two compacts, although they are not legally binding, marked a historic change, representing a near-universal consensus on the issues requiring sustained international cooperation and commitment. Whether countries will seize that opportunity to implement them is still to be known.[19] In this context, it is worth noting the very half-hearted acceptance of the global compacts by some UN member states and the fact that some important countries refused to sign the compact.

The changes in institutional settings within the United Nations system relate mainly to supporting states' implementation of the Global Compact for Migration. IOM has entered the United Nations system, and the interagency Global Migration Group has been succeeded by the United Nations Network on Migration.

5.0 United Nations Network on Migration

The United Nations Network on Migration (UNNM)[20] was established with a main purpose of ensuring effective and coherent system-wide support of the implementation of the Global Compact for Migration. IOM was assigned as Network Coordinator and Secretariat. The Network's Executive Committee comprises eight agencies: International Organization for Migration (IOM), the United Nations Department of Economic and Social Affairs (UN DESA), International Labour Organization (ILO), the Office of the United Nations High Commissioner for Human Rights (OHCHR), the United Nations Children's Fund (UNICEF), the United Nations Development Programme (UNDP), UNHCR, and the United Nations Office on Drugs and Crime (UNODC). The extended Network membership includes the Executive Committee entities plus an additional thirty United Nations entities.[21] No single United Nations entity has the necessary expertise and capacity; these entities will need to join forces in implementing actions and projects. Some projects will be supported by the Migration Multi-Partner Trust Fund.[22]

6.0 The Normative and Institutional Architecture of the Global Governance of Migration

A useful typology for studying the roles of the main actors in global governance and the interfaces between them was proposed in the WHO publication on Health Diplomacy.[23] It addresses three main governance domains:

1) *Global migration governance*, which refers to those venues and actors that specifically have a mandate in migration. The two principal organizations are IOM and UNHCR.

2) *Global governance for migration*, which refers to those institutions and venues whose mandate is outside of migration but who directly impact on migration. This includes the International Labour Organization (ILO), Office of the United Nations High Commissioner for Human Rights (OHCHR), United Nations International Children's Emergency Fund (UNICEF), the United Nations General Assembly, the United Nations Security Council, and the World Health Organization (WHO). Even though none of these have migration specifically in their remit and none apart from WHO are dedicated to health, all show a strong nexus of health and migration within their respective mandates.

3) *Governance for migration*, which refers to institutions, rules, norms, actors, and processes at the national and regional (subregional) levels. Entities such as the European Commission, the European Parliament, the Organization for Economic Cooperation and Development (OECD), and the Eurasian Economic Union frequently have developed policies, directives, and strategies concerning migration. In the European Union, the migration/refugee crisis that reached a dramatic peak in 2015, mainly due to the Syrian war, prompted a series of strategic and legislative initiatives to manage the situation. This was particularly challenging because of the significantly diverse interests of its member states in migration policy, and thus it was difficult to create a strong framework. Two main strategic approaches on migration by the EU could be identified: The first was developed within the framework of the EU policy on migration and entailed measures of managing migration flows and measures of controlling and averting migration. The second tackles migration as a source of danger for the security of the EU member states and the safety of their people and was developed within the framework of the Common Security and Defence Policy.[24] It is worth noting that in 2020, the European Commission adopted a New Pact on Migration and Asylum,[25,26] which aimed "to build a (legislative)

system that manages and normalises migration for the long term and which is fully grounded in European values and international law." It is meant to provide a comprehensive approach, bringing together policy in the areas of migration, asylum, integration, and border management, offering a common framework for solidarity and responsibility sharing. It puts special emphasis on the special needs of vulnerable groups and identifies the needs and the rights and interests of children as a priority, as boys and girls in migration are particularly vulnerable. The integration of migrants and their families will be a key aspect of creating inclusive societies. The framework will draw on all relevant policies and tools in key areas such as social inclusion, employment, education, health, equality, culture, and sport. Despite its significance, however, this new pact has been criticized widely for failing to reach a new EU-wide consensus and thus for maintaining the pillars of the existing EU Migration Policy (i.e., the rule of the responsibility of the first EU state of entry to examine asylum requests from migrants and the flexibility of the other EU member states' obligation to determine themselves how are they going to provide support to the first EU states of entry).[27] For the countries of South America, the MERCOSUR Residence Agreement provides the basic framework for migration governance in the region.[28] It is regarded as a cornerstone in the advances of migration policy worldwide because regional migrants only have to prove to be a national of one of the signatory states to access temporary or permanent residence in another signatory state. This was a stark difference from the traditional criteria of migratory legislation worldwide, where generally a residence permit has to be linked to labor, family reunification, or studies.[29]

The three international organizations with the strongest normative and/ or operational mandates related to the global governance of migration are the IMO, the UNHCR, and the ILO.

7.0 International Organization for Migration

In 2016, the IOM[30] formally joined the UN family. The IOM coordinates the UN Network on Migration and has the lead responsibility for the implementation of the GCM.[31] IOM's Migration Governance Framework[32] (MiGOF) articulates three objectives: (1) advance the socioeconomic well-being of migrants and society; (2) effectively address the mobility dimensions of crises; and (3) ensure that migration takes place in a safe, orderly, and dignified manner.

8.0 United Nations High Commissioner for Refugees

The United Nations High Commissioner for Refugees[33] (UNHCR) is the lead agency for the implementation of the GCR. It is the primary global institution responsible for protection and assistance to refugees, asylum seekers, and stateless persons. It is tasked with providing legal protection over time in the context of evolving political and mobility landscapes and humanitarian exigencies. UNHCR's key duty is to supervise the convention's application, and its mandate evolves based on policy directives from the UN General Assembly and the UN Economic and Social Council (ECOSOC).

9.0 International Labour Organization

The ILO[34] has three sets of actors that make up its governing structure: governments, employers, and trade unions. The ILO's operational role in the domain of migrants is much narrower than either of the other two organizations, but it continues to play an important normative function. ILO works with other agencies either in the context of the United Nations Network on Migration (UNNM) (of which ILO is a member of its Executive Committee) or through several bilateral cooperation agreements with UN agencies. The ILO's focus on migration is based on the nonbinding Multilateral Framework on Labour Migration,[35] adopted in 2006. Its aim is to assist states "in implementing more effective policies on labour migration, including on rights, employment and protection of migrant workers."[36] ILO supports programs to enhance social protection of migrants; prevent human trafficking; improve migrant labor recruitment practices; enhance skills recognition of migrants; support reintegration of migrants; and protect domestic workers.

10.0 Non-State Actors

Non-state actors have enormously important roles (formal or informal) in all aspects of the global governance of migration (whole of society approach), offering flexibility and knowledge of conditions and promoting equity and inclusion on the ground as well as services and resources to support migrants and refugees in vulnerable conditions.[37] Several nongovernmental organizations (NGOs) dealing with migrants and refugees are represented at the UN. It is important to mention the NGO Committee on Migration,[38] which was established in 2006 and has consultative status with the ECOSOC, brings together over fifty NGOs. Its purpose is to encourage the promotion and protection of migrants and their human rights.

In 2007, the Global Forum on Migration and Development[39] (GFMD) was established, which allows governments—in partnership with civil society, the private sector, the UN system, and other relevant stakeholders—to analyze and discuss sensitive issues, create consensus, pose innovative solutions, and share policy and practices. Today, it represents an important means to support the GCM implementation.

11.0 Migration Governance Interfaces with Health

There are several bridges linking the roles of international institutions and global governance (formal and informal) frameworks for migration with the health of migrants and refugees and its determinants. The landscape of actors and relevant instruments is complex and multilayered. The key features of this landscape are the overarching significance of the Sustainable Development Goals agenda (SDGs);[40] the Global Compact for Safe, Orderly and Regular Migration and the Global Compact on Refugees; a series of WHO World Health Assembly (WHA) resolutions, strategies, and plans addressing migrants and refugee's health; the role of international institutions; and the role of non-state actors.

The SDGs suggest multiple entry points to bring the migration, development, and health sectors together to develop and implement unified and coordinated responses. Five targets (4, 5, 8, 10, and 16) explicitly mention migration, and several targets have an impact on health outcomes for migrants including those on poverty (target 1), hunger (2), gender (5), water (6), employment (8), inequality (10), peace (16), and implementation (17).[41] Under the third health target, the most important is target 3.8, which calls for universal health coverage (UHC)—a key SDG target to meet global commitments on UHC for refugees and migrants, ensuring access to health systems throughout the different stages of migration.

12.0 The Compacts Process and Health

The compacts process created a significant impetus for pursuing migrants' health goals that can be achieved through the concerted action of several agencies facilitated by the creation of the United Nations Network on Migration.

The Global Migration Compact features health and well-being and gender equality as cross-cutting priorities in ten out of the twenty-three objectives. Most importantly, under the fifteenth objective, the emphasis is on the development of national and local health-care policies and plans that address the health needs of migrants. The provision of access to affordable and culturally sensitive health services and the promotion of the physical and mental health of migrants and local communities are in line with the World Health Organization Framework of Priorities and Guiding Principles to Promote the Health of Refugees and Migrants.[42]

Other issues covered in the GMC objectives include developing gender-responsive country profiles on all aspects of migration including health and vulnerabilities, eliminating the adverse drivers and structural factors that compel people to leave their countries, ensuring the highest attainable standard of physical and mental health for migrant workers, protecting unaccompanied and separated children and providing access to health-care and mental-health services, reducing the negative effects of detention on migrants, ensuring access to education and health care to children, and promoting social inclusion on education and health. The Global Compact for Refugees[43] has devoted a special section to health (paragraphs 72 and 73) calling on states and relevant stakeholders to enhance access to national health systems to refugees and host communities including women, girls, children, young and older persons, those with disabilities, those suffering from chronic diseases, TB, and HIV, and all those who have survived trafficking, torture, and violence. In addition, the compact encourages capacity development and training for refugees who would be engaged as health workers.

13.0 The Health Focus of Key UN Agencies and Nongovernmental Organizations (NGOs)

The principal global organization with a strong policy and with a strategic and technical focus on migrants' health is WHO. WHO, especially in recent years, has issued a number of resolutions and developed strategies and action plans on migrants' and refugees' health at both global and regional levels. Furthermore, the health of migrants and refugees is addressed in numerous other documents dealing with specific technical areas, such as equity and the social determinants of health, vulnerability and health, the health of women and children, patient-centered health systems development, and so on.

WHO frameworks that provide guidance and indicate strategic opportunities to support migration and health interventions include:

1) The 2008 WHA resolution "Health of Migrants."[44]
2) The 2017 WHA resolution "Promoting the Health of Refugees and Migrants."[45]
3) The declarations made at two Global Consultations on Migration and Health.[46]
4) The WHO (draft) Global Action Plan "Promoting the Health of Refugees and Migrants" (2019–2023).[47]
5) The Global Compact for Safe, Orderly and Regular Migration, which features health as a cross-cutting priority.
6) UHC2030 Global Compact for Progress towards Universal Health Coverage.[48]
7) Disease prevention and control programs, including for malaria, HIV, and TB.
8) The Global Health Security Agenda (GHSA).[49]

With regard to other organizations, it is important to first mention IMO, which has significant institutional technical capacity devoted to preventive and curative health programs for migrants and mobile populations, and the UNHCR, in whose programmatic activities health is frequently integrated. Similarly, with its mandate on human rights, the United Nations Office of the OHCHR has a solid system of charter- and treaty-based instruments that relate to both migration and health. UNICEF's work on child protection and inclusion allows for a systematic inclusion of the health dimension. The Agenda for Action for Refugee and Migrant Children specifically addresses the interface of health and migration.[50] ILO relies strongly on its normative function and has, therefore, a number of conventions that relate to labor migration and to health. In addition, ILO adopted a global framework on labor migration in 2006 that reflects a strong rights-based approach and refers to occupational health and safety and access to health care.[51]

In the global health domain, blocs, clubs, alliances, and informal networks gain importance and by default are geared toward positive outcomes in improving health and well-being. The only health-specific forum that has so far had a fully dedicated political dialogue on migrant health is the Global Consultation on Migrant Health. This was a platform for countries created by IOM, WHO, and the government of Sri Lanka for multi-sectoral dialogue and political commitment. The Second Global Consultation was held in 2017 in Colombo, Sri Lanka, and gave rise to the

Colombo Statement.[52] It would be an omission from this chapter not to acknowledge the tremendous role international and national NGOs are playing in countries, not only in terms of advocacy of migrants and refugees rights, but also by providing essential health services, shelter, and social support. Important to mention here are three organizations: Doctors without Borders (Médecins sans Frontieres), Doctors of the World, and SOS Children's Villages. International networks of local authorities also represent important platforms for promoting awareness, political commitment, and action for the health and well-being of migrants and refugees. The WHO Healthy Cities networks, for example, consistently include on their action agenda the special needs of migrants and the key role of local governments in addressing them.[53]

14.0 Conclusion

Migration has always been part of human societies, and there is compelling evidence that people who move can contribute powerfully to human development, with new ideas and innovations that drive economic and social progress. Clearly, to do this they must be in good health, which is where the human right to health and universal health coverage come in. Global governance for migration needs to be continuously strengthened through dialogue, inclusive processes, normative frameworks, transparency, coherent strategies, and strong leadership. Yet so often in today's political and social dialogue, this is not where we are. There are many negative attitudes and stereotypes. Focusing on the health of refugees and migrants can perhaps change this negative narrative. Supporting the relevant schemes with the necessary committed appropriations is a significant prerequisite, as the case of the EU has demonstrated with the increase of the resources committed for the management of external borders, migration, and asylum, from €13 billion for the period 2014–2020 to almost €35 billion for the period 2021–2027.[54]

The institutional transformations in the past two years mainly within the UN system and the adoption of the two compacts have generated a positive momentum for international cooperation on the multiple and complex issues relating to migration, increased awareness of the vulnerabilities of migrants, refugees, and asylum seekers, and the employment of whole-of-government and whole-of-society approaches. The success of all the new measures is yet to be demonstrated and is subject to the will of countries to implement the provisions of the compacts and the ability of the United Nations Migration Network under the leadership of IOM to effectively support change. The various instruments that have been put in place must succeed in guaranteeing human rights, including the right to health.

Undermining human rights and the right to health can have devastating consequences on the health and well-being of migrants during crises such as the Covid-19 pandemic. The pandemic has exacerbated the existing vulnerabilities of the world's migrants and refugees. Travel bans, closed borders, lockdowns, and living conditions in cramped camps all amplified the risks to migrants and slowed down migration processing. Basic public health measures, such as social distancing, proper hand hygiene, and self-isolation, are thus not possible or extremely difficult to implement in refugee camps. Migrant workers who were employed in temporary, informal, or unprotected work were especially vulnerable to job loss and wage reductions during the Covid-19 pandemic. Preparedness plans should therefore be inclusive and consider migrants and refugees and their special needs, with emphasis on adequate access to health services, protection, prevention, and social support.[55,56,57]

Migration is a highly politicized subject that needs to be better understood in all its facets, including its positive effects for countries of origin and destination, the causes and the driving forces of migration today and in the future, the vulnerabilities of migrants and refugees, and the need for balancing issues of state sovereignty and identity with global solidarity and international cooperation. There is a need for whole-of-government and whole-of-society approaches, as well as a need to employ migration diplomacy and health diplomacy in inclusive processes.[58]

CHAPTER NINE

Migration and Changing Global Patterns of Infectious Diseases

Nicolas Vignier

1.0 Introduction

The link between infectious diseases and migration is both a public health issue and, for some, a political concern that has often been a part of debates about migration. The objective of this chapter is to discuss the role played by migration in the international spread of infectious diseases and the burden of infectious diseases among migrant populations.

2.0 Migration and Risk of Importation of Infectious Diseases

As global demographic patterns change and migration increases in volume, we can assume that global patterns of infectious diseases will follow the same dynamic with global disease trajectories, pandemics, and pathogen mutations.

Several emerging infectious diseases (EID) have been identified since the end of the twentieth century.[1] These EID are due to new agents; they include, for example, HIV-1 (1980), Severe Acute Respiratory Syndrome CoronaVirus (SARS-CoV 1 and 2, 2003 and 2019), avian influenza virus H5N1 (2005), and H1N1 (2009). EID are also due to extension of their geographic area, including for example West Nile, dengue, chikungunya, and Zika viruses, increased incidence of infectious disease (e.g., HIV, tuberculosis, plague), modification of virulence (e.g., *Neisseria meningitidis*), or acquisition of bacterial resistance (extended-spectrum beta-lactamases

[ESBL] or carbapenemase producing Enterobacteriaceae and multidrug-resistant [MDR] tuberculosis).[2] There have also been several cases of re-emerging infections, including polio virus (2014) and Ebola virus (2014). EIDs threaten public health and are sustained by increasing global commerce, travel, the disruption of ecological systems, and urbanization. However, their interactions with travel and migration are less well known. International travelers could indeed play a role in importing EIDs and could be a sentinel of major epidemics. We have seen the (re)emergence of diseases imported by travelers in Europe, such as chikungunya and dengue in France and Italy, and malaria in Greece.[3]

However, migrants are not the cause of emerging infectious diseases. EIDs are generally acute infectious diseases occurring after a short incubation and evolving over a few days. Migration takes place over a long period of time; therefore, the incubation time of an emerging infectious disease is most often exceeded when the migrant settles in a country. Most infectious diseases to which migrants are exposed do not expose the host population to a risk of transmission and are nonemergent infectious diseases. The only disease for which this is a clear concern is tuberculosis, a bacterial infection with respiratory transmission and with a long incubation period. However, this theoretical risk is rarely observed in the field, even if rare cases of transmission, in particular to health or social professionals, have been observed.[4]

3.0 Migrants, a Population Overexposed to Infectious Diseases

The concern around infectious diseases and migration is much less a concern for the host population than it is for migrants themselves, as they are disproportionately exposed to infectious and tropical diseases. This is linked to the epidemiology of infectious diseases in the countries of origin, but also to poor conditions of migration resulting in exposure to infectious diseases and, in some countries, to the lack of access to a health-care system and to insurance coverage among migrants.[5] As a result, migrants are at higher risk for a range of infectious diseases, including COVID-19, HIV, hepatitis B, tuberculosis, schistosomiasis, and malaria.[6] Existing evidence from different countries highlights the difficulties that migrants face in accessing health services,[7] which contributes to the burden of excess mortality faced by migrants.[8]

Some infectious diseases affecting the health of migrants deserve to be highlighted.

3.1 Hepatitis B and C

Hepatitis B is a vaccine-preventable and treatable communicable disease that is highly prevalent in several areas of the world, notably Africa and Asia. It is a chronic, often asymptomatic infectious disease that can be complicated by cirrhosis and liver cancer. It is often discovered late in the countries of destination due to a lack of screening policy in many countries. The average prevalence of chronic hepatitis B among migrants born in a country with high prevalence is 5.5 percent in Europe and is higher among refugees and asylum seekers.[9] Moreover, it is estimated that three in four persons with hepatitis B or C are not aware of their status. Hepatitis C is less prevalent but is not rarely diagnosed in migrants from countries at risk. Egypt and central Africa are particular countries of concern for the origins of hepatitis C. Screening is all the more useful, as a curative treatment is now available.

3.2 HIV and Sexually Transmitted Infection

Migrants are a key population affected by HIV.[10] While the prevalence of HIV infection is linked to the prevalence in the country of origin, it has been shown that precariousness and poor migration conditions increase the risk of acquiring HIV after arrival in the country of destination.[11] Two profiles of HIV post-migration acquisition exist: one concerns newly arrived migrants and the other involves long-settled migrants and is related to the acquisition of multiple partnerships.[12] Prevention programs should ensure that all migrants are provided with free and facilitated access to repeated HIV (and HBV and HCV) testing, linkage to care and treatment if they are HIV positive, and Pre-Exposure Prophylaxis (PrEP) for HIV-negative persons if relevant.

3.3 Tuberculosis

Tuberculosis is becoming a rare disease in low-incidence countries. Migrants represent a significant number of residual cases.[13] Tuberculosis in migrants is commonly the result of reactivation of latent infection with the bacteria *Mycobacterium tuberculosis* acquired outside the host country. Without treatment, it is a possibly a serious illness. It is also the most advanced disease that can become contagious; an early diagnosis and guaranteed access to health care are therefore essential. Variations in levels and trends in TB notifications among the foreign-born are likely explained by differences

and fluctuations in the number and profile of migrants, as well as by variations in TB control and the health and social policies in the host countries.[14]
Tuberculosis can be detected before the onset of the disease by screening
for latent tuberculosis infection (skin test or blood test).

3.4 Parasites

Parasitic diseases are frequent among migrants from endemic countries
and can reveal themselves through symptoms, in particular digestive symptoms. Malaria is an important febrile disease that is mainly observed in
travelers visiting migrants to non-endemic countries.[15] Other parasitic diseases can be asymptomatic but carry significant morbidity, such as bilhar-
zia (also called schistosomiasis) and anguillulosis (also called strongyloi-
diasis).[16] The latter requires screening by serology, which, if it is positive,
allows treatment and cure.

3.5 HTLV-1

HTLV-1 is an RNA retrovirus discovered in 1980 that can be transmitted
sexually (during repeated intercourse over a long period of time), through
blood (IV drug addiction, blood transfusion), and from mother to child,
particularly via breastfeeding. As with HIV and hepatitis, infection with
HTLV-1 is most often asymptomatic. However, it is associated with the
development of two main diseases: the adult T-cell leukemia/lymphoma
called ATLL with high mortality and myelopathy associated with HTLV-1,
also called tropical spastic paraparesis (TSP/HAM), with significant morbidity. The cumulative risk of developing one of these two diseases is
estimated at 3 to 8 percent. The number of people living with HTLV-1
worldwide is estimated at five to ten million, with predominance in Japan,
tropical Africa, the West Indies, and South America.[17] It is a disease that
is neglected among migrants, yet its screening by serology would prevent
maternal–fetal and sexual transmission.

3.6 Covid-19 and Migration

With the exception of a Chinese study showing an association between
rural-to-urban internal migration and the Covid-19 outbreak in the thirty-
nine cities of China, most studies have not found a link between migration
(understood as the movement of a population from one country to an-

other to settle there) and the spread of the SARS-CoV-2 pandemic.[18] The global spread of the pandemic has mainly relied on international travel by travelers and workers.

Conversely, populations of immigrant origin have borne a disproportionate burden of Covid-19. Several studies report excess mortality among migrant or racial/ethnic minority populations.[19] In particular, persons who live in shared facilities such as homeless shelters have been shown to be at high risk of getting infected.[20] Moreover, migrants from low- or middle-income countries have also been shown to have high levels of Covid-19 morbidity and mortality,[21] and for those who live in homeless shelters, the risks may be compounded. Elevated levels of Covid-19 morbidity and mortality among persons who experience socioeconomic disadvantage and migrants likely reflect a high prevalence of risk factors of severe Covid-19 infection (i.e., diabetes, hypertension) and insufficient information access to the health-care system.[22] Persons residing in homeless shelters and migrants may constitute relevant target groups for Covid-19 vaccination.

4.0 Infectious Disease and Migrants, a Screening Issue

The data on infectious disease transmission among migrants justify the systematic screening for infectious diseases in asymptomatic migrants. A prerequisite for carrying out this assessment is information and collection of informed consent, which presupposes that it is carried out in an unconstrained framework. Its access should be unconditional regardless of the administrative and legal status of migrants. The content of this health checkup is detailed in table 9.1.

5.0 Infectious Disease and Migrants, a Health-Care Access Issue

The main pillars of infectious disease prevention and control are early diagnosis and case management, which are essential both for the successful treatment of patients and for controlling infectious disease as a public health problem. Access to health care for migrants is thus a major public health tool that is largely discussed in this book. As some infectious diseases can be acquired in the destination country, prevention is also essential. It is based in particular on vaccination, promotion of sexual health,

TABLE 9.1 **Systematic health check-up recommended according to the country of origin for an asymptomatic migrant**

	Sub-Saharan Africa	North Africa	Central and Southeast Asia	Latin America	Caribbean
Medical background	X	X	X	X	X
History of violence	X	X	X	X	X
Sexual vulnerability	X	X	X	X	X
Mental health, post-traumatic health	X	X	X	X	X
Complete clinical examination with blood pressure	X	X	X	X	X
Dipstick (blood in the urine?)	X				
Capillary blood sugar	If ≥ 45 years old				
Chest X-ray (tuberculosis screening)	X	X	X	X	Haiti/ Dominican Republic
Tuberculin skin test or IGRA*	X	X	X	X	Haiti/ Dominican Republic
CBC, renal and hepatic function	X	X	X	X	X
HIV, hepatitis B and C serology	X	X	X	X	X
Syphilis serology	± If risk exposure	± If risk exposure	± If risk exposure	± If risk exposure	± If risk exposure
PCR Chlamydiae / gonococcus urinary or vaginal self-sampling	±	±	±	±	±
Schistosomiasis and strongyloidiasis serology	X				
Parasitological examination of stool	±		±	±	
Parasitological examination of urine	±				
HTLV1 serology	X			X	X
Chagas disease serology				X If risk§	
Sickle cell screening	±		±		±
Post-vaccination serologies	X	X	X	X	X
Chicken pox serology	±				
National screening programs according to national recommendations (cervical smear, mammography, blood in stool)	X	X	X	X	X

Note: *IGRA: interferon gamma release assay specific of *Mycobacterium tuberculosis*; §: from poor rural areas with precarious housing (especially Bolivia) and respect for human rights. More generally, the prevention of infectious diseases and their consequences among migrants is based on a reduction of poverty and social exclusion, the equitable access to health care, prevention measures, and social services, and a culturally sensitive patient-centered approach.

6.0 Conclusion

Infectious diseases threaten public health and are sustained by increasing global commerce, travel, and the disruption of ecological systems. Travelers could be a source of major epidemics. Conversely, there is little evidence to support the theories by which migrants would expose the host population to significant infectious risk. Migrants are unlikely to be responsible for the diffusion of emerging infectious diseases. Migrants are overexposed to infectious diseases that threaten their own health and therefore represent a population that can benefit from systematic screening and early treatment for infectious disease.

CHAPTER TEN

Mental Illness and Substance Use and Migration

Traumatic Exposures during High-Risk Migration

Sergio Aguilar-Gaxiola, María Elena Medina-Mora, and
Gustavo Loera

1.0 Introduction

This chapter frames migration in two perspectives: psychiatric epidemiology and cross-cultural psychiatry. These two perspectives speak to migration as a mixed movement involving people migrating to escape armed conflicts, violence, and persecution threatening their lives, to seek economic opportunity, and to reunify with parents and other family members. While some migrants are successful when migrating to the United States, many are exposed to traumatic experiences during their migration journey. According to the Programa de las Naciones Unidas para el Desarrollo (United Nations Program for Development), only one in five migrants from Central America reach the United States. Meanwhile, 80 percent are retained in Mexico and are often victims of discrimination and exploitation and may be subjected to violence and various types of abuse.[1]

2.0 Two Perspectives

2.1 Psychiatric Epidemiology

This perspective examines the causes and prevalence of mental disorders—depression, anxiety, adaptation difficulties, substance use, post-traumatic stress disorder (PTSD), paranoid reactions—in societies and vulnerable communities. Most researchers agree that the causes of mental disorders are multidirectional across psychobiological processes.[2] Kenneth S. Kendler contends that the pathways that lead to mental disorders cannot be understood through simple linear causations that rarely translate into meaningful solutions. This is particularly relevant to migration. Migration in itself is not synonymous with mental disorders; it is the vulnerability and risks associated with migration that place migrants at risk of poor mental health.[3] Therefore, this calls for the study of migration and mental health to consider the driving forces that shape the migration process and how these forces may influence mental health. Other researchers have also advocated for the broadening of psychiatric epidemiology through innovative discoveries that are directly relevant to genetic and biological research.[4,5] This illustrates the utility of broad-lens epidemiological research to understanding the underpinnings of disease and population-based solutions to improve the overall health of migrant populations.

2.2 Cross-Cultural Psychiatry
(Transcultural Psychiatry and Ethno-psychiatry)

This perspective highlights social factors that affect health, the importance of context, and migration bereavement (e.g., chronic stress). Achotegui explained the migratory mourning or bereavement that is often linked to stress and childhood experiences and affects a migrant's identity.[6] He highlights, for example, the migrants' transition through Mexico and how this exposes them to new contexts, making them more vulnerable to stressors, anxieties, violence, and fear for themselves, family members traveling with them, and their families left behind. Multiple experiences with migratory bereavement increase the migrants' vulnerability and difficulty making adjustments when confronted with hostile experiences from the host culture.

Forced migration may involve a sense of hopelessness for failure in the migration journey, an absence of opportunities, the fight to survive, traumas experienced, and a lack of rights. This translates to multiple chronic stressors lasting months and even years and the perception that no matter what they do, they cannot change their situation; this leads to learned helplessness,[7] poor self-efficacy,[8] deficits of social support,[9] and systemic racism and xenophobia. For many migrants, the dream of coming to a host country in search of a better life too often turns into a sustained nightmare.

3.0 Reasons for Migration

It is estimated that around 42.7 million people live in a country different
from the one they were born in and approximately 1.6 million people migrate from north Central America to Mexico and to the United States, making it the biggest migration corridor in the world.[10] Additionally, of the nearly
265,000 migrants in transit from El Salvador, Guatemala, and Honduras,
only 20 percent are successful in reaching the United States.[11] The often-
cited reasons for migration include: (1) poverty and inequality in economic
growth; (2) high population growth in cities and rural settings; (3) vulnerability to climate change; (4) high levels of violence; (5) economic and educational opportunities in the United States; and (6) family reunification.[12]
For example, in Honduras and Guatemala, 74 percent and 67 percent of
the population lives below the poverty income threshold, among the highest in Latin America. While poverty is much lower in El Salvador (41.6%
of the population), it is still much higher than the average poverty rate in
Latin America. With both Mexico and the United States closing their borders to nonessential travel to contain the spread of Covid-19, it has only
exacerbated the inequities and living conditions of migrants back home and
among refugees and asylum seekers at the Mexico-US border.

3.1 A Migrant's Journey, Risk Factors, and Voices

In an effort to provide evidence-based best practices, we must first be at-
tuned to the migratory factors or human conditions that tend to alter life
trajectories in the course of entering and remaining in the host country.
We use here some examples about Mexican and Central American immigrants to the United States. The inability to attain an education or enter
the workforce and feel like a productive member of society may increase
a migrants' dependency on public assistance and lead to higher rates
of substance use. Below are four voices of migrants who immigrated to
the United States as children and youth and who illustrate the impact of
trauma and PTSD. These four migrant persons were in the United States
between one and three years and attending a high school in Los Angeles,
California, when they were interviewed.

Lourdes (seventeen-year-old from Mexico):

> Due to poverty, a deteriorating economy, and violence in my country, my parents
> decided to separate so that my father could immigrate to the US.... I was just five

years old and trying to make sense why my father was leaving us. . . . Every night I would pray to God to have my two parents back together and be a happy family. . . . Every day I was consumed with sadness. . . . After twelve years of not seeing my father and with the living conditions in my country getting worse, I was now at greater risk and a potential victim to the gangs. . . . My mother and I decided to reunite with my father and migrate to the US. After two years in the US reunited with my father, I find myself in a similar situation, our future is in the hands of the US government and my mother and I may soon be deported back to my country. Being separated from my father was very painful. . . . I struggle with anxiety and depression thinking of being separated again . . . often I question the purpose of living.

Isabel (seventeen-year-old from El Salvador):

As a child migrating to this country, I experienced things that no adolescent should experience. I'm talking about abuse at all levels. . . . My little brother suffered much more crossing the border. My brother was twelve when he migrated to the US. . . . He went days without eating and experienced repeated abuse along the way. . . . He still suffers from those traumatic experiences. Instead of feeling sorry for myself, the inner turmoil helped me build strength and resiliency. Even though stressors are high, as a young immigrant, I learned to fight for myself and not be embarrassed for who I am . . . I use this resiliency to help my little brother deal with his trauma.

Enrique (eighteen-year-old from Guatemala):

When it comes to traumatic experiences, I've had several that shook me at my core. One morning I was preparing for school, I heard gunshots right outside the front gates that leads into our apartment . . . on the sidewalk I saw a body with a gun wound and cops pointing their guns toward me. . . . We were asked to return to our apartments. . . . This huge guy with tattoos . . . the shooter . . . asked that I let him into the apartment. . . . I was so scared. . . . Somehow . . . the cops got to him. That same morning, I went to school and I was trembling all day . . . [the experience] was surreal. . . . I was shaken pretty bad. For two weeks my family and I did not leave our apartment. Since then, I've witnessed many more shootings [and deaths]. You see so many that you learn to get used to it.

Luis (seventeen-year-old from Honduras):

There is a lot of trauma that one goes through when migrating to the US. I remember being harassed and beaten by the federal police in Mexico and almost

died ... going days without eating and just trying to survive. Whatever little money
I had (Mexican pesos), I hid from the Mexican police ... they would beat you and
rob you. When making the long journey to the US, I saw and experienced a lot of
crime [and violence] from gangs and drug cartels. My trauma was so bad that when
I settled in the US, I was constantly waking up to a helicopter hovering above our
apartment. . . . I would get scared and start reliving the traumatic encounters with
the Mexican police and gangs. . . . I would hide under my bed because I thought
they were coming for me. Where we live, there are a lot of shootings, so the police
helicopter is constantly circling at night with its high-powered searchlight coming
through our apartment window. . . . I relive my traumas every day.

Migrants from Mexico with children born in the United States are often
faced with the excruciating decision to leave their US-born children behind or bring them with them to Mexico. For parents it is a double trauma
of leaving the United States and having to adapt to the Mexican context;
the trauma and discrimination that many US-born children face in Mexico
has long-lasting effects on their ability to stay connected with community
life[13] and ultimately leads to poor health outcomes and substance use.[14]

3.2 Substance Use

Studies have found that migrants in transit across or along the Mexico-US
border are exposed to physical, psychological, and sexual violence and exhibit high levels of substance and illicit drug use behaviors.[15,16] Researchers have found alcohol dependence to be higher among migrants who
were robbed and experienced physical violence in the context of their migration journey.[17,18] This association between substance use behaviors and
exposure to violence of any kind can be seen as a significant risk factor
for migrants' mental health that needs more attention. With the Covid-
19 pandemic, this concern is more evident, as many migrants will experience hardships due to job loss, housing instability/inability to pay rent, not
enough food, social isolation, and other social, economic, and structural
determinants that will impact their mental-health status.

4.0 The Mental-Health Status of Migrants during Covid-19

The Covid-19 crisis and 2020–2021 fires in the US West Coast provide a
contemporary illustration of how social and economic stressors influence

the mental health of migrants who are already at greater risk of poor mental health. Covid-19 and the recent fires have added new layers of stressors and anxiety to the social, economic, environmental, political, and emotional burdens already present in the daily lives of underserved migrant communities. The pandemic has amplified systemic structural inequities affecting migrants and their mental health and increased their risk of contracting Covid-19 that led to excessive mortality.[19] For example, Garcia and colleagues reported that the mortality ratio for foreign-born Latinos ages twenty to sixty-four with a high school degree or less was 10.73 times the Covid-19 death rate for Whites.[20]

Migrants trapped in shelter camps at the US southern border and denied entry or an opportunity to request sanctuary are more vulnerable to Covid-19 and to multiple stressors and traumatic experiences and resulting mental-health conditions. Moreover, without adequate access to preventive care, migrants are at greater risk of health conditions such as obesity, hypertension, asthma,[21] and diabetes,[22] which, when combined with anxiety, depression, substance abuse, and PTSD, can lead to more severe cases of Covid-19 and sometimes death.

Coupled with recent data from the US Centers for Disease Control and Prevention (CDC) showing Latino persons, both adults and children, have a greater likelihood than White persons of contracting Covid-19, past research on health disparities demonstrates a treatment gap and other indicators of systemic structural inequities and vulnerabilities that can explain the increased risk and higher rates of Covid-19 infections, hospitalizations, and deaths among Latino migrants.[23] Poverty, a social determinant strongly linked to mental disorders, is more prevalent among migrant communities and has made migrants more vulnerable to Covid-19 and behavioral health conditions. Migrants tend to be essential workers who are more likely to keep working despite the high risks of Covid-19 illness, lack of access to adequate personal protection equipment (PPE), and infection due to workplace exposure[24] because they are not able to access unemployment benefits, paid sick leave, or enough food or economic relief without a significant income loss. Migrant workers are disproportionally represented in economic sectors severely affected by Covid-19, such as agriculture and food, domestic and care work, construction, manufacturing, transportation, hospitality, and travel and tourism. Job losses are usually exacerbated by the limited access to safety-net systems and may have a downward impact on wages in the long term.[25] Many migrants are not able to work remotely or generally rely on any form of a safety net.[26] Overall, the pandemic has affected the earning power of 164 million migrant workers who support through remittances at least 800 million relatives in less affluent countries.[27,28] For example, El Salvador reported a drop of 40 percent in remittance flows in the first five months of 2020 compared to the same months in 2019.[29]

5.0 Resilience as a Protective Factor

Protective factors that align to an individual's perseverance and ability to manage adversities can lead to positive mental-health outcomes. Resilience, in the simplest form, is defined as the process of positive adaptation to a new environment, achieving social belonging, gaining fulfillment out of life, and recovering from trauma or adversity.[30] Strong resilience consists of protective factors like having a positive caregiver, supportive family and community relationships, and a spiritual/religious connection. Religious beliefs and supports have been interpreted as a source of strength associated with resilience. Researchers examining the strengths and resilience of a group of migrant women in Tijuana, Mexico, for example, found that internal strengths (i.e., religious beliefs, courage, endurance, and goal setting) and external factors (i.e., support received from people, institutions, and families) played a key role in their survival.[31] Personal characteristics such as self-efficacy and personal agency[32,33] are also linked to resilience. Migrants with low self-efficacy are at greater risk of quickly being consumed by their past traumas and present stressors from adverse circumstances. That is, individuals with poor self-efficacy and agency may have low resilience and difficulties dealing with adversity and are at higher risk for mental health and substance use conditions.[34,35] Researchers have found a strong association between the adversity of migration and resilience, well-being, and positive behavioral health outcomes.[36]

Migrants' perceived sense of control over their environment and belief that they can alter their life course and meet challenging societal and environmental demands represent individual resiliency and self-efficacy.[37] Perceived self-efficacy plays a major role in a person's resilience and recovery from adverse experiences or trauma. For example, Benight and Bandura found that people who believe they can defeat past traumas tend to demonstrate effective coping abilities to regain control over their lives rather than having their lives dictated by adverse conditions or environments.[38] Efficacy beliefs influence an individual's level of perseverance when facing adversities.

6.0 Interventions: Best Practices to Building Resilience

In this section, we define *best practices* as community-defined interventions that, when appropriately tailored to migrants' culture, language, and life histories, lead to evidence substantiating effectiveness. In Bronfenbrenner's ecological perspective,[39,40] resilience in the face of adversity can also facilitate the development of well-being under stressful conditions. Migrant people's experiences are resilience landscapes that emerge from the depths of their individual migration journey—as are their life course experiences as they adjust to a new life in the United States. For children and adolescents, the amount of exposure to traumatic experiences shapes their life trajectories and mental-health status. This is consistent with the three frameworks (social-ecological, life course, and migration) described in chapter 2.

6.1 Mindfulness toward Well-Being

Using mindfulness as an intervention for migrants can help them acknowledge and accept their experiences—even the most painful ones—rather than suppress them or avoid them. For example, Anna Reebs and colleagues[41] developed a trauma-sensitive intervention called Mindfulness-Based Trauma Recovery for Refugees (MBTR-R) to help migrants and refugees suffering from PTSD recover and heal after enduring the physical and mental ordeal of their migration journey. These researchers found that 52 percent of asylum seekers who received this intervention recovered from PTSD. Researchers have found mindfulness-based interventions to be scalable community-accessible interventions that can be used as treatments for depressive symptoms in adults experiencing stress and trauma.[42]

With Isabel, the case study introduced earlier, while she acknowledges and accepts her traumatic experiences as part of who she is and as a foundation to become stronger and persist, she is affected by her brother's pervasive fears and altered life course. Practicing mindfulness as a recovery tool to achieve mental well-being can help Isabel to continue recognizing her own thoughts as they reappear and to use her story to offer support to her brother and other migrants who may be suppressing their experiences. Previous work in the area of mindfulness has associated mindfulness as an intervention tool with improving empathy and communication skills.[43] This may explain Isabel's ability to notice her own thoughts, release herself from a vicious cycle of negative thinking and demonstrate empathy toward her brother to achieve his mental well-being.

For Enrique and Luis, their multiple exposure to traumatic violent and assaultive events signals a greater risk of PTSD. This is consistent with prior research showing the effects of previous assaultive violence in childhood increasing the risk of PTSD in adulthood.[44] A recent study found that mindfulness-based treatments help restore connections between large-scale brain networks among individuals with PTSD.[45] Mindfulness is a "present-centered" technique that targets symptoms of avoidance and negative cognitions, including self-blame, shame, and guilt among individuals with PTSD.[46]

6.2 Sense of Belonging (Pertenencia) and Well-Being

With intergenerational trauma, as seen among the offspring of survivors of the Holocaust and other atrocities of war, community trust and cohesiveness are also eroded. Individuals and families become isolated and less able to connect with others. This hits particularly hard on disadvantaged communities and marginalized populations, such as refugees and immigrants who struggle with making a life in new and unfamiliar surroundings and for whom, historically, security and advancement has depended on their capacity for collaborative effort and a sense of belonging. For Lourdes, the United States represented a place of belonging and having her family together. There are many immigrant youths with a similar story who are just wanting to feel safe and use their human capacity to contribute to the US workforce. A key building block of resilience that maximizes protective factors and minimizes risk factors is *pertenencia*. When migrants are uprooted, they lose what they value the most when they migrate—family and country.[47] When their traumas have been overwhelming from their journey and they face more debilitating risk factors or multiple secondary adversities[48] and conflicted environments, they may feel displaced, marginalized, and unable to reclaim *pertenencia*. For many migrants, survival has become a way of life; they are experts in preparing for and overcoming hardships that define their life course and resilience.[49] For Lourdes, Isabel, Enrique, and Luis, being recognized as survivors and resilient people and helped to feel productive and to reach a level of acceptance and sense of community that will not paralyze their creativity, their hopes, and their human capabilities to contribute and feel a part of community life are important. These are protective strategies to support Lourdes, Isabel, Enrique, Luis, and other migrants overcome all risks and continue preparing for the worst, whatever crisis may be next. Simply put, when people with an immigrant background tap into their protective factors, they are more likely to self-manage prior and new traumas and slowly regain what they value most—a sense of purpose and belonging and, ultimately, family and country.

7.0 Conclusion

Migration increases the risk for poor mental-health outcomes. For example, the World Health Organization (WHO) estimates that 22 percent of migrants will develop a mental disorder.[50] Mental disorders tend to persist, so interventions must not only respond to emergencies, but must also be maintained as part of the community care system. Diagnostic tools and evidence-based psychosocial and clinical interventions to mitigate disparities, support well-being, and foster life skills, coping strategies, and resilience are needed. The challenge is to find effective ways to take evidence-based interventions to the communities and people in need like Lourdes, Isabel, Enrique, and Luis. The aim must be to promote inclusivity, dignity, respect, and safety and to learn from the resilience of migrants. Through these efforts, we can reduce the mental-health burden of migration, protect the dignity of migrant populations, and contribute to the fulfillment of the United Nations Sustainable Development Goals.

CHAPTER ELEVEN

Urbanization and Theoretical Perspectives on Migration and Mental Health

Yang Xiao

1.0 Introduction

Migration is one of the sentinel global demographic shifts of the early twentieth century.[1] The evolution of migration as a global concern for public health echoes the global rise in urban living. In 2008, global urbanization exceeded 50 percent for the first time. Moreover, urbanization is expected to reach 70 percent by 2050, with the number of urban residents increasing by 3.1 billion between now and then. While urbanization brings political, cultural, economic, medical, and educational opportunities, it also can present challenges to the health of migrants and host populations.[2,3] Rates of illness tend to be more common in areas with higher urbanization; for example, Peen and colleagues compared the prevalence of mental disorders in five different areas and found that the cities with the highest level of urbanization had a 77 percent greater incidence of mental illness than those with the lowest level of urbanization.[4]

2.0 Mental Illness

Within a new era of global economic and social change, mental illness has become the world's third most common disease, after only heart disease and cancer. In the United States, more than forty-four million adults (18%

of the total population) suffer from mental illness. In England, one in six people between sixteen and sixty-four years old have symptoms consistent with mental illness. In China, fifty-four million people—accounting for 4.2 percent of the country's population—suffered from depression in 2017. There is an extensive literature summarizing the factors that lead to mental problems.[5] For example, multiple elements of the social, economic, and physical environment at different life stages[6] may be associated with mental health. There is abundant reason to think that migration—accompanied as it is with a range of stressors experienced before, during, and after migration—affects mental health. However, some scholars have found that immigrants have equal or even better health outcomes than nonmigrants, despite migrants' lower socioeconomic status and limited access to health services. This is known as the "healthy migrant effect."[7,8] It means that newly arrived migrants tend to have better health status than the local population and that healthier individuals are more likely to migrate and move further away from home.[9,10] However, this observation may not be fully applicable for mental health.[11,12] For example, Xiao, Miao, and Sarkar found that interprovincial migrants can have worse mental-health status than intra-provincial migrants in China.[13]

Upon arrival at their destination, migrants may face challenges of adaptation and integration, including competition and conflicts among individuals, groups, and different cultures. These challenges are all associated with potential psychological burden,[14] which has been associated with mental illness, including mood-anxiety disorders.[15] Differences in economic structure, society, culture, behavior, and lifestyle between places of origin and destination often result in challenges for migrant integration, making migrants permanent outsiders in their new context. Several theories suggest that mental-health challenges faced by migrants are centrally tied to their challenges with social integration, influenced by difficulties in gaining advantages in the labor market, and made worse by social isolation and discrimination. This has been at the core of scholarship that aims to better understand the forces that shape mental health among migrants. Existing literature around migrant mental health in the United States and Europe can be summarized in two categories: studies concerned with spatial scale and studies addressing the migration process.

First, in terms of spatial scale (fig. 11.1), several studies emphasize the mental-health effects of social integration in migrants' host cities. Theoretical and empirical research has been conducted on the health of migrants at different spatial scales. We summarize some key observations from these studies:

Research frameworks

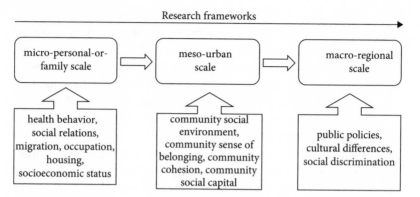

FIGURE 11.1. Breadth of research frameworks on the mental health of the migrants

1) At the macro-regional scale, several studies have shown that policies that may impede social integration between countries and regions, together with structural factors that promote social and racial discrimination, can pose mental-health risks for migrants. For example, Malmusi conducted research on the relationship between immigration integration policies of fourteen European Union (EU) countries and the mental health of immigrants.[16] This work showed that compared with those from countries where there was an explicit effort to accept multiple cultures, immigrants to countries where different cultures were excluded had poorer health. By way of another example, Alegría, Álvarez, and DiMarzio found that racial discrimination had a negative impact on the mental health of first-generation immigrants in the United States.[17]

2) At the meso-urban scale, communities are an important geographic lens to consider forces that influence inclusion and the mental health of migrants.[18] Community integration can promote mental health by enhancing trust between neighbors and providing an environment of emotional support and mutual respect for disadvantaged groups.[19] At the same time, an individual's mental-health status is strongly influenced by community values, including social support, social participation, social capital, social network at the community level, and the safety of the community environment.[20,21] Gale and colleagues found that in multiple deprivation areas in the United Kingdom, community cohesion improved the mental health of residents.[22]

3) At the micro (personal or family) scale, the impact of social integration on mental health is more complex, involving health behavior, social relations, migration, occupation, housing, and economic and social status. Status syndrome rests

on the health differences between people in different positions in society. The higher the socioeconomic status of the group, the better the average mental-health status. Ling Na notes that people also receive social support and social capital through social interaction and participation in cultural or spontaneous activities.[23] Both intragroup bonding social capital and intergroup bridging social capital can promote the acquisition of healthy resources and opportunities and improve mental health.

Second, other studies focus on the migration process. The extant literature, some of which is summarized in figure 11.2, shows that the health of migrants is influenced through the entire process of migration. This can be divided into four stages: "before migration," "arriving at the destination," "staying in the destination," and "returning to country of origin."[24,25] Shuval suggests that three types of changes related to migration exist: physiological changes (changes in lifestyles such as climate and eating habits), social changes (changes in social status, economic status, roles, and social relationships), and cultural changes (changes in cultural norms and cultural values).[26] The more changes migrants experience, the more difficult it can be for them to adapt to the new environment,[27,28] which, in turn, is associated with mental-health problems.[29,30] As migration has increased in prevalence and importance worldwide, scholarship on the forces that shape migration and its health consequences has increased. Studies in the field may consider the link between migration and mental health through the lens of three theoretical perspectives: social isolation theory, goal pressure theory, and acculturation theory.

Social isolation theory suggests that the separation of the original social network during the migration process and the serious obstacles to contact and communication between the migrants and their destination community will lead to the occurrence of mental illness. Meanwhile, the goal pressure theory suggests that the gap between the expectations before migration and the acquisition of assets and status after migration is the main cause of mental illness.[31]

Acculturation suggests that the most serious adaptation problems faced by the migration process are caused by cultural differences, including the differences in cultural norms, cultural practices, and the values that exist between migrants' hometown and destination city. Those who have difficulty accepting or adapting to cultural differences are more likely to have mental illness.[32,33] Immigrants who are able to integrate more successfully are, by contrast, less likely to have poor mental health.

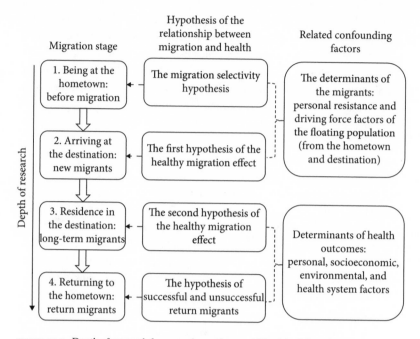

FIGURE 11.2. Depth of research frameworks on the mental health of the migrants

The investigation of the relationship between acculturation and mental health has received increasing attention, as it has become more apparent that social integration is not binary, but a process that emerges over the migrants' lifecourse.[34,35,36] In many local municipalities, social integration policies do not account for differences in the origin of migrants and the challenges that underlie acculturation over time. Hunt, Schneider, and Comer reviewed sixty-nine academic papers on acculturation[37] and found that Salabarría-Peña's definition of acculturation was the clearest and most widely accepted: "When hometown culture comes into contact with mainstream culture, the process of people adapting to the latter is acculturation. In this process of acculturation, people accept mainstream culture while maintaining or abandoning their hometown culture."[38] Based on this definition, the impact of acculturation on mental health includes the following two aspects:

1) Unidirectional model. In this process, immigrants gradually change from their hometown culture to their mainstream culture and finally adapt to only one

culture.[39] This suggests that acculturation only affects migrants themselves as they change cultures but does not affect other groups. Therefore, the hometown culture brought by migrants has no influence on the mainstream culture of the destination.[40]

2) Two-dimensional model. It has also been suggested that acculturation should include two dimensions—namely, the degree of contact with and participation in the mainstream culture and the degree of maintaining the hometown culture. These two dimensions are independent but complementary.[41,42] This model suggests that immigrants can choose the values, languages, attitudes, and behaviors of different cultures when they are faced with different acculturation challenges. Based on this, Berry further summarized a two-dimensional model (fig. 11.3) for the two-dimensional influence mechanism, which includes four levels of acculturation status: "assimilation," or high adoption of the host culture and low maintenance of the origin culture; "separation," or low adoption of the host culture and high maintenance of the origin culture; "marginalization," or low adoption of the host culture and less maintenance of the origin culture; and "integration," or high adoption of the host culture and maintenance of the culture of origin.[43,44,45] The different status of acculturation mainly depends both on people's willingness, actions, and preferences to participate in mainstream culture[46] and on the tolerance of mainstream culture and the attitude of mainstream culture toward cultural differences that will also affect the process of

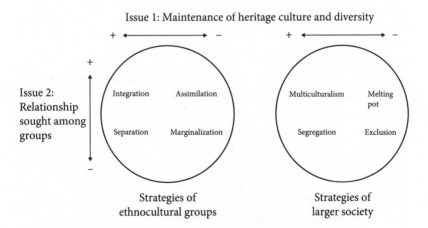

FIGURE 11.3. John Berry's two-dimensional model of acculturation

Source: Berry, J. W., 1980, "Social and Cultural Change," *African Studies Review* 17, no. 2: 79–88.

acculturation.[47,48] Under the dual influence of the individual's willingness to acculturate and the openness of the destination country to welcome newcomers, immigrants will eventually settle into one of the four acculturation strategies.[49]

Many researchers have further theoretically supplemented and empirically verified Berry's two-dimensional model of acculturation and found that the effects of different acculturation strategies on people's mental health are not consistent.[50] For example, the empirical research of Gaertner and Dovidio shows that integration may be best associated with mental health, because immigrants in the state of integration have a better sense of integration into the destination society and also maintain a sense of hometown cultural uniqueness.[51] Golding and Burnam found that acculturation had no effect on the risk of depression.[52] Using data from a large-scale community survey, Kaplan and Marks found that the relationship between acculturation and depression varies with age groups.[53] Their research showed that acculturation has little influence on depression levels of young people. However, they also suggest that acculturation can effectively help alleviate depression for the elderly. Salant and Lauderdale found that immigrants from Asia had low health conditions due to their difficulty in integrating into the mainstream Western culture and lifestyle.[54] Other studies have also found that for certain groups of people, acculturation does not have any significant effect on their mental health, such as Hispanic college students,[55] Puerto Rican persons in the United States,[56] and elderly Korean immigrants.[57]

3.0 Conclusion

The dual forces of globalization and urbanization are likely to continue to drive migration for decades to come. This calls for attention to the structure of the migrant experience and how this may affect the mental health of migrants in coming decades. There are substantial differences in the migrant experience across groups, characterized by the level of the migrant's socioeconomic advantage, the receptivity of the destination country, and the resources available to help buffer the impact of migration. These forces influence migrants' integration into destination cities and countries and ultimately shape migrant mental health.

CHAPTER TWELVE

Nutrition and Migrant Health

Erin Hoare, Adrienne O'Neil, and Felice Jacka

1.0 Introduction

Diet and nutrition are central to health and well-being. However, nutrition and consequent health are far more complex than simply the foods consumed by the individual. As nutrition research has evolved, it has become clear that environmental and social factors are major contributors to population over- and undernutrition and subsequent health outcomes. Migration—the geographic movement and settlement of people—is driven by factors such as threats to safety, lack of economic opportunities, and natural events including drought and famine and poses unique risks and opportunities. While the issue of nutrition in the migration context is broad, the focus of this chapter is on newly arrived migrants from abroad in the context of Western countries. Accessibility and availability of foods high in nutritional quality, in addition to wider social and environmental challenges such as safe and clean housing, poor educational and employment outcomes, and disproportionate risk of chronic physical conditions, have significant and concurrent impact on migrant nutrition. Conversely, the economic, social, and health service opportunities afforded to individuals upon migrating may also have positive impacts on nutrition. The nutrition of host populations is of interest with the arrival and integration of migrant populations. This chapter examines migrant nutrition and highlights some key issues impacting nutrition among migrant populations.

2.0 Nutrition and Health

2.1 Migrant Health

It is estimated that there are more than 272 million international migrants, defined as foreign-born individuals or the foreign population obtained from nationally representative surveys.[1] Migration poses a significant public health challenge, with access to health services often denied to individuals and a broad and varied set of social determinants increasing the risk of poorer health outcomes. For example, it has been recognized that communication barriers, structural and cultural issues, and a lack of employment and education opportunities disproportionately affect migrant groups. While migrant groups are broad in terms of demographics and other characteristics, a range of poor health indicators—including, for example, a higher risk of poor maternity and perinatal outcomes and higher levels of mental illness—have been identified among migrants.[2] The health of migrant communities has been acknowledged to be largely affected by the health policies and legal rights of the specific jurisdiction afforded to migrant groups upon relocation and settlement[3] based on their legal status. Health outcomes are recognized to be shaped by the interacting and evolving drivers unique to different migrant groups. Critically, it is accepted that it is not migration itself, but the social determinants that accompany migration and resettlement environments that interact to affect health outcomes.[4]

2.2 Human Nutrition

Nutrition is the obtainment and provision of foods and drink required for health and development. A nutritious diet is comprised of adequate intake of foods with necessary nutritional content to support good human health.[5] Nutrition, including nutritional needs and intake, is assumed to be affected by various interacting and complex factors such as age, genetics, and other biological factors, as well as nonbiological factors such as culture, poverty, and social status.[6] Given the complexity of underlying determinants in human nutrition, it is unsurprising that nutritional needs and optimal nutritional intake vary across individuals, societies, and communities worldwide. Indeed, malnutrition, undernutrition, and overnutrition represent a leading cause of the disease burden globally, and the cost of the industrialized food system to global health and the environment is estimated at US$12 trillion annually.[7]

Broadly speaking, nutritious diets include a variety of high-quality, unrefined or minimally processed foods, including fruit, vegetables, whole grains, protein, and healthy fats.[8] A high intake of water and limited intake of sugary, high-fat, processed foods and snacks are also recommended as part of a healthful diet. Nutritional deficiencies are typically characterized by a reduced intake of foods considered to be part of optimal nutrition and/or an increased intake of foods with little to no nutritional benefit.

Malnutrition caused by lack of optimal nutrition has adverse immediate and long-term health consequences. Undernutrition can lead to low weights, stunting and wasting, and disease. Illnesses resulting from undernutrition are most common among children under five.[9] Micronutrient-related malnutrition refers to the inadequate intake of particular micronutrients found in foods and can lead to the body's inability to develop and thrive.[10] Noncommunicable disease resulting from poor nutrition includes cardiovascular diseases, type 2 diabetes, high blood pressure, unhealthy weight, and some cancers.[11] In 2017, the Global Burden Of Disease study found that eleven million deaths and 255 million disability-adjusted life years were attributable to dietary risk factors.[12] Diet therefore represents a major leading risk factor for the prevention of chronic diseases and illness and is of major interest to global health.

2.3 Migrant Nutrition

As established, migrant communities face a disproportionate risk of adverse health outcomes including poor nutrition.[13] The global migrant population is highly heterogenous based on factors such as push or pull migration (referring to the adverse factors that contribute to individuals leaving their community of origin and the improved opportunities encouraging movement and settlement), and the nutrition status of migrant communities is therefore widely variable. However, it is accepted that the resettlement process and changing social, structural, family, and other environments can adversely impact individuals' opportunities to engage in healthful behaviors, including adherence to nutritious diets.[14] Conversely, the employment and economic opportunities provided upon migration may increase household income, improve access to health care, and enable healthy behaviors, including healthful diets. Among migrants, poor nutritional quality has been observed.[15] As examples, low consumption of foods rich in calcium and vitamin D were observed among children settled in Canada.[16] A high engagement in Western diets (characterized

by low consumption of fruits, vegetables, and whole foods and high consumption of processed, sugary foods that are high in saturated fats) has
been observed in women who migrated to the United States from Somali.[17] Reduced diet diversity was observed among Iraqi refugees in
Lebanon, including low consumption of fruits and other whole foods and
high consumption of processed high-fat foods.[18] There is also evidence
to show maintenance of premigration diet upon arrival and settlement
in host countries and balanced healthful dietary knowledge and practice
among migrant groups upon settlement, further highlighting heterogeneity in migrant nutrition.[19] A recent study in the development of metabolic
diseases post-migration demonstrated that migration from non-Western
countries to the United States was associated with immediate loss of gut
microbiome diversity, which is itself influenced by both long-term diet and
significant dietary changes.[20]

Migrant communities may experience increased risk of the double burden of nutrition, which refers to the coexistence of undernutrition risk and
overweight and obesity risk.[21,22] The adverse consequences of this double
burden are significant—undernutrition early in life can be a predisposing
factor to overweight and other noncommunicable diseases, such as type 2
diabetes and cardiovascular disease.[23] Nutrition-related factors, in particular undernutrition, are a major contributor to global child mortality, with
approximately 45 percent of the burden explained by nutrition-related
factors.[24] The myriad of social, economic, and acculturative factors experienced by migrant communities increases the risk of the double burden of
nutrition, which in turn increases the risk of various medical, developmental, and other serious and long-lasting outcomes.

Given this heterogeneity, here we consider some dynamic factors
influencing the relationship between migration and nutrition, including food
access and availability, cultural food practices, and broader issues facing migrant communities, such as climate change and the impact on nutrition.

3.0 Key Issues in Migration and Nutrition

3.1 Food Security

The availability and accessibility of nutritious foods is a major driver of
nutrition behaviors. In fact, the obesogenic environment—the factors
in the social and community environment that promote and sustain unhealthy behaviors leading to unhealthy weight—is the major driver of

global overweight and obesity rates.[25] Food security—the availability, accessibility, and reliability of foods high in nutritional value—plays a complex role in migration and nutrition. First, research suggests that food insecurity is a major determinant of migration. A study in 2019 of almost thirty thousand individuals across sub-Saharan Africa found that the severity of food insecurity increased with the probability of intentions to migrate internationally.[26] However, this study also found that the decision and actual action to migrate internationally decreased with increasing levels of food insecurity. The most severe food insecurity is typically found among the most disadvantaged and impoverished communities. Therefore, this study highlighted the major role of food insecurity in migration, but also the ongoing additional challenges that those most disadvantaged face in carrying out migration, even when intentions and desires to migrate exist.

Given the major role food insecurity plays in the intention and decision to migrate, it is not surprising that migration has been shown to have positive impacts on food security. A series of case studies published in 2010 examined the impact of migration on food and nutrition security and found that positive effects on nutrition have been observed as a result of increased remittance upon migration.[27] Improved opportunities for food access as well as improved sanitation and health-care facilities have been identified among migrant communities. However, improved health outcomes following improved food security is not a straightforward causal pathway. Availability and access to both nutrition and nonnutritional foods (e.g., through obesogenic environments), have been observed.[28,29,30,31] Further, changing family dynamics upon migration, reduced time for meal preparation (e.g., increased employment opportunities and subsequent reduced time at home), and unfamiliarity with foods in shops and meal formats have also been reported.[32,33] Forced migration has been shown to increase food insecurity, reflecting an additional global public health problem.[34] These findings, taken together, show that food insecurity appears to be a major determinant of intentions and subsequent migration; however, the nutritional health outcomes of improved food security are not straightforward.

3.2 Cultural Food Practices

The maintenance of traditional food practices has been self-reported by migrants arriving in host countries as a priority, and supporting these practices is an important enabler of health and well-being.[35,36,37] The ability to maintain cultural food practices is influenced by a number of factors. Migrant groups may bring traditional skills and practices that allow food preparation and subsequently impact nutrition. The availability of traditional food ingredients in the local setting can impact the extent to which cultural food practices are maintained, as can the integration of host country dietary habits. The maintenance of traditional beliefs and food practices widely recognized as key components of cultural identity may make adaptation to new cultures less likely.[38,39,40]

However, migration typically leads, at least partly, to the exposure and subsequent uptake of the host population diet.[41,42] A systematic review examining the changes in food habits post-migration identified that dietary acculturation in Western countries is associated with increased diets high in fat and sugar and low consumption of fruits and vegetables.[43] This review also identified eating out and increased portion sizes as outcomes of this process. Further, increased exposure to food advertising—primarily for unhealthy fast foods in Western countries—has also been associated with an uptake of unhealthful dietary practices.[44,45] Additional social and economic challenges further exacerbate such risks for newly arrived individuals in host countries, including language barriers, ease in accessing such foods, and the cost of foods.[46]

3.3 Climate Change

An evaluation of nutrition and migrant health cannot ignore the role and impact of a changing global climate. A study of Guatemala, Peru, Ghana, Tanzania, Bangladesh, India, Thailand, and Vietnam identified that changing agricultural activity due to climate factors and the subsequent impact on food produce was the major driver for migration.[47] In addition to agricultural conditions, there are other environmental pressures leading to migration, including natural disasters and rising sea levels. The impact of such environmental pressures on nutrition and dietary habits is significant—food availability is affected, as are social, economic, and general livelihoods, as they are often dependent on natural resources.

It has been posited that migrants can experience improved health compared to nonmigrants in host populations.[48] However, the climate strains on countries worldwide are expected to grow and intensify, and the nutrition- and food-related challenges typically observed in countries of origin are also now evident in host countries.[49] In other words, issues such as sustainable food systems and effectively planning and implementing structures to allow for adequate food availability are globally relevant and independent of income or economic status.[50] While migrant nutrition is assumed to be influenced by traditional dietary practices closely connected to cultural identity, as well as to host population practices and environments, it is acknowledged that an increasingly and rapidly changing climate will underpin further changes to the dietary habits of migrants and host populations.[51]

4.0 Conclusion

This chapter explored what is known on nutrition and migrant health, focusing specifically on the social determinants of migrant health among newly arrived migrants from abroad in the context of Western countries. Among other complexities, food availability is a major driver of the decision to migrate. Migrant nutrition is heterogenous, and dietary habits have been reported to both improve and worsen among migrant populations upon resettlement. The factors driving these outcomes include increased remittance, the ability to maintain traditional dietary practices, exposure to and the integration of host population dietary habits, and wider environmental challenges on food systems driven largely by a changing global climate. With dietary risks representing a major cause of the global burden of disease and migrant populations facing unique and disproportionate health challenges, the nutrition of migrant groups is of significant ongoing importance in global public health.

CHAPTER THIRTEEN

Sexual, Reproductive, and Maternal Health in the Context of Migration

Sónia Dias, Ana Gama, and Patrícia Marques

1.0 Introduction

S exual, reproductive, and maternal health (SRMH) is essential for human development and quality of life. It is central to a global commitment to improving population health, enhancing gender equality, and reducing poverty and social inequalities. SRMH is targeted in the Sustainable Development Goals (SDGs) as part of the 2030 Agenda for Sustainable Development explicitly under the third goal: ensuring healthy lives and promoting well-being for all at all ages, ensuring universal access to sexual and reproductive health-care services including for family planning, information, and education, and reducing maternal and infant mortality.[1] SRMH is also addressed in other SDGs that aim to ensure that all men and women have equal rights to economic resources and access to basic services and to end all forms of discrimination and violence against women and girls.

Sexual health is defined as a state of physical, emotional, mental, and social well-being in relation to sexuality; it is not merely the absence of disease, dysfunction, or infirmity. Sexual health requires a positive and respectful approach to sexuality and sexual relationships. Reproductive health is "a state of complete physical, mental and social wellbeing and not merely the absence of disease or infirmity in all matters related to the reproductive system and to its functions and processes."[2] Maternal health includes the overall health status of women across pregnancy, child delivery, and postpartum and the right to access appropriate health-care services to safely plan and pursue pregnancy and childbirth.

Concerns about SRMH among migrants have been growing as international migration intensifies worldwide. According to the International Organization for Migration, international migration is "the movement of persons away from their place of usual residence and across an international border to a country of which they are not nationals."[3] Almost half of all migrants are women, and most are of reproductive age. Multiple and complex determinants play a key role in SRMH vulnerability and contribute to health inequalities among these populations, yet their impact in health varies across different groups. The increasing heterogeneity of the population resulting from human mobility constitutes a challenge to health systems. This calls for culturally competent health services that address population diversity and needs extending across cultural backgrounds, migratory experiences, and demographic characteristics.[4]

2.0 Vulnerability to SRMH in the Context of Migration

SRMH is influenced by a range of determinants, including behavior, attitudes, societal and cultural factors, and biological risk. The migratory process entails potential exposure to health risks that heighten migrants' vulnerability in SRMH. In the pre-migratory context, poor social and housing conditions, low literacy, and under-resourced health systems in many countries of origin can result in limited SRMH knowledge and reduced patterns of preventive practices—for example, in terms of family planning and sexually transmitted infections prevention.[5] Cultural background also strongly influences beliefs and attitudes toward sexuality, reproductive function, and sexual and reproductive health and therefore plays an important role in health practices. In a qualitative study conducted in Portugal, some African migrant women referred to beliefs that oral contraceptives were ineffective and harmful to their health, which discouraged use of them.[6]

During transit and upon arrival to the destination country, many migrants face social hardships in new cultural and socioeconomic contexts, including legal and political restrictions on their rights, social discrimination, and marginalization. Social exclusion resulting partially from low income, poor labor conditions and unemployment potentially limits individuals' capacity and resources for adopting preventive measures. In addition, separation from partners and social isolation from family, friends, or community have been found to increase engagement in risky sexual behaviors, such as multiple partnerships and unprotected sex.[7]

Moreover, evidence suggests that migrants, mostly women, can be exposed to gender-based violence throughout their migratory process, including domestic violence and sexual abuse, with serious impacts on physical and mental health.[8] A German study highlighted that 49 percent of married Turkish women living in Germany have experienced some type of violence.[9] In certain cultures, domestic violence is tolerated, and often women are ashamed or afraid of exposing these events.[10] This can be exacerbated in the migration context, where women are often dependent on their partners financially or for residence permit, experience low social support, or have limited access to assistance to report incidents to authorities.[11] A literature review on intimate partner violence among Latino, Asian, Middle Eastern, and North African communities in the United States documented similar constraints, as well as a lack of knowledge about the social resources available, language, lack of culturally appropriate services and a fear of discrimination and negative stereotypes that hinders help seeking.[12]

Contexts of economic constraints, legal barriers related to undocumented status, and lack of employment alternatives often limit migrants' options to informal and unregulated jobs. In such contexts of high socioeconomic vulnerability, sex work often emerges as an activity to which some migrants, particularly women, are coerced into. Data indicate that in European countries, between 41 percent and 90 percent of sex workers have migrant backgrounds.[13] Sex work is associated with a wide range of high health risks, including violence and sexual abuse.[14] Migration-related factors such as irregular status and social exclusion may further affect migrant sex workers' power to assert control over their working environments and negotiate safer sex, besides limiting access to health services, thereby putting them at risk of HIV and other sexually transmitted infections (STIs).[15]

3.0 Current Evidence on SRMH among Migrants

Overall, research suggests that some groups of migrants tend to have poor SRMH outcomes compared to native populations and face barriers in access to SRMH services.[16]

Regarding family planning, evidence has shown that knowledge about contraceptive methods and its use among some migrant women are lower compared to their native counterparts.[17] A study in Fiji and New Zealand with iTaukei women pointed out as possible explanations for their reduced knowledge and use of contraceptives such factors as socio-cultural taboos and sensitivities (e.g., reproduction is perceived to be a natural process that contraception could interfere with), gender roles that dictate relationship norms and limit communication about family planning, and low proficiency of the host country language that hinders access to family planning information, among others.[18] The lower use of contraception results in a higher risk of unintended pregnancies and consequent induced abortions, which have been shown to be more frequent among migrant women.[19]

Literature on disparities in maternal health outcomes between migrant and native populations has been conflicting. Several studies indicate that pregnant migrant women are generally more likely to have poor maternal health outcomes.[20] Research has shown that migrant women are at increased risk for stillbirth, preterm birth, neonatal and infant mortality, and congenital abnormalities compared with native women.[21] It has been documented that the social and economic difficulties faced by many migrant women can have adverse effects on their physical and mental health, particularly during pregnancy, and compromise their well-being during and after this period.[22] By contrast, other evidence has shown similar or even better perinatal outcomes among migrant women compared to natives— for example, a reduced risk of low birth weight has been found among migrants.[23] This latter set of findings can be attributed to the "healthy migrant effect," where some migrant groups on arrival to the host country appear to have better health outcomes; during pregnancy, for example, this could be due to healthier behaviors, such as lower intake of alcohol and nicotine.

The field of STIs is a much-studied area where migrants have been considered particularly vulnerable. Research on this area has mainly focused on HIV and shows that migrants, especially those originating from countries with generalized HIV epidemics, are disproportionally vulnerable to HIV/AIDS, and a significant portion of them acquire HIV after arrival in the host country.[24] Engagement in concurrent partnerships with regular and occasional partners and inconsistent condom use have been frequently reported in studies with sub-Saharan African migrants, particularly among men.[25] Indeed, evidence suggests a gender differential, with migrant women being particularly vulnerable to STIs due to frequent difficulty in negotiating condom use and low power to refuse unprotected sex with their partners.[26] Also, migrant women tend to be more exposed to sexual assault and sex work, which increases the risk of STIs.

4.0 Access to SRMH Care

As widely documented, migrant populations face increased obstacles to health services at all stages of migration. In many destination countries, migrants have reduced access and use of health services compared to native populations.[27] The use of health services among migrant populations is particularly low when it comes to preventive care. Evidence shows that access to screening programs to detect breast and cervical cancer—two of the most common cancers among women—tends to be lower among migrant women, which potentially results in delayed diagnosis and treatment of sexual and reproductive pathologies.[28] Low uptake of STIs screening among migrants has also been reported, contributing to the underdiagnosis of infections and delayed diagnosis and treatment.[29] Later initiation of antenatal care and the underutilization of maternal health services have also been described among some migrants.[30]

Several barriers hindering migrants' access to SRMH services can be found at multiple levels, including individual, social, economic, cultural, system-related, and policy levels. Some of these barriers include individuals' low health literacy and lack of knowledge about SRMH, the prioritization of practical and social needs over health-care needs, and the inability to afford the cost of care or health insurance. Irregular migration status is a major barrier. Undocumented migrants have more limited access to health services due to legal constraints, and in contexts where access to care is legally assured regardless of immigration status, there is often a lack of knowledge about migrants' health rights among services staff and migrants, which can hinder migrants from seeking care.[31] Unawareness of the health services available and a lack of information and support to navigate through the health system also play a role. In addition, language and communication difficulties often lead migrant women to resort to their spouses as translators during consultations, jeopardizing their privacy and limiting their openness about their health needs and concerns, potentially discouraging them from seeking SRH care.[32] Other discouraging factors include a lack of trust in services and professionals and past negative experiences with professionals with limited sensitivity to the challenges faced by migrants.

Cultural values, religious beliefs, and social stigmas associated with seeking sexual and reproductive health services, together with feelings of embarrassment and an unwillingness to be attended by male doctors routed in gender-based norms can also deter some migrant women from using SRMH services.[33] Gender roles may influence the use of contraception and family planning services. In many cultural contexts, such as Islamic cultures and patriarchal societies, the husband's perception that these services are not relevant or needed can be another barrier. Additionally, migrants from cultures where home birth is traditional may avoid obstetrical care, potentially jeopardizing their quality of care and compromising maternal and neonatal health outcomes.[34] Complicated administrative and bureaucratic procedures to register patients and legal constraints related to irregular migration status deter many migrants from accessing SRMH care.[35] In addition, the lack of translated and culturally adapted medical information and the absence of qualified interpreters in health services, as well as insufficient cultural competencies among health-care providers to deal with culturally diverse populations and address their SRMH needs, intensify the gap between these populations and the health services. For example, women who went through harmful traditional practices such as female genital mutilation (FGM) (i.e., partial or complete removal of female external genital organs, with a wide range of adverse physical and mental health effects) may have additional health needs.[36] Yet, the provision of adequate health care to these women may be hindered by professionals' lack of knowledge and technical expertise around the health needs that are particular to FGM.[37]

5.0 Conclusions

Overall, poor socioeconomic conditions, undocumented status, social exclusion, gender inequity, cultural-based values and attitudes, and obstacles in access to health services contribute to SRMH inequities affecting many migrants. Addressing migrants' SRMH needs will require an understanding of patterns of health inequities and how different determinants influence these inequities. For all aspects of SRMH, a multidisciplinary approach that allies social sciences to medical research and epidemiology is essential to understanding the nature, the magnitude, and the physical, psychological, social, cultural, and economic consequences of poor SRMH outcomes among migrant populations.[38]

SRMH is a particularly sensitive research topic that can be challenging to investigate. An efficient strategy to study and address these sensitive issues, especially among vulnerable and hard-to-reach populations such as migrants, requires the adoption of a participatory research approach.[39] Involving communities in the research process can increase their trust and acceptance of the research, contributing to knowledge that can incorporate migrant perspectives and is translatable into effective, tailored health policies and strategies. Engaging all key stakeholders, including community leaders, migrant communities, health-care providers, and policy makers, can be crucial to achieving more research that contributes to tackling health inequities, developing migrant-friendly health-care systems, and improving SRMH outcomes among migrant populations.

CHAPTER FOURTEEN

Unique Health Considerations during Forced Displacement

Sabrina Hermosilla and Janna Metzler

1.0 Forced Displacement and Health

Fleeing conflict, disaster, and persecution, over seventy-nine million people were forcibly displaced globally by the end of 2019, a near doubling in just the past decade.[1] Forcibly displaced populations are a large component of the migrant experience, and their stories are integrated throughout this book. This chapter synthesizes and highlights the unique challenges that forcibly displaced populations face across their migration journey.

Codified in the 1951 Geneva Convention, the United Nations High Commissioner for Refugees (UNHCR) is responsible for three primary categories of forcibly displaced populations: *refugees*, who have crossed international geopolitical borders during their flight to safety; *internally displaced*, who have not crossed international borders but have been forced to flee from their homes; and *asylum seekers*, people who have crossed international borders and legally sought asylum in another country.[2] The past twenty years have seen continued civil unrest and climate-driven disasters that have fueled the forced movement of the largest populations ever seen in human history. The number of those internally displaced, one of the hardest to innumerate groups, has increased significantly during this time (see fig. 14.1).[3] Almost seventy percent (68%) of the currently displaced population originate from just five countries: Syrian Arab Republic (6.6. million), Venezuela (Bolivarian Republic of) (3.7 million), Afghanistan (2.7 million), South Sudan (2.2 million), and Myanmar (1.1 million).[4]

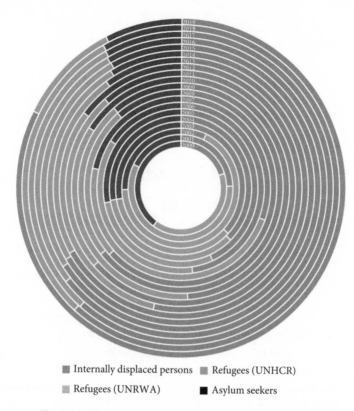

■ Internally displaced persons   ■ Refugees (UNHCR)

▨ Refugees (UNRWA)   ■ Asylum seekers

FIGURE 14.1. Trends of global displacement by percentage of total displaced (2000–2019)

Forcibly displaced populations are often the most vulnerable in any community. Their health and well-being are influenced by the geopolitical history and the legal, structural, and environmental realities in their home country and all the places they pass through on their route to permanent settlement. This chapter highlights the unique health considerations, influenced by the intersection of the changing contextual realities of displaced populations across their migration journey.

2.0 Health across the Forced Displacement Journey

At each phase of the migration journey, forcibly displaced populations are exposed to unique threats and potential resources that influence their health and well-being. This chapter will highlight key drivers of health, a population of interest, common health profiles, and interventions across each of the five phases: predeparture, flight, temporary settlement: acute, temporary settlement: protracted, and resettlement. While there are some universalities to the health consequences of forced displacement, each phase presents unique challenges and opportunities that influence population health. While not all forcibly displaced individuals will travel through all these phases, the majority will.

2.1 Predeparture

One of the most important stages in the migration journey is also one of the hardest to measure. We often cannot predict who will and will not migrate before a mass migration event. However, from studying populations who have already started on their forced migration journey, we can retrospectively recreate an understanding of individuals' and communities' predeparture context that can guide our understanding of their current and future health needs. The literature has repeatedly shown, however, that those who are most vulnerable before displacement are most vulnerable during and after displacement.[5]

The overall root causes of forced displacement are beyond the scope of this chapter, but it is essential to highlight that structural, economic, and gender inequalities fuel domestic conflict by inhibiting effective and equitable responses to disasters, thus driving the health of populations before they leave their country of origin.[6] Exploring the top five countries contributing to displaced populations today—Syrian Arab Republic, Venezuela, Afghanistan, South Sudan, and Myanmar[7]—all except Venezuela (high) and Myanmar (medium) have low human development indexes,[8] reflecting health threats such as poor nutrition (with subsequent risk of starvation); few health providers; poor access to health care (with resultant low vaccination coverage and other long-term consequences); poor sanitation; and high mortality, especially among vulnerable children under five years old, and maternal mortality.[9] Thus, even before starting on the arduous journey of migration, these populations are often already suffering long-term public health emergencies. In fact, improved health and futures are often a primary driver of displaced populations.

2.1.1 AT RISK OF DISPLACEMENT WITH DISABILITIES.   Within this context of premigration inequalities, women, children, and those with pre-existing conditions are at greater risk of exploitation and negative health outcomes.

Only recently has the international community meaningfully focused on migrants with disabilities, and in general, there is a still a dearth of data around this group.[10] About fifteen percent of the global population has a disability, and some 6.7 million persons with disabilities were forcibly displaced in 2016 (the most recent data available).[11] Within this premovement context, the relation between physical and mental disability and displacement is complicated. Individuals living with disabilities often risk being abandoned in their homes or communities, with limited access to basic food, water, and sanitation when mass migration events occur.[12]

2.2 Flight

Populations face increased risks and negative health outcomes during the first mobile phase of their displacement, *flight*. During the flight phase, displaced populations are at risk of exploitation, physical harm, mental stress and exhaustion, violence victimization, and death. The health impact of flight on displaced populations is directly related to the terrain, distance, duration, season, and fellow migrants with whom displaced people travel with. By definition, most leave in extreme emergency conditions, with few supplies or personal resources beyond those they are able to physically carry.

2.2.1 CROSSING THE MEDITERRANEAN.   Take refugees crossing the Mediterranean to seek asylum in Europe, for example. While over one hundred thousand people cross the Mediterranean each year, from 2014 to 2016, that average peaked with over one million refugees crossing in 2015 and over five thousand dead or missing in 2016.[13] During this one- to four-month arduous voyage, people suffer physical violence (30% in some reports) from border guards and experience extreme mental health problems (80% in some reports).[14] On the way, refugees lack access to hygienic sanitation facilities, proper nutrition, shelter, and clothing and are exposed to psychological and physical violence.[15]

Women and girls face considerable obstacles during their migration journey, owing to their traditional gender roles, which often limit their economic resources and thus financial resources during flight; caretaking responsibilities for children and extended family members; and, especially in this context, restrictions to traveling alone from both a cultural and security perspective. Before reaching the sea crossing, most women have been exposed to some form of sexual and gender-based violence (SGBV), often by smugglers, to secure seats for their family, avoid torture, or in exchange for other goods and illegal services.[16] Once the journey across the sea has started, women are often forced to take the most dangerous seats on overcrowded and unsafe boats, leading to increased mortality when those boats eventually capsize and sink.[17]

2.3 Temporary Settlement—Acute Phase

As a proportion of their population (excluding Palestinians under UNRWA), Aruba (156/1,000), Lebanon (134/1,000), Curacao (99/1,000), Jordan (69/ 1,000), and Turkey (43/1,000) host the largest proportion of refugees in the world.[18] In 2019, 40 percent of displaced people were hosted in lower-middle- and low-income countries,[19] adding additional challenges to areas already struggling with economic hardship. While all member states of the United Nations are meant to share responsibility related to immediate protection for displaced populations (hosting or providing resources), in practice, high-income countries have hosted between thirteen and nineteen percent of refugees in the past ten years.[20]

Once displaced individuals have fled their homes—and crossed an international border in this case—their first place of refuge is often within a local host community (60%) or formal refugee camp.[21] Camps provide much-needed access to resources (basic food, shelter, access to health care and education), international aid, security, and stability and facilitate communication and coordination with host communities. In camp settings, the primary health concerns in the early acute arrival phase center around infectious disease (aggravated by crowded living conditions and hastily constructed infrastructure and housing), addressing poor nutrition (often a direct consequence of the protracted disruption of access to adequate and healthy food and water during both the premigration and flight phases), and addressing chronic and reproductive health issues. Unfortunately, conditions in camps themselves (either refugee or internally displaced) often increase the risk of infectious diseases and, when not appropriately managed, spark concerns that can increase physical and psychological insecurity, which can lead to increases in SGBV and deterioration in psychological well-being.[22]

2.3.1 DISPLACED CHILDREN.   Almost half (thirty to forty million) of all forcibly displaced individuals are children under eighteen years old.[23] Living in acute humanitarian crises exposes children to life-threatening events and

risks such as abduction, child labor, mental health and psychosocial distress, physical dangers and injuries, physical and emotional neglect and
maltreatment, and SGBV, as well as risks inherent with armed group association or from separation or lack of accompaniment.[24] Unintentional
injuries are responsible for as much as 25 percent of deaths among young
children (five to fourteen years old) and are the primary cause of death
and permanent impairment among older children (fifteen to nineteen).[25]
The type and impact of an injury differs by children's age, context, disability, gender, role, and socioeconomic status. Humanitarian crises increase
everyday hazards and risk and introduce new ones, such as land mine and
infectious disease exposures.[26]

2.4 Temporary Settlement—Protracted

More than three-quarters (77%) of refugees are currently living in a
"protracted refugee situation." As defined by the UNHCR, a protracted
refugee situation is one where at least twenty-five thousand refugees
sharing the same nationality have been exiled for over five consecutive
years in the same host country.[27] As crises move from the acute to protracted phase, displaced populations must contend with complex and intersecting threats to their health. Most acute emergency settlements are
not designed for long-term residence, leading to challenges with infrastructure that can impact water and sanitation, security, and protection
against environmental conditions. As funds from emergency response
dry up, securing funds for longer-term improvements can prove difficult
and increase insecurity in these settings. Even in places where physical
conditions have been secured, displaced populations often have restrictions placed on their physical movement and access to local employment,
education, and health systems, increasing their fragility and forcing many
into adopting more dangerous coping mechanisms to address their daily
needs.[28]

2.4.1 MENTAL HEALTH CONCERNS. As the relief and hope that are often
present in the acute phase start to wane, displaced populations begin to contend with their futures, the long-term consequences of their experiences—
predeparture, during transit, and in their new environment—and mental
health issues and psychosocial distress begin to increase. In contexts as
diverse as Rwanda, Uganda, Nepal, Venezuela, and Jordan, frustration
and deterioration of hope for a better future, mixed with the long-term

consequences of torture and abuse, have led to increases in depression, post-traumatic stress symptoms, and, in the extreme, deaths by suicide.[29] Protracted forced displacement situations amplify the risk of refugees with disabilities of experiencing violence, including sexual and domestic abuse, exploitation by family members, discrimination, and exclusion from access to education, livelihoods, a nationality, and other public services.[30]

2.5 Resettlement and Return

Permanent resettlement, either to another country or through voluntary repatriation, is the final step on the forced displacement journey. In 2019, 5.7 million displaced people found permanent solutions through voluntary repatriation to their country (or region for internally displaced) of origin and resettlement. Afghanistan, Syria, and Cote d'Ivoire saw the largest returns. Refugees were resettled to twenty-six different countries; however, for every one resettlement spot available, there are twenty refugees in need of placement. Of those fortunate to be resettled, with the assistance of the UNHCR, over seventy-five percent were survivors of torture or experienced violence, and over half were children. During the decade from 2010 to 2019, the United States of the America (55%), Canada (20%), and Australia (11%) became home to most of the resettled refugees.[31]

Resettled refugees often struggle to assimilate and access local resources and frequently experience discrimination in their new countries. These stressors, combined with their pre-existing conditions from their forced migration experience, often lead to higher morbidity and mortality, as compared to their non-resettled neighbors.[32]

2.5.1 RESETTLED BHUTANESE REFUGEE SUICIDES.   Bhutanese refugees, both in Nepal and resettled to the United States, die by suicide almost twice as much as their neighbors in the United States (Nepal camps: 20.8; resettled: 20.3; United States: 10.6 per 100,000 people).[33] Resettled refugees struggle to negotiate the separation from their family, the cultural and linguistic isolation from their resettlement communities, and the loss of ethnic and refugee group identity, all of which contribute to a sense of thwarted belongingness and can lead to suicidal ideation and death by suicide. For Bhutanese specifically, the sense of being a burden on society and their families is a primary stressor.[34] As with all resettled populations, culturally sensitive and proactive interventions and access to education, health, and economic opportunities are essential to support these communities' integration into host societies.

2.6. Moving from Temporary to Durable Solutions

Understanding the drivers and health profiles of displaced populations provides a useful lens through which we can better understand how to augment existing approaches throughout the humanitarian program cycle toward more durable solutions that promote the lasting health and well-being of the forcibly displaced. The following section presents ideas to evolve existing practice—presented by phase—in addressing these multifaceted drivers of gender inequality and health inequities while working toward durable solutions across the migration journey.

2.6.1 PREDEPARTURE: EMERGENCY PREPAREDNESS TO MITIGATE RISK. Complex emergencies and disasters that generate forced migration events are defined by the multifaceted acute needs and priorities of the affected populations but also offer opportunities for long-term sustainable solutions that leave communities stronger and more equitable than before the crisis. Disaster risk-reduction activities that are focused on strengthening the capacity of communities to support the response and recovery efforts in emergencies can greatly impact the sexual and reproductive health outcomes of women and girls. Building on existing tools, such as the *Facilitator's Kit for Community Preparedness for Reproductive Health and Gender*,[35] communities can evolve a localized and inclusive SRH response while identifying key barriers and supports required for successful implementation of disaster management plans. These localized plans require the direct buy-in of local, regional, and national governments to ensure these are integrated into national systems that mitigate risk, reduce vulnerabilities, and strengthen existing capacities for a comprehensive and coordinated response. Ensuring that persons with disabilities, older persons, and those with pre-existing conditions remain central during the design of and also within these plans reduces vulnerabilities that may lead to greater risk of exploitation and negative health outcomes.

2.6.2 FLIGHT: KEEPING SAFE ON THE ROAD TO SAFETY. The last decade has seen tremendous economic hardship, widespread violent crime, and extreme social inequities within many Central American countries. As a result of these conditions, coupled with a lack of safe and legal channels to claim asylum, many have been forced to flee their countries of origin in search of safety, only to be denied entry upon arrival at the US border. The migrant caravan drew international attention in 2018 for the shortcomings of Mexican and US immigration policy and its newly imposed *metering* and Migration Protection Protocols as a way of wait-listing entry and further denying asylum seekers with valid claims.[36] Addressing the root causes of this forced displacement and its related health impacts requires the development of an inclusive, rights-based regional strategy that meets the needs of those most at risk, particularly women and girls, and promotes a robust humanitarian relief agenda in coordination with reform in domestic and international laws to support and protect refugees and migrants.[37] In the wake of the global pandemic, a new surge in the caravan related to securing life-saving medical care has emerged with much less global attention to the humanitarian imperative. For stability and prosperity in the region, it is critical to reestablish adequate funding for the United Nations Population Fund (UNFPA) and for the World Health Organization (WHO) to ensure appropriate, human rights–centered responses during the health pandemic.[38]

2.6.3 TEMPORARY SETTLEMENT—ACUTE: EARLY INTERVENTION FOR CHILDREN.   Child Friendly Spaces are widely touted as a staple of the primary response to mental health and psychosocial support used to meet the acute needs of refugee and displaced children. These community-based programs provide a safe learning environment for children to resume a sense of normalcy using structured and free play activities to mitigate the harmful effects of trauma and improve overall psychosocial well-being. When run effectively, Child Friendly Spaces are a conduit through which a range of services for children that are critical to their health and development remain available and accessible, although further research is required to establish their lasting impact across diverse contexts.[39]

2.6.4 TEMPORARY SETTLEMENT–PROTRACTED: ONGOING RESPONSE AND RECOVERY INTERVENTIONS.   Economic insecurity is a primary driver of child marriages in emergencies.[40] In protracted crises, household economies rely heavily on external aid, education, and livelihood opportunities to lessen the financial strain that is known to contribute to decisions to marry their daughters as children. Local initiatives—created and driven by refugee youth themselves—combine physical activity, education, and psychosocial support to improve economic and health conditions for children and their families.[41] Durable solutions to prevent and mitigate the risk of child marriage include gender transformative and equity-driven programming approaches that also strengthen the national health and protection systems to meet the needs of adolescent girls and their families. This could include enhancing access and the availability of education beyond the primary level, ensuring that vocational training is available for adolescents and their caregivers, or ensuring that refugees legally have the right to work and contribute to and receive benefits from the national social and health system.

2.6.5 RESETTLEMENT AND RETURN: LONG-TERM SOLUTIONS. To support long-term integration of resettled and repatriated populations, local, community-centered programs should offer a wide variety of services, from job placement to language instruction to psychological services. With nonprofit, governmental, and international support, resettlement centers like The Center (Utica, New York) have the opportunity to not only support resettled refugees, but also to restart local economies and provide health and social services, improving the population health of both resettled refugees and their new neighbors.[42] During voluntary repatriation, cash grants can provide a flexible tool to be used as part of a broader support package to meet the needs of refugees upon arrival in their country of origin.

3.0 Forced Displacement and Health: Where to Next?

Topics such as stigma, gender discrimination, access to services (health, economic, legal), and geopolitical historical contexts (including colonial legacies) that influence migrant and host communities' health are seen in the extreme among forcibly displaced populations. If we can learn to address the needs of the displaced throughout their migration journey, we can learn to improve the population health of everyone affected by migration.

CHAPTER FIFTEEN

Older People, Health, and Migration

Tony Warnes

1.0 Introduction

This chapter examines relationships between old age, migration, and health in relatively affluent populations and ends with reflections on changes that may stem from the Covid-19 pandemic. The exposition reflects the author's long interest in and considerable research on the topics, beginning with a 1970s project with Chris Law on the movement of retirees from English metropolitan areas to the North Wales coast[1] and including a 1995–1997 study of UK citizens who had migrated for retirement to regions of Spain, Portugal, Italy, and Malta that was conceived and conducted with Russell King and Alan Williams.[2] This led to follow-up projects with researchers in several European countries who were also studying retirement migration by their compatriots to Mediterranean destinations.[3,4]

2.0 Migration and Age

Most dictionaries give a timeless definition of *migrate*: to move from one country or locality to another. The moving objects can be people, animals, birds, or inanimate objects, including now data transferred between devices. This straightforward meaning is accepted by most analysts and modelers of human migration, although some prefer *residential mobility* for the short moves that are frequent in cities, especially by renters. These *partial displacement* migrations occur without wholesale changes in workplaces, children's schools, or social networks. In contrast, many long-distance moves are *total displacements* and over time may change even language and religion, especially for descendants. Population *migration* has been applied to the mass transportation of Africans to the Americas from the sixteenth to the nineteenth centuries, to the shift of people from economically declining rural areas to expanding towns and cities (rural-urban migration), to displacements from high-density inner cities to peripheral suburbs (suburban migration), and to the southward shift of older people from northern Europe and North America to warmer latitudes (sunbelt migration). The common usage of *migrant* is less clear-cut. Journalists and people at large now associate *migrant* with people that are foreign born; indeed, being such a migrant is a legally recognized civil status in France and Germany. This meaning is spreading. The European office of the World Health Organization (WHO) maintains a "Migration and Health" website, which states that "currently, approximately 10% of the population of the WHO European Region are migrants." If "ever changed usual residence" was the criterion, the figure exceeds 80 percent. The WHO's meaning is apparent from the focus of its website on policy and welfare issues concerning "refugees and foreign migrants."[5]

Direct counts of migrations were rare before the 1950s, so estimates relied on birthplace and population change statistics.[6,7] Subsequently, some national censuses included questions on place of residence one or five years previously, but this refinement has declined since 1990 as governments economize. Representative migration data continues to be collected by one-off and repeated large government-funded social surveys. The demographers, population geographers, and other social scientists that analyze the data customarily adopt the definition of a migration as a change in the usual place of residence over one or five years.

The relationship between age and migration has a consistent broad form. Young adults are most migratory, and children and the young-old the least. The main features are exemplified by US census data for 2000. From 1995 to 2000, the peak migration rate was 70.2 percent for those aged twenty-five to twenty-nine and the lowest (19.9%) for those aged seventy to seventy-four (table 15.1). Earlier and fuller analyses have been published.[8,9] An early-adult peak has been found in all societies, but its age shifts over time as marriage, partnering, fertility, education, employment, and retirement practices change. The peak is tied to the age at which children leave their parents' home for work or education, become financially independent, and form new households. Around the middle of the last

TABLE 15.1 **Migrants 1995–2000, United States of America**

Age	5–9	10–14	15–19	20–24	25–29	30–34	35–39	40–44	45–49	50–54	55–59	60–64	65–69	70–74	75–79	80–84	85+
%	51.4	42.2	41.3	63.3	70.2	62.2	50.5	40.8	33.9	29.9	26.7	24.7	22.1	19.9	20.4	23.9	32.1

Notes: Age: age-groups in years. %: percentage migrated.
Source: Census 2000 PHC-T-23, *Migration by Sex and Age for the Population 5 Years and Over for the United States, Regions, States, and Puerto Rico: 2000*, https://www.census.gov/data/tables /2000/dec/phc-t-23.html.

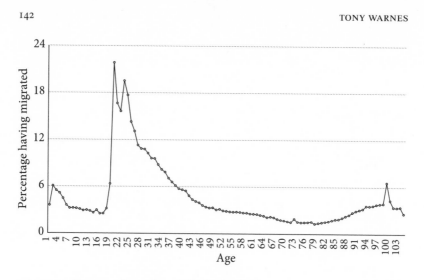

FIGURE 15.1. One year migrants in 2018, England and Wales

Source: Office for National Statistics (UK), *Internal Migration: Local Authority and Region Moves by Sex and Single Year of Age Totals, Year Ending June 2018*, ONS.

century in affluent countries, the peak age was around five years younger than now, and in low-income agricultural societies, it has timelessly been twelve to sixteen years. In the United States from 1995 to 2000, with increasing age above seventy-five, the rate of migration increased, reflecting moves to be nearer family support, to enter nursing homes and assisted living, and to enable home downsizing. Many of these late-life moves follow a partner's death or the onset of disabling illness.

During the later 2000s, there was a migration spike around the modal retirement age in many affluent countries. In the 1960s, it was approximately sixty-three years, a result of the high rates of male full-time employment and the eligibility rules for state and private-insurance old-age benefits. This spike was pronounced in Sunbelt migrations, as into Florida and Arizona, and from Northern Europe to Mediterranean resorts. As changes in the labor market altered the age-specific and sex-specific schedules of engagement in paid work, the peak flattened and has now disappeared. Other characteristics of the relationship between age and migration are revealed by single year-of-age data for England and Wales for 2017 to 2018. A usual feature is the rise in the migration rate among those in their nineties (fig. 15.1). Many of these moves are short distance and into supported settings, including children's homes. While not the prime concerns of this paper, two other features of the plotted rates merit explanation. The decreasing rate of migration among children as they age from two to seventeen years is another usual feature, reflecting the parents' declining migration rate with increasing age. In contrast, a novel feature is the twinned-peak at eighteen to nineteen and twenty-one to twenty-two years, neatly corresponding with the enrolled ages on higher education courses.

3.0 Associations between Age, Health, and Migration

Migration has been a leading research topic among population geographers, sociologists, and social demographers, and there is a large, dedicated literature.[10] Some have specialized in older people's migration, although the connections with health have been a minority interest. We have seen that the relationship between age and the propensity to migrate has a consistent broad form and intricacies that change over time and that generalizations about the form are valid. In contrast, it is more difficult to capture concisely the relationship between older people's health and migration. It is useful to distinguish two aspects: the influence of good and poor health on the likelihood of moving and the health consequences of undertaking a migration. In broad terms, good health among the young-old promotes innovative, long-distance migrations, while poor health in advanced old age encourages short-distance moves to access family or institutional support. Poor health and disabling conditions increase the likelihood of moving to a location or property that is more convenient, manageable, or supportive but in some cases reduce the ability or willingness to undertake the disruptive and energy-sapping business of moving. Those with poor health may be motivated to move to an area that they or their advisors perceive to be heathier or to offer better health care. Equally, those in good health may be the most likely to move to areas that offer new experiences or more active lifestyles involving walking, climbing, yachting, or property improvement. Environmentally attractive destinations are favored for the direct benefits to the migrants and because they encourage visits by close friends and family members, thereby promoting family cohesion, social life, and morale.[11]

Health conditions, particularly respiratory disorders, arthritis, and neurological disorders, have for centuries led physicians to advise their patients to move to warmer, drier, or less polluted areas. The practice grew considerably following the German physician Hermann Brehmer's recommendation in 1859 of high-altitude treatment for tuberculosis, which spawned the sanatorium movement. By 1923 in the United States, there were 656, and by 1953, there were 839, with over 136,000 beds. Many countries have spa resorts developed around springs of mineralized water with allegedly curative properties, and a few have for centuries attracted older people for convalescence and long-term residence (e.g., Saratoga Springs in New York State and Bath in England). From the middle of the nineteenth century, Cannes and Nice were favored destinations among older, affluent Northern Europeans for winter or permanent residence, instigating international retirement migration, but the custom has a long history. The philosopher John Locke suffered greatly from asthma and spent 1676 to 1677 in Montpellier, France. Its renowned medical school and hospitable city also attracted Laurence Sterne, the author of *Tristram Shandy* and a consumptive, for the winter of 1762 to 1763. The healthiness of the Mediterranean climate and diet is widely presumed among Europeans and North Americans but inseparable from the truism that Mediterranean winters are more comfortable than those at higher latitudes and more conducive to outdoor activity and socializing, boosting morale and well-being. The cachet applies to Southern Europe, the Californian and contiguous Mexican Pacific coasts, and the Gold Coast of Queensland, Australia.

It should be noted that over five years, only a minority of people change permanent residence and only a small fraction of every age group undertakes a "total displacement" migration. Even through the ages of most retirements, say from fifty to sixty-nine years, probably no more than one-quarter of New Yorkers and Londoners engage in the more common long-distance migrations, which involve either returns to the areas of birth and early life or movements to scenically attractive areas in the same country or abroad. Put another way, it is only a minority that think it practicable and potentially beneficial to retire away from large cities. The attraction of such moves varies with people's interests, ambitions, and the importance they place on family, friendship, and activity connections in the origin area.

4.0 The Health Implications of Migration in Later Life

The health implications of a migration are conditioned by a person's age, prior health, family support, and socioeconomic status. These personal attributes and miscellaneous contingencies are the dominant influences on the outcome of moving or staying. An early nostrum of geriatric medicine was that to move a patient was often harmful. While this idea arose for within-hospital moves, it influenced family doctors' advice to frail patients. In contrast, most ethnographies and social surveys of long distance "amenity-seeking" moves by older people find overwhelmingly positive reports, primarily on cost-of-living (including medication) and lifestyle grounds. It must be remembered, however, that most disenchanted movers will have returned to their origin areas or moved again. A minority experience increasing difficulties, brought about by interactions between diminishing resources bereavement, and increasing care needs.[12,13]

Several researchers have attempted to determine the health consequences of migrations from large, representative data sets, but the exercise is problematic. There are few longitudinal inquiries (that collect data repeatedly from the same respondents); few large social surveys incorporate clinical assessments, and the definitions of *poor* or *good* health and of disability are variable and difficult to implement consistently. A commendably rich UK data set was developed by Maria Evandrou, Jane Falkingham, and Marcus Green from seventeen successive annual waves (1991–2007) of the longitudinal British Household Panel Survey (BHPS).[14] The Wave 1 BHPS panel began in 1991 with 5,500 households and 10,300 individuals drawn from 250 areas of Great Britain. Samples for Scotland, Wales, and Northern Ireland were added later. Respondents in adjacent waves (T1 and T2) were linked and the sixteen paired-year subsets merged. The analysis sample of 71,356 was restricted to respondents aged fifty-plus at T1 and did not include people living in institutional accommodation. The BHPS measure of self-reported health status over the past year used a five-point Likert scale (excellent, good, fair, poor, and very poor). Improved health was defined as a rise by more than one category between T1 and T2. Similarly, health decline was defined as a decline by more than one category. The data set also coded long-term illness that limits activity (LLTI). Variables were created for key lifecourse events, such as getting married or divorced, being widowed, becoming unemployed, or retiring.

Table 15.2 shows that the percentage migrating tended to rise for all older age groups as health worsened (and migration was much higher for men and women aged eighty-plus with a LLTI). This suggests that it is simplistic to assume that all migration among the young-old is amenity driven; rather, migration in these age groups is a mixture of amenity- and

TABLE 15.2 **Percentage migrating over one year during 1991–2007 by self-reported health status and age group, United Kingdom.**

	Age group (years)			
	Health status			
T1 and T2	50–59	60–69	70–79	80–89
Men				
Excellent	4.5	3.3	2.0	2.2
Good	3.7	2.7	2.1	2.1
Fair	3.5	3.6	2.6	3.9
Poor	4.5	3.8	3.9	2.6
Very poor	9.5	6.3	5.0	—
Women				
Excellent	4.0	2.7	2.1	4.0
Good	3.1	2.8	2.2	4.2
Fair	4.3	2.9	3.2	4.6
Poor	5.0	3.7	3.7	6.3
Very poor	3.4	3.5	2.8	7.3

Source: British Household Panel Survey data 1991–2007, analyzed by Evandrou et al., "Migration in Later Life" (cf. endnote 14), table 6.

health-related moves. Further analysis showed that for men and women aged fifty to sixty-nine years, migration rates were similar among those whose health had deteriorated and improved, but at ages seventy to seventy-nine, migration was highest among those whose health had improved. The direction of causation was unclear; changing residence may have raised self-perceived health and well-being, or improved health may have facilitated the migration. Hence, the relationship between health status and migration is more complex than at first appears. The authors emphasized that late-life migration is strongly associated with the formation and dissolution of partnerships and that partnership dissolution has enduring effects, for older people who had been divorced or separated were more likely to move than the never-married even after the first year of the breakdown.

Returning to the United States, Karen Conway and Jonathan Rock analyzed data from the Integrated Public Use Microdata Series (IPUMS) for 1970 to 2000.[15] It was built from 4 to 5 percent samples of the decennial census data on interstate five-year migrants and included armed services veteran status and a disability measure (whether the respondents had a lasting physical or mental health condition that compromised functioning). A return migration was defined as a move back to the state of birth. Measures for income, employment status, education level, marital status, ethnicity, and gender were included. Only a few of their findings can be reported. The nonelderly migrated across state lines at more than twice the rate of the elderly (10 to 11% vs. ≈4%). Migration rates were a little higher among the oldest. Veterans aged sixty-five and up had greater interstate mobility than nonveterans. The return proportion of moves increased with age. Migrants typically had higher rates of disability, and the disability gap was larger the older the age group and grew over time. The multivariate analyses verified these patterns after controlling for background characteristics. Among older people, reporting a disability significantly increased the likelihood of migrating and increasingly so with age. Furthermore, the magnitude of the effect grew substantially over time. In 1980, a person over eighty-five or with a disability was 1.4 times more likely to have migrated than one free of disability, and by 2000, the comparable ratio was 1.9. Disability was a strong predictor of interstate migrations across all age groups. Veteran and socioeconomic status diminished or remained constant in their importance while disability grew. The findings strongly suggested that elderly migration decisions had tilted toward the need for assistance.

5.0 The Impact of the Covid-19 Pandemic

For over a century in Western countries, epidemiological conditions have rarely entered assessments of the desirability of a migration. The arrival early in 2020 of the Covid-19 pandemic was unprecedented for most Europeans and Americans. Will it change older people's migrations? It is too early to know, but possible effects can be outlined. Over the centuries, a common response to pestilence has been for the footloose to leave infection hot spots, particularly the most populous cities. Daniel Defoe's *Journal of the Plague Year* (based on notes by his uncle) relates that in London, the plague took hold from February 1664 and resurged vigorously in June, when "the nobility and gentry ... thronged out of town."[16] Media coverage of the current pandemic reported similar escapes to second homes in the United States and the United Kingdom and other adjustments to daily habits (e.g., shopping increasingly occurring online and shifting from major central business districts to outer suburbs and small towns). For many people, the most irksome consequences of the pestilence have been restrictions on face-to-face interactions. Whether evaluations of the desirability of migration will change depends on how long it takes to develop effective, affordable, and long-lasting prophylactic and curative treatments and instant testing. If this takes longer than, say, two years, I expect entrepreneurs to develop Covid-secure retirement and assisted-living gated complexes with mandatory testing for residents, visitors, and tradespeople as they enter. They will enable family, social, and business gatherings that continue to be hazardous elsewhere. Variants to encourage both amenity-seeking and supportive moves can be envisaged.

CHAPTER SIXTEEN

The Health of Migrant Children

Ayesha Kadir and Anders Hjern

1.0 Introduction

Childhood is a time of transitions. As children grow and develop, their health, cognitive, and social skills are molded through interactions with their physical and social environment. Identity and understandings of the world are forged, which in turn influence how children engage with their environment.[1] These early experiences follow children throughout the lifecourse, impacting their physical health, mental health, who they grow up to become, and what opportunities they will have. For migrant children, in addition to the traditional and biological transitions of childhood and adolescence, there is a transition of place.

The UN Convention on the Rights of the Child (CRC) defines children as all people under eighteen years of age.[2] By this definition, one in eight international migrants are children—a total of thirty-six million children.[3] These children bear a disproportionately high risk of being forced from their homes, accounting for half of all refugees and 42 percent of forcibly displaced people. In 2019, 153,300 unaccompanied or separated children were counted across the globe.[4] Migration also affects children indirectly when parents migrate for education or work. The number of children in this circumstance is unknown but is thought to be in the hundreds of millions.[5] In China alone, 69.7 million children are separated from one or both parents in this way.[6]

Migrant children have specific health needs and risks that are related to the circumstances of migration and each phase of their journey. The journey is often prolonged, and children may pass through several countries.

TABLE 16.1 **Key articles from the Convention on the Rights of the Child that relate to migrant child health**

The Convention on the Rights of the Child is a helpful tool when considering migrant children's health as it addresses the interdependent effects of children's physical, social, political, and economic milieu on child health, development, and well-being

Article 2.1	States Parties shall respect and ensure the rights set forth in the present Convention to each child within their jurisdiction without discrimination of any kind, irrespective of the child's or his or her parent's or legal guardian's race, colour, sex, language, religion, political or other opinion, national, ethnic or social origin, property, disability, birth or other status.
Article 9.1	States Parties shall ensure that a child shall not be separated from his or her parents against their will, except when competent authorities subject to judicial review determine, in accordance with applicable law and procedures, that such separation is necessary for the best interests of the child.
Article 20.1–20.2	A child temporarily or permanently deprived of his or her family environment, or in whose own best interests cannot be allowed to remain in that environment, shall be entitled to special protection and assistance provided by the State. States Parties shall in accordance with their national laws ensure alternative care for such a child.
Article 22.1	States Parties shall take appropriate measures to ensure that a child who is seeking refugee status or who is considered a refugee in accordance with applicable international or domestic law and procedures shall, whether unaccompanied or accompanied by his or her parents or by any other person, receive appropriate protection and humanitarian assistance in the enjoyment of applicable rights set forth in the present Convention and in other international human rights or humanitarian instruments to which the said States are Parties.
Article 24.1	States Parties recognize the right of the child to the enjoyment of the highest attainable standard of health and to facilities for the treatment of illness and rehabilitation of health. States Parties shall strive to ensure that no child is deprived of his or her right of access to such health care services.
Article 27.1	States Parties recognize the right of every child to a standard of living adequate for the child's physical, mental, spiritual, moral and social development.
Article 28.1	States Parties recognize the right of the child to education, and with a view to achieving this right progressively and on the basis of equal opportunity, they shall, in particular: (a) Make primary education compulsory and available free to all; (b) Encourage the development of different forms of secondary education, including general and vocational education, make them available and accessible to every child, and take appropriate measures such as the introduction of free education and offering financial assistance in case of need; (c) Make higher education accessible to all on the basis of capacity by every appropriate means; (d) Make educational and vocational information and guidance available and accessible to all children; (e) Take measures to encourage regular attendance at schools and the reduction of drop-out rates.
Article 39	States Parties shall take all appropriate measures to promote physical and psychological recovery and social reintegration of a child victim of: any form of neglect, exploitation, or abuse; torture or any other form of cruel, inhuman or degrading treatment or punishment; or armed conflicts. Such recovery and reintegration shall take place in an environment which fosters the health, self-respect and dignity of the child.

Source: United Nations, 1989, Convention on the Rights of the Child, edited by United Nations and ISSOP Migration Working Group.

Children face an increased risk of violence and exploitation even after settlement in their new home. Acknowledging their vulnerability, the CRC gives special attention to the rights of migrant children (table 16.1). This chapter will review the influence of migration on child health from a child rights perspective.

2.0 Health Needs and Risks

The health of migrant children is related to a number of contextual factors, including their age, the health risks in the country of origin, their premigration health status, the reason they left their home, the conditions during the journey and after arrival, and their experiences throughout the migration process (fig. 16.1). Over the course of migration and settlement, children are at increased risk for experiencing multiple kinds of adversity, including food insecurity, inadequate shelter, separation from a caregiver, violence, exploitation, injury, their own illness, and/or caregiver illness.[7] Although arrival in the destination country may result in the removal of some forms of adversity, these adverse childhood experiences can have cumulatively harmful effects on children's psychomotor development, immune function, and long-term physical and mental health.[8]

While more than 60 percent of international migrant children live in low- and middle-income countries,[9] the overwhelming majority of studies on migrant child health are observational studies undertaken in high-income settings and often focusing on specific conditions or diseases. In order to highlight the importance of context, we will review what is known about migration and child health based on the phase of the children's journey, with further discussion on topics of particular importance. Figure 16.1 provides an overview of the risks associated with migrating during childhood.

2.1 In the Country of Origin

The reasons that children leave their homes, with or without caregivers, have an important impact on their health. They may have experienced armed conflict or extreme poverty. They may be seeking safety or better opportunities for their future. Political persecution and armed conflict are major causes of forced displacement of children and, in particular, of children traveling unaccompanied or being separated from caregivers.[10] Inadequate

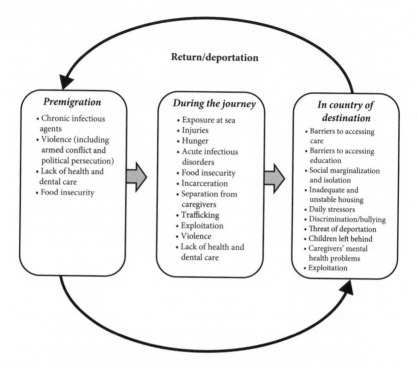

FIGURE 16.1. Risk factors for migrant child health in relation to phases of the journey

Source: Hjern, Anders, and Ayesha Kadir, 2018, *Health of Refugee and Migrant Children,* WHO Regional Office for Europe.

living conditions and limited access to health care are associated with increased risk of communicable diseases such as tuberculosis, malaria, diarrheal diseases, viral hepatitis, intestinal helminths, leishmaniasis, and vaccine-preventable diseases like measles and pneumonia.[11] Children may be undernourished or, conversely, obese. Iron and other micronutrient deficiencies are common among children with limited access to food, with intestinal parasites, and/or with recurrent infections such as diarrhea and pneumonia. Recent studies from Europe found 2 to 12 percent of asylum-seeking children from low-income settings had latent tuberculosis (TB); less than 1 percent had active TB disease.[12] Infants may have been born without access to antenatal care during pregnancy or skilled birth attendants at delivery, thus bearing increased risk of birth complications and long-term sequelae.[13,14] It is important to note that most studies have been undertaken in children after arrival in their destination country. Conditions during the journey and after arrival may also place migrant children at risk of contracting communicable diseases.

2.2 During the Journey

The route and means of travel have important impacts on child health. Prolonged journeys with risky means of travel put children at risk of separation from caregivers, injury, illness, exploitation, and death. Programs tracking migrant deaths in the Mediterranean Sea regularly report children among the fatalities.[15] Overcrowding, inadequate shelter, and limited access to hygiene and sanitation facilities place children at risk for viral respiratory infections, pneumonia, tuberculosis, diarrheal diseases, and skin infections. Differing resistance patterns for bacterial infections may require tailored antibiotic therapy that differs from the protocols of the transit country health system. Infants born during the journey are at high risk for complications such as asphyxia, hypothermia, and infection. Breastfeeding can be difficult for mothers on the move due to lack of privacy and safety; the associated poor infant nutritional status places the child at risk for developmental delay as well as a number of physical health problems.[16,17,18]

2.3 In the Destination Country

A recent systematic review on the health of migrant children in reception centers showed heterogeneous findings for a number of health conditions, again highlighting the importance of context in determining child health outcomes.[19] Language barriers, unfamiliar surroundings, lack of information about how to access basic services, lack of knowledge about their rights, and fear of incarceration or deportation are barriers in access to shelter, health care, education, and legal assistance. Limited knowledge of safety risks in the new environment is associated with increased rates of unintentional injuries, including motor vehicle injuries, poisoning, suffocation, and scald burns.[20] Structural, cultural, and language barriers and a lack of knowledge among health workers about the health risks and needs of migrant children are associated with delays in diagnosis and barriers to adequate and effective health care.[21] Overcrowding in accommodation facilities in Europe has been associated with Hepatitis A outbreaks, with particularly high prevalence in children.[22] High rates of dental caries across studies suggest that migration is associated with barriers in access to dental hygiene products and maintenance dental care at some or all stages of the journey.[23,24,25]

3.0 Violence and Exploitation

Violence in childhood is associated with a host of immediate health effects, including injury, illness, psychological trauma, and death. Migrant children are at risk for experiencing a broad range of typologies of violence, including armed conflict, community violence, domestic violence, physical abuse, trafficking, structural violence, racism, and xenophobia. Structural violence refers to the harm caused to individuals and groups from social structures and arrangements. For migrant children, this may include the reasons for the migration, barriers in access to health care and education, restrictions in movement, and social isolation, to name a few. Unaccompanied and separated children are at particularly high risk for exploitation and trafficking. More than one in nine unaccompanied children who applied for asylum in Europe in 2015 have gone missing.[26] Caregiver trauma and mental ill health predispose children to violence in the home. A recent study found that children whose caregiver suffers from post-traumatic stress disorder are more likely to experience harsh parenting.[27] It is important to note that a systematic review of the literature found no evidence for increased risk of child maltreatment in the general population of immigrant and refugee children.[28] At the level of the community and the society, racism and xenophobia are associated with interpersonal violence, social isolation, and barriers in access to basic needs.[29] Table 16.2 discusses detention and child trafficking of migrant children.

4.0 Mental Health

Migrant children are exposed to a complex web of risk factors that creates a high burden of mental health problems (fig. 16.2), including anxiety, depression, post-traumatic stress disorder, sleep disturbances, internalizing behaviors, and externalizing behaviors. Uprooting, even when the journey is intentional, is associated with loss and stress in children. Traumatic experiences such as violence, near drowning, and detention may continue to affect children after arrival in their new home. Migrant children who experience multiple adversities are at risk for anxiety, depression, self-harm, and substance abuse.[30]

TABLE 16.2 **Violence against children: Special risks for migrant children**

1. Child trafficking
    Trafficking of migrant children takes many forms, including child labor, sexual exploitation, forced criminal activities, street begging, and illegal adoption. Unaccompanied and separated children are at highest risk; however, accompanied children are also at increased risk for trafficking compared with children in the local population. Children may also experience trafficking of a caregiver. The risk of trafficking is present throughout the journey and even after arrival in the destination country.
2. Detention of migrant children
    Refugee children may be systematically detained together with or separated from caregivers upon arrival in a country or while waiting for deportation. A recent example is the large-scale detention of migrant children in the United States. Reports describe separation of children from caregivers, overcrowding, inadequate clothing, inadequate water and sanitation facilities, limited access to health care, and twenty-four-hour light exposure. Outbreaks of communicable diseases, psychological trauma, and at least seven deaths have been attributed to detention conditions. Although the detention of children and separation from caregivers are violations of children's rights according to international law, they are commonly practiced across the globe.

Sources: Hjern, Anders, and Ayesha Kadir, 2018, *Health of Refugee and Migrant Children,* WHO Regional Office for Europe (Copenhagen); Mishori, R., "US Policies and Their Effects on Immigrant Children's Health," *American Family Physician* 101, no. 4 (2020): 202–4.

It is important to stress that not all children who experience trauma become traumatized or psychologically distressed. The support of parents is the most important protective factor for most migrant children. Likewise, children whose caregivers suffer a mental health disorder have increased rates of mental health, behavioral, and somatic health problems.[31,32]

The social and legal situation of the child and family has important consequences for mental health. A large body of research demonstrates the importance of social support systems for maintaining good mental health. Most migrant families leave important parts—or perhaps all—of their social support system in their country of origin. This makes them particularly dependent on the support of their nuclear family and their ability to create new social networks. Further, many migrant families live in difficult socioeconomic circumstances in the early years in their new country, often experiencing low-income and crowded transitional housing conditions. A lack of child-friendly immigration procedures is common; indeed, some studies describe immigration procedures that are more harmful than the child's experiences before migration. The asylum application process may last years and include multiple relocations, creating significant and chronic stress for parents and children alike and contributing to poor mental health outcomes in refugee children.[33]

While children's experiences during the journey and in the early period after arrival have significant impact on their physical and mental health in the short term, available evidence from interview studies suggests that psychological symptoms related to the migration process wane over time

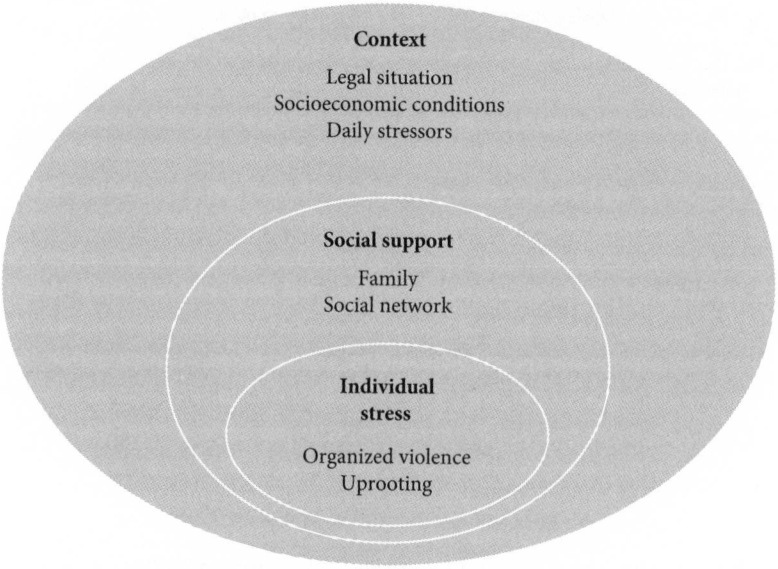

FIGURE 16.2. An ecological model of the psychosocial situation of refugee children in exile

Sources: Hjern, Anders, and Ayesha Kadir, 2018, *Health of Refugee and Migrant Children*, WHO Regional Office for Europe; Hjern, A., and O. Jeppson, "Mental Health Care for Refugee Children," in *Forced Migration and Mental Health: Rethinking the Care of Refugees and Displaced Persons*, edited by D. Ingleby, Amsterdam: Springer, 2005.

in most children. The social determinants of health take precedence in the long-term, with factors such as racism, social inequalities, structural violence, and uncertain legal status having increasing importance for children's physical and mental health.[34,35]

5.0 Unaccompanied and Separated Children

Children are increasingly traveling unaccompanied or separated from their caregivers. During the last decade, four hundred thousand unaccompanied children were documented worldwide; this is thought to be a significant underestimate.[36] Up to 20 percent of children arriving in the European Economic Area from 2015 to 2017 arrived without a parent or legal guardian.[37] The vast majority of studies on unaccompanied and separated children have been undertaken in Europe and Australia.

A lack of protection and support from a caregiver makes unaccompanied children particularly vulnerable to exploitation as well as poor

mental health and well-being.[38] Large epidemiological studies of unaccompanied teenage asylum seekers in Belgium and the Netherlands have
demonstrated high rates of depression and post-traumatic stress disorder
during the first years after resettlement. While studies have consistently
shown that unaccompanied children bear high risk for poor mental health
outcomes, these young people are often resourceful and arrive with a
clear vision of a positive future in their new country, despite the suffering
many of them have endured.[39] A key determinant of long-term healthy
adjustment is the maintenance of relationships with substitute caretakers during the first years after resettlement through school and continuity
of care.[40] Longitudinal studies in the United States and Norway indicate
that the mental health burden of unaccompanied minors fades over time,
much as it does for accompanied children.[41,42]

In most countries, the support provided for young asylum seekers is determined based on their chronological age. Unaccompanied children under
eighteen are usually provided with substitute caretakers, and their cases
are handled with priority during the asylum process, based on the rights afforded to them in the CRC. However, many children lack documents with
an exact birth date. With the arrival of greater numbers of asylum-seeking
unaccompanied minors in Europe, methods to assess age have become controversial. The majority of European Union member states rely on medical
technology to determine age in children who lack official documentation
of their birth date. X-rays—and more recently magnetic resonance imaging (MRI)—of the hand/wrist, collarbone, and/or teeth are commonly used
to approximate age. These techniques have marked individual variation in
age-specific maturity during the later teen years. Further, the variation in
skeletal maturation between children from high- and low-income countries
is unknown. As such, medical imaging is unsuitable for assessing whether
a young person is below or above eighteen years of age.[43,44] Acknowledging these pitfalls, a few countries have begun to primarily rely on psychosocial evaluations of age using structured interviews and observations of the
young people in the first reception facilities to determine maturity.[45]

6.0 Intervention and Health Promotion

Children develop through interactions with their physical and social environment, including their families, communities, and neighborhoods, and
with the governmental and nongovernmental institutions and organizations that shape society. Each of these factors can be supported to protect

and promote migrant children's health and well-being. Meeting the basic needs of children and families is a prerequisite to promoting health and preventing illness; all children need and have the right to safety, secure and adequate housing, access to potable water and sanitation, food security, education, and health care.[46] Once basic needs have been met, attention can be turned to other factors to promote and protect migrant child health and well-being.

Resilience theory describes a dynamic process that leads to positive and healthy adaptation to experiences of threats or adversity.[47] Factors that enhance resilience in migrant children include a supportive home environment, the mental health of caregivers, social inclusion, and positive experiences in school.[48] Education is not only a basic need and right of migrant children, it is also a protective factor and a means to promote healthy adaptation to their new environment.[49] Positive contact with peers in school and in the community helps to counteract social isolation and promotes the development of social support networks for children and families. Stability and continuity are important: prolonged asylum processes, multiple relocations, multiple school changes, and barriers in access to education all place children at risk for poor mental health outcomes.[50]

A major focus of advocacy and interventions has been on restoring a sense of stability and structure to daily life. Keeping families together and reunifying separated children with their families is a critical part of this; attachment to caregivers provides support and a sense of safety and protection, which in turn fosters healthy development of the child. When children are separated from their caregivers, this attachment is threatened and a host of maladaptive biological and psychological processes take place, with harmful consequences for the individual child's health throughout the lifecourse. Separation from parents during childhood is associated with developmental delay, altered stress physiology, and increased risk of mental illness.[51,52] Keeping families together and reuniting separated families, where possible, can mitigate trauma experienced during migration and prevent further harm to children's health.

Language barriers, different cultural understandings of health, and different expectations for health-care encounters can lead to delays in diagnosis, unnecessary investigations and/or treatments, and problems with administering and adhering to treatment.[53] Training health professionals to provide competent cross-cultural care and using professional interpreters for language-discordant encounters can improve the quality of care and health outcomes.[54]

7.0 Summary and a Way Forward

The health of migrant children is influenced by complex and intersecting factors, including the state of their health before travel, their experiences and conditions during the journey and after settlement in the country of destination, the health of caregivers, and children's understandings of and adaptation to the challenges they face. While health trends are seen for certain migration patterns, the outcomes of individual children vary according to the child's experiences and how they respond to them. The evidence base on migrant child health is primarily from observational reports in high-income settings with a heavy focus on infectious diseases and, to a lesser extent, mental health. Our understanding of chronic diseases and disability in migrant children remains limited. Further, few rigorous studies have examined the context-specific effects of migration on children's health or the impact of specific interventions to protect and promote health, well-being, and child development. Knowledge gaps include a theoretical understanding of resilience, intersectionality, and how children's experiences of different kinds of violence affect their health and development in different contexts. As we have discussed, children's health status before the journey as well as the conditions and their experiences during and afterward impact their health. Cultural, social, political, and economic factors all contribute to how children make sense of and engage with their experiences, and this in turn affects their sense of identity, their behavior, and their outcomes in the longer term. Future research should include children and caregivers in the study of risk and protective factors across contexts to better explore how the transitions migrant children experience can influence, both negatively and positively, their health trajectories and life opportunities.

CHAPTER SEVENTEEN

Violence, Migration, and Mental Health

Jutta Lindert

1.0 Introduction

Violence is a common and serious health and human rights problem. Little is known about the pattern of violence exposure of migrants during the migration process, including premigration, movement, and post-migration stages, and the potential violence-migration nexus. Reasons for the lack of knowledge are manifold; one of the main reasons might be that violence has been recognized as one of the major factors influencing health only recently. Understanding of the violence-migration nexus is needed to assist researchers, mental health professionals, service providers, and policy makers in developing informed approaches to policy and psychosocial services addressing migrants. The relationship between migration and violence depends on risk factors at societal, community, and family levels during the migration process, including social, cultural, and gender norms, exposure to conflicts and forced displacement, family violence, and exploitation. Exposure to violence during migration can lead to mental disorders, cognitive distortions, somatic complaints, sexual and relationship problems, attempted suicide, alcohol and drug abuse, and violent behavior. In this chapter, first the migration and violence nexus are described. Second, potential exposures to violence during migration are identified. Third, mental health consequences of exposures to violence are reviewed; and finally, challenges for a better understanding of violence against migrants to design effective, appropriate, and targeted interventions are proposed.

2.0 Migration — A Global Movement

The number of people in migration is enormous. In 2020, there were 272 million people worldwide living outside their country of birth (3.5% of the
world population; median age: thirty-nine) out of a global population of
7.7 billion. Of those, 47.9 percent were females, 13.9 percent were children
below the age of eighteen, and 10.6 percent (25.9 million) were refugees,
with 20.4 million falling under the United Nations High Commissioner
for Refugees (UNHCRs) mandate.[1] The overwhelming majority of people migrate internationally for reasons of work. There is no universally
agreed upon definition of migration or migrant. The United Nations
Recommendations of International Migration defines "an international
migrant" as any person who has changed his or her country of usual residence.[2] Accordingly, migration patterns are diverse. Although often there
is a distinction made between labor migrants and forced migrants, the
distinction between groups is difficult, and groups may have mixed motives for migrating. It is not necessarily hardiness that leads to migration;
people might be forced to migrate to avoid armed conflicts, persecution,
the fallout of natural disasters, and economic instability. More than 40 percent of all migrants worldwide in 2019 were born in Asia, primarily in
India, China, and other South Asian countries. Mexico was the second
largest country of origin. Migrating from hardship, migrants regularly
cross (multiple) international borders on difficult journeys. Previous studies have shown that violence is a threat at different stages of migration.[3]
It is difficult, however, to quantify the precise magnitude of exposure to
violence against migrants.

3.0 Violence — A Global Public Health Problem

Violence is a global public health and human rights problem. Violence has
been recognized as a human rights problem for a long time, but the recognition of violence as a public health problem is more recent.[4,5] In 1996,
the forty-ninth World Health Assembly adopted a resolution declaring violence a major public health problem. As defined by the World Health Organization (WHO), violence can be understood in a broad sense as "the
intentional use of physical force or power, threatened or actual, against
oneself, another person, or against a group or community, that either results

in or has a high likelihood of resulting in injury, death, psychological harm, maldevelopment or deprivation."[6] Following this definition of violence, I investigate the various forms of violence in this chapter in an ecological model—at the individual, relationship, community, and societal level.[7] In this analysis, structural and physical violence, sexual and psychological violence, and financial exploitation are included. The forms and severity of violence vary historically, geographically, and in population groups. Following the WHO definition and the ecological model of violence, the violence-migration nexus across selected different levels and types will be described.

4.0 Violence and Migration

When individuals migrate, they come from different environments with certain health risks and enter new environments that have different health risks. Migration can be a movement away from health risks, including moving away from physical or structural violence.

Studies suggest that migrants are exposed to various types of violence during the different stages of migration (premigration, movement, arrival). Premigration migrants may witness and experience atrocities of war, persecution, community violence, and domestic violence. This exposure to violence may play a role in decision-making and motivations to migrate, and transnational migration may serve as a strategy to escape violence (table 17.1).[8] In addition, migration may be a strategy used to escape the social and cultural norms that promote violence in the country of origin. Unfortunately, violence does not necessarily end when migrants leave their home country. During movement, high rates of violence are possible.[9] In the country of arrival, migrants may face structural violence and domestic violence. A review of family violence in migrant families found associations of family violence in the country of arrival with exposure to violence in the premigration country.[10]

As table 17.1 suggests, practically all types of violence can occur during the different migration stages. In the following section, the migration-violence nexus is described in more detail.

5.0 Premigration Violence

Migrants include refugees, persons seeking asylum, and undocumented migrants. The historical contexts of these migrants differ very much and

TABLE 17.1 **Potential types of violence and migration phases**

	Migration phase		
	Premigration	Movement	Arrival
Type of violence			
Societal			
Structural violence	x	x	X
Conflicts	x		X
War	x		
Human trafficking	x	x	X
Community			
Gang violence	x	x	X
Sexual exploitation	x	x	X
Domestic violence			
Child physical abuse	x	x	X
Child sexual abuse	x	x	X
Child emotional abuse	x	x	X
Child marriage	x	x	
Intimate partner violence	x	x	X
Financial exploitation	x	x	X

might include cultural acceptance of violence, human rights violations, life-threatening violence as a means for solving conflicts in wars, or acceptance of violence against children and violence against women.[11,12]

5.1 Premigration Societal Violence

In a study on migrants in France originating from North and West Africa with a median age of twenty-nine, high levels of exposure to societal violence were reported. In most cases (58%), the reason for seeking asylum was political persecution. Almost all attendees (94%) presented with scars. The most common mechanisms of injury were beatings (84%), burns (32%), and cuts/stab wounds (15%). Sexual violence was reported for 37 percent of women (10/27) and 4 percent of men (9/213).[13] The overall high prevalence of war-related events of sexual violence was highlighted in several other studies,[14] including among women fleeing from the Democratic Republic of the Congo.[15]

5.2 Premigration Family Violence

Violence against girls and women is prevalent in many countries, including in countries from where migrants come.[16,17,18] A review on violence against children, which included thirty-seven studies conducted with data from fifty-nine countries, examined this type of violence. Firstly, in contexts where there was a strong norm in support of violence against children, parents and teachers practiced violence because the violence was normalized, and parents thought it was expected of them. Stark et al. (2017) presented a detailed description of violence against adolescent girls in the Democratic Republic Congo. More than half of the sample reported victimization in the previous twelve months (54.4%); a majority suffered multiple incidents of victimization. The most frequently reported type of victimization was psychological violence (38%). Approximately one-fifth of the girls reported sexual violence. This report highlighted the fact that the most frequent perpetrators of all forms of violence, including sexual abuse, were family members or intimate partners (husbands or boyfriends). For children, the most frequent perpetrators before migration were caregivers and not members of an armed group or other officials.[19]

Childhood sexual abuse (CSA) is one of the most common types of childhood violence exposure (median prevalence: 20.4%),[20] especially among females.[21] Approximately one in five women reports a history of CSA. Females are at a two- or threefold higher risk of CSA compared to males. In a meta-analysis, the overall pooled rate of CSA was 24 percent; however, there was considerable heterogeneity among the studies. On subgroup analyses, the CSA rate was different between different geographic regions and sample sources with lower medians of female CSA in estimates for Europe (17%) and Asia (18%)[22] and higher rates in the African region—50.8 percent (36% to 73.8%) for girls and 60.2 percent (43% to 84.9%) for boys.

5.3 Intimate Partner Violence

Women in many countries all over the world report violence in their home countries as a normalized part of life, supported by patriarchal gender norms and socialization.[23] Intimate partner violence (IPV) is committed by a current or former spouse, boyfriend or girlfriend, or dating partner.[24] Some factors increase or decrease exposure to domestic violence; a higher education level decreases the probability of domestic violence across all ages. Unemployment increases the probability of IPV in adult women (physical/sexual IPV, PR: 1.7; psychological IPV, PR: 1.3).

Unstable environments increase the probability of sexual violence (SV). Globally, about 35.6 percent of women have experienced SV, with varying prevalence estimates.[25] Men can also be subjected to SV, though it may be difficult to provide general prevalence estimates, as SV is generally underreported, with an elevated amount of non-reporting the in case of violence against men and boys. Findings suggest that SV against men and boys may not be rare. Frequently reported forms of violence in these settings were genital violence, forced witnessing of sexual violence, and rape. Violence often occurred during the movement phases.[26]

Most studies on SV among men have examined the above index in affected communities and war-torn areas. The prevalence of SV among refugees around the world was largely variable, from zero to 99.8 percent: in Africa, it has been reported from 1.3 to 99.8 percent; in Asia, the prevalence is variable from zero to 84.6 percent; and in America and Europe, it is 3.5 percent and 3.3 percent, respectively. Therefore, the exposure to SV in the region of origin especially among forcibly displaced persons may be high.[27]

In addition to considerations of violence as an impetus for migration and the risk of violence during migration, many women face further violence and exploitation during movement. A meta-analysis of studies in humanitarian settings suggested that 21 percent of female refugees or displaced women in complex humanitarian emergencies experienced sexual violence, a probable underestimation. Some women report an escalation or initiation of violence and abuse by same or new partners after migrating to the host country, despite efforts to escape battering in the home country.

6.0 Violence during the Movement Phase

Violence exposure during movement is frequent, especially for refugees and asylum seekers. A study on refugees in a refugee camp reported that 80 percent of Sudanese migrants came from Darfur, 78 percent of Syrians were from either Deraa or Aleppo, 44 percent of Afghans were from Pashto tribal areas, and 30 percent of Iraqis were from Kirkuk or Mosul. Of those, 65.6 percent (95% CI 60.3–70.6) reported experiencing exposure to violence during their journey or in the refugee camp at Calais at least once. Among those who reported at least one violent event, 30.8 percent (95% CI 25.1–37.2) said the violence occurred in Libya and 25.3 percent (95% CI 19.9–31.6) in Calais. The most common type of violence reported was assault and battery (45.7% [95% CI 39.9–52.2]), while 26.9 percent (95% CI 21.4–33.4) reported facing tear gas and 14.2 percent (95% CI 10.1–19.6) reported experiencing repeated violence with forced detention.

The overall proportion of participants having suffered from violence was 96.4 percent among men and 88.2 percent among women. The prevalence of physical, deprivation, and sexual violence for men and women were 94.2, 81.7, and 18 percent and 80, 86.7, and 53.3 percent, respectively.[28]

Violence during the movement phase is a hallmark of human trafficking. Human trafficking is estimated to affect the lives of over twenty-seven million people worldwide; however, estimates are difficult due to the covert nature of trafficking. Human trafficking involves recruitment, transportation, and the harboring or receipt of persons, usually by coercion. Individuals are trafficked for sexual exploitation but also for domestic servitude and forced labor in a range of industries, including factory work, agriculture, construction, commercial fishing, and street begging.[29] The violence, abusive living conditions, and restrictions on movement commonly associated with trafficking pose serious risks to trafficked people's health. A systematic review conducted in 2012 identified nineteen studies reporting on the health risks experienced by women and girls trafficked for sexual exploitation and found a high prevalence of physical and sexual abuse. The review also highlighted the near-complete absence of evidence at that time on the health of trafficked men and of individuals trafficked for labor exploitation. The prevalence of sexual violence was estimated at 10 percent during predeparture, 35 percent during the traveling period, 58.1 percent at destination, and 19.5 percent in detention stages.[30]

7.0 Violence in the Host Country

Unfortunately, violence does not necessarily end in the host country. Migrants may face structural violence, such as lack of access to employment opportunities or violence at the hand of family members.[31]

8.0 Migration, Violence, and Mental Health

The WHO defines good health as "a state of complete physical, mental, and social well-being, and not merely the absence of disease or infirmity."[32] This recognition of mental health emphasizes the importance of viewing health holistically. As such, mental health is shaped by a multitude of factors, including gender, age, and socioeconomic factors and structural, community, and interpersonal violence.[33] The adverse health outcomes of violence are diverse and include a variety of mental health consequences.[34,35]

The impact and consequences of violence on mental health are pervasive among adults and youth[36] and include feelings of loss assumptions that others and the outside world are dangerous and threatening. Because of victimization before, during, and after migration, migrants have an elevated risk of developing mental health problems.[37,38,39] A review and meta-analysis of 181 surveys from forty countries, comprising 81,866 refugees and people affected by torture and conflict found that the unadjusted weighted prevalence rate was 30.6 percent for post-traumatic stress disorder and 30.8 percent for depression. Compared with labor migrants, refugees had approximately double the prevalence of depression and anxiety. However, it might be that violence exposure for migrants is reduced in the host countries; therefore, a better understanding of the positive impact of migration on violence-affected persons is needed.

9.0 Challenges

Generally, there is a lack of data to understand the full migration-violence and health nexus. Instruments to assess violence across the migration stages are missing. Most assessment instruments have been developed in English-speaking countries. Some have been translated into the languages of and validated for high-income countries. Translations into the languages of countries where migrants come from are often not available. Therefore, instruments that assess exposure to violence across the migration process are needed. It might be that we often miss the full picture of violence exposure, as the acceptability of the disclosure of violence varies. The lack of population norms for instruments is yet another challenge. Depending on the context of experiencing violence, norms should probably refer to either the population in the country of origin or the host population.

Sources of information may be another difficulty. The validity and reliability of sources of information on violence are an issue for migrants and nonmigrants. Violence exposure is often not reported to authorities, particularly in the context of war and conflicts and in countries with norms of solving conflicts by using violence. Additionally, victims may have motives to withhold or elaborate information. Sampling procedures and study design are yet another source of variability between studies. The outcome measures vary markedly. For example, lifetime prevalence of violence does not clearly distinguish between the causes and outcomes of war atrocities in the country of origin or the risks and sequelae of family violence in the country of arrival.

10.0 Conclusion

Overall, there is a dearth of epidemiological data on violence against migrants.[40] This coincides with the lack of data in the field of migration, health, and violence.[41] Available epidemiological data differ in terms of concepts, severity of violence, methods, and, consequently, outcomes. To increase comparability of data and improve research on violence and migrants, an empirical base is needed.

In order to account for the violence-migration nexus, research should incorporate the different phases of migration. To avoid problems in the comparison of violence, all studies should describe and differentiate between types of violence during migration, perpetrators (caregivers, peers, strangers), and settings of violence (country of origin, on the move, country of arrival). A lifecourse approach should be adopted, and short-, medium-, and long-term effects of the migration-violence nexus should be investigated. Finally, given the prevalence of violence against women and girls, gender-specific data should be provided.

CHAPTER EIGHTEEN

Remittances, Health Access, and Outcomes

Melissa Siegel

1.0 Introduction

While this book looks at migration and health more generally, this chapter specifically looks at the effects of remittances on access to health care and health outcomes. First, this chapter will clarify what is meant by remittances. There are three main types of remittances: monetary/financial, in-kind, and social. Monetary or financial remittances are money that is sent by migrants back to their friends, family, or community generally in their origin (country). In-kind remittances are things or goods that are generally sent back to the migrant's country of origin. These typically consist of clothes, electronics, medicine, food, and other goods. Social remittances refer to values, norms, and knowledge that can be transferred from one place to another. Remittances can be sent within a country (internal remittances) or between countries (international remittances). While all three types of remittances can have an effect on health access and outcomes, this chapter focuses specifically on monetary remittances with an emphasis on international monetary remittances (hereafter referred to only as *remittances*).

Internationally, remittances make up an important, relatively stable source of external finance for many countries and have grown substantially in recent decades. In 2020, remittances to low- and middle-income countries were US$540 million. This is only 1.6 percent below what was sent in 2019, in direct contrast to predictions by the World Bank of a 20 percent reduction on 2019. In many counties, remittances were more important than both foreign direct investment and official development assistance combined. India, China, Mexico, the Philippines, and Egypt were the top five remittance receivers in 2020 in absolute terms; Tonga, Lebanon, Kyrgyz Republic, Tajikistan, and El Salvador were the top five receivers in relative terms (as a percentage of GDP). The top four source countries for remittances in 2020 were the United States, the United Arab Emirates, Saudi Arabia, and the Russian Federation.[1]

Even with the Covid-19 pandemic, when remittances were predicted to fall dramatically due to the economic downturn in most countries and the precarious and often more vulnerable situation of migrants, remittances were more resilient than expected. This resilience was mainly due to migrants' strong desire and willingness to help their families even by reducing their own well-being in countries of destination and drawing on savings. According to the World Bank, other factors, like economic stimulus packages that were introduced in major countries of destination and which migrants also benefited from, some better-than-expected economic performances in migrant hosting countries, migrants shifting to more formal channels to send their remittances (making it easier to count them officially), and cyclical movement in oil prices and currency exchange rates, all played a role in the remittance resilience during 2020.[2]

There are a number of ways in which remittances affect health-care access and health outcomes. The first is having more available monetary resources in the household to put toward preventative health care, being able to pay for health services and access to medicine when needed, and buying more and better-quality food. Another way that remittances could affect health outcomes is that the additional money in the household could mean that children or other members of the household no longer need to work or no longer have to work in dangerous jobs that are detrimental to their health. A third mechanism through with remittances could affect health is through investment in education. Increased education is generally correlated with better health outcomes. Additionally, via education, the recipients can gain new information about better health practices.

Remittances can also, theoretically, affect health negatively. If remittances are spent on excessive or worse quality food, this could lead to worse health outcomes. For instance, take the example of a mother abroad sending back money to her children. Perhaps the children now decide to buy more candy and eat more fast food because they now have the resources to do so and perhaps less parental oversight. This could decrease health outcomes.

This chapter first looks at the evidence on how remittances affect health outcomes and then turns to the evidence on how remittances affect health-care access and expenditures by reviewing a number of studies in the field.

2.0 Remittance Effects on Health Outcomes

Turning to the evidence on how remittances have affected health access and outcomes around the world, this chapter will begin with health outcomes. Luis Miguel Tovar Cuevas and colleagues[3] recently reviewed the available literature of remittances and health outcomes. They found positive, negative, and mixed effects of remittances on health outcomes. However, they found that many more studies have detected positive effects than negative or mixed results. Table 18.1 gives an overview of the effects of the main studies consulted as well as others reviewed by the author.

There are very few studies that find negative effects of remittances on health outcomes. One notable study in this regard is from Fernando Riosmena and colleagues (2012),[4] who look specifically at Mexico. They focus on migration from Mexico to the United States and the acceleration of the nutrition transition in Mexico, where an increase in obesity is observed. They find that the additional income via remittances is an important channel for the weight changes they observe. It is important to note that it is not only the money (or financial remittances) that are sent back, but also the social remittances (or norms) that are sent back at the same time that contribute to this shift.

Many studies find much more mixed evidence with more nuance into time effects (e.g., Frank 2005)[5] and specific situations when remittances do seem to have an impact. For example, Antón (2010)[6] found a positive short- and medium-term impact but no long-term impact on children's nutrition outcomes. Even with these more mixed results, there are notably more positive than negative outcomes. There is often either a positive effect or no noticeable effect (Sunil et al. 2012)[7]. Sometimes we see a positive effect in one area while we see a negative effect in another (Castillo-Hernández et al. 2009).[8] For instance, Hamilton and Choi (2015)[9] found that remittances and return migration decrease the risk of low birth weight but increase incidence of macrosomia. In another study, which reviewed twenty studies around the world looking at the effects of remittances on diet and nutrition, Thow, Fanzo, and Negin (2016)[10] found that studies showed an increase in access to food and food security, but remittances did not seem

TABLE 18.1 **The effect of remittances on health outcomes**

Author	Effect	Country
Positive effect		
Kan (2020)[1]	Found a positive relationship between remittances and health expenditures, days unable to work due to chronic illness, days unable to work due to sudden illness, the share of healthy household members, medicine consumption for those who chose not to seek medical care, and a decrease in the frequency of acute illness.	Tajikistan
Azzarri and Zezza (2011)[2]	Found that remittances were associated with better nutritional outcomes among children, mainly through households' improved access to food.	Tajikistan
Kroeger and Anderson (2014)[3]	Thinness of children was reduced over time thanks to remittances.	Kyrgystan
Lu (2013)[4]	The results showed that adults in (labor) emigrant households were significantly less susceptible to being underweight than those in nonmigrant households and did not have an increased risk of being overweight.	Indonesia
Howard and Stanley (2016)[5]	Receiving remittances accounted for 16 percent of the higher observed weight and height of children, with remittances-receiving households spending more on food (i.e., meat and fish in Honduras) and education.	Honduras
Bebczuk and Battistón (2010)[6]	Remittances improved anthropometric measures.	Ecuador, Honduras, Mexico, and Nicaragua
de Brauw (2011)[7]	Children in households with international migrants performed better in height/age scores compared to children in nonmigrant households.	El Salvador
Zhunio, Vishwasrao, and Chiang (2012)[8]	1 percent increase in real remittances per capita resulted in a 0.03 percent increase in life expectancy and a 0.15 percent reduction in infant mortality.	67 low- and middle-income countries
Carletto, Covarrubias, and Maluccio (2011)[9]	Found that migration and remittances improved child growth.	Guatemala
Gerber and Torosyan (2013)[10]	Remittance-receiving households had a decreased probability of poor health among household members.	Georgia
Terrelonge (2014)[11]	Found a significant positive effect of remittances on reduction of child mortality and malnutrition. An extra US$100 of remittance receipts per capita led to a reduction of 7.8 child deaths per 1,000 live births and a reduction of 5.7 infant deaths per 1,000 live births.	138 developing countries
Chauvet, Gubert, and Mesplé-Somps (2013)[12]	Remittances positively contributed to reducing child mortality, in particular for children belonging to the upper quintile classes.	84 and 46 developing countries
Amakom and Iheoma (2014)[13]	A 10 percent increase in remittances improved health outcome (measured as life expectancy at birth) by 1.2 percent on average.	18 SSA countries
Amega (2018)[14]	Remittances lowered infant and adult mortality and prolonged the percentage of newly born infants who lived up to age sixty-five (survival to age sixty-five) and the overall life expectancy of the population.	46 sub-Saharan African countries

TABLE 18.1 *(continued)*

Author	Effect	Country
Positive effect		
Acosta and Vizcarra-Bordi (2009)[15]	Children in remittance-receiving households had better health outcomes that those who did not receive remittances in the areas of weight-for-age and height-for-weight.	Latin American Countries
Terrelonge (2014)[16]	Increasing remittances reduced malnutrition measures and decreased the intensity of hunger.	Developing countries
Böhme et al. (2015)[17]	Remittances improved the diets of older people.	Moldova
Negative effect		
Riosmena et al. (2012)[18]	This study focused on the relationship between Mexican migration to the United States and the acceleration of nutritional transition in Mexico, where increases in obesity rates were observed due to receiving remittances.	Mexico
Mixed effects		
Hamilton and Choi (2015)[19]	This study found that remittances and return migration decreased the risk of low birth weight but increased incidence of macrosomia.	Mexico
Frank (2005)[20]	This study showed a positive effect of remittances on infant health but with a time effect. Only women who received remittances for over a year showed a decrease in the risk of giving birth to a low-weight child.	Mexico
Antón (2010)[21]	This study found positive short- and medium-term impact, but no long-term impact on children's nutrition outcomes.	Ecuador
Thow, Fanzo, and Negin (2016)[22]	In this literature review of twenty studies on the effects of remittances on diet and nutrition, the studies showed an increase in access to food and food security, but remittances did not seem to have an effect on undernourishment, and remittances may have led to buying less healthy food.	Global
Sunil et al. (2012)[23]	Migrant households that did not receive remittances had lower probability of having low-weight births, and there were not significant results for households that received remittances.	Mexico
Castillo-Hernández et al. (2009)[24]	Receiving remittances seemed to be associated with the absence of short duration maturation in children under five. The risk of malnutrition in women between the ages of twelve and forty-nine was higher among those who did not receive remittances. For children between five and eleven, the risk of malnutrition was lower in households that did not receive remittances than in those that did.	Mexico

Sources: [1] Sophia Kan, "Is an Ounce of Remittance Worth a Pound of Health? The Case of Tajikistan," *International Migration Review* 55, no. 2 (June 1, 2020), https://doi.org/10.1177/0197918320926891.
[2] Carlo Azzarri and Alberto Zezza, "International Migration and Nutritional Outcomes in Tajikistan," *Food Policy* 36, no. 1 (February 1, 2011): 54–70, https://doi.org/10.1016/j.foodpol.2010.11.004.

(continues)

TABLE 18.1 *(continued)*

[3] Antje Kroeger and Kathryn H. Anderson, "Remittances and the Human Capital of Children: New Evidence from Kyrgyzstan during Revolution and Financial Crisis, 2005–2009," *Journal of Comparative Economics* 42, no. 3 (August 1, 2014): 770–85, https://doi.org/10.1016/j.jce.2013.06.001.

[4] Yao Lu, "Household Migration, Remittances and Their Impact on Health in Indonesia," *International Migration* 51, no. s1 (2013): e202–15, https://doi.org/10.1111/j.1468-2435.2012.00761.x.

[5] Larry L. Howard and Denise L. Stanley, "Remittances Channels and the Physical Growth of Honduran Children," *International Review of Applied Economics* 31, no. 3 (November 21, 2016): 376–96.

[6] Ricardo Bebczuk and Diego Battistón, "Remittances and Life Cycle Deficits in Latin America," CEDLAS, Working Papers 0094 (CEDLAS, Universidad Nacional de La Plata, February 2010), https://ideas.repec.org/p/dls/wpaper/0094.html.

[7] Alan de Brauw, "Migration and Child Development during the Food Price Crisis in El Salvador," *Food Policy* 36, no. 1 (February 1, 2011): 28–40, https://doi.org/10.1016/j.foodpol.2010.11.002.

[8] Maria Cristina Zhunio, Sharmila Vishwasrao, and Eric P. Chiang, "The Influence of Remittances on Education and Health Outcomes: A Cross Country Study," *Applied Economics* 44, no. 35 (December 1, 2012): 4605–16, https://doi.org/10.1080/00036846.2011.593499.

[9] Calogero Carletto, Katia Covarrubias, and John A. Maluccio, "Migration and Child Growth in Rural Guatemala," *Food Policy* 36, no. 1 (February 1, 2011): 16–27, https://doi.org/10.1016/j.foodpol.2010.12.002.

[10] Theodore P. Gerber and Karine Torosyan, "Remittances in the Republic of Georgia: Correlates, Economic Impact, and Social Capital Formation," *Demography* 50, no. 4 (August 1, 2013): 1279–301, https://doi.org/10.1007/s13524-013-0195-3.

[11] Sophia C. Terrelonge, "For Health, Strength, and Daily Food: The Dual Impact of Remittances and Public Health Expenditure on Household Health Spending and Child Health Outcomes," *Journal of Development Studies* 50, no. 10 (October 3, 2014): 1397–410, https://doi.org/10.1080/00220388.2014.940911.

[12] Lisa Chauvet, Flore Gubert, and Sandrine Mesplé-Somps, "Aid, Remittances, Medical Brain Drain and Child Mortality: Evidence Using Inter and Intra-Country Data," *Journal of Development Studies* 49, no. 6 (June 1, 2013): 801–18, https://doi.org/10.1080/00220388.2012.742508.

[13] Uzochukwu Amakom and Chukwunonso Gerald Iheoma, "Impact of Migrant Remittances on Health and Education Outcomes in Sub-Saharan Africa," *IOSR Journal of Humanities and Social Science* 19, no. 8 (2014): 33–44, https://doi.org/10.9790/0837-19813344.

[14] Komla Amega, "Remittances, Education and Health in Sub-Saharan Africa," ed. Francesco Tajani, *Cogent Economics and Finance* 6, no. 1 (January 1, 2018): 1516488, https://doi.org/10.1080/23322039.2018.1516488.

[15] L. D. Acosta and I. Vizcarra-Bordi, "Desnutrición infantil en comunidades mazahuas con migración masculina internacional en México Central," *Poblac y Salud en Mesoamérica* 6, no. 2 (2009): 118.

[16] S. C. Terrelonge, "For Health, Strength and Daily Food: The Dual Impact of Remittances and Public Health Expenditure on Household Health Spending and Child Health Outcomes," *Journal of Development Studies* 50, no. 10 (2014): 1397–410.

[17] M. H. Böhme, R. Persian, and T. Stöhr, "Alone but Better Off? Adult Child Migration and Health of Elderly Parents in Moldova," *Journal of Health Economics* 39 (2015): 211–27.

[18] Fernando Riosmena et al., "U.S. Migration, Translocality, and the Acceleration of the Nutrition Transition in Mexico," *Annals of the Association of American Geographers* 102, no. 5 (September 1, 2012): 1209–18, https://doi.org/10.1080/00045608.2012.659629.

[19] Erin R. Hamilton and Kate H. Choi, "The Mixed Effects of Migration: Community-Level Migration and Birthweight in Mexico," *Social Science and Medicine* 132 (May 2015): 278–86, https://doi.org/10.1016/j.socscimed.2014.08.031.

[20] Reanne Frank, "International Migration and Infant Health in Mexico," *Journal of Immigrant Health* 7, no. 1 (January 1, 2005): 11–22, https://doi.org/10.1007/s10903-005-1386-9.

[21] José-Ignacio Antón, "The Impact of Remittances on Nutritional Status of Children in Ecuador," *International Migration Review* 44, no. 2 (2010): 269–99.

[22] Anne Marie Thow, Jessica Fanzo, and Joel Negin, "A Systematic Review of the Effect of Remittances on Diet and Nutrition," *Food and Nutrition Bulletin* (February 25, 2016), https://doi.org/10.1177/0379572116631651.

[23] T. S. Sunil, M. Flores, and G. E. Garcia, "New Evidence on the Effects of International Migration on the Risk of Low Birthweight in Mexico," *Maternal and Child Nutrition* 8, no. 2 (2012): 185–98.

[24] J. L. Castillo Hernández, M. M. Álvarez Ramírez, E. Y. Romero Hernández, S. C. Cortés, R. Zenteno-Cuevas, and L. N. Berrún-Castañón, "Asociación de las remesas con el estado nutricio y la adecuación de la dieta en habitantes de la localidad El Espinal, municipio de Naolinco, Veracruz, México," *Rev. Avanc. Seg. Alim. y Nutr.* 1, no. 1 (2009): 77–87.

to have an effect on undernourishment and may have led to the purchase of less healthy food. From a location perspective, the majority of studies with mixed results were conducted in Mexico and Latin America.

The majority of studies found showed clear positive benefits of remittances on different health outcomes from nutrition (Azzarri and Zezza 2011[11]; Böhme et al. 2015[12]), to infant, child, and adult weight (Kroeger and Anderson 2014[13]; Lu 2013[14]; Terrelonge 2014[15]), to better growth of children (Howard and Stanley 2016[16]; Bebczuk and Battistón 2010[17]; de Brauw 2011[18]; Carletto et al. 2011[19]; Acosta and Vizcarra-Bordi 2009[20]), to better life expectancy (Amakom and Iheoma 2014[21]), to reducing infant mortality (Terrelonge 2014[22]) and increasing general life expectancy in the case of low- and middle-income countries (Zhunio et al. 2012[23]; Chauvet et al. 2013[24]; Amega 2018[25]), to generally decreasing poor health (Gerber and Torosyan 2013[26]). Many of these studies that show more positive outcomes are also conducted on large numbers of low- and middle-income countries all over the world.

The evidence is clear that the positive effects of remittances on health outcome greatly outweigh any possible negative effects. However, the country context and outcomes that have been studied in the past are limited, with most country-level studies focused on Latin American countries and the majority of outcomes focused on child health indicators.

3.0 Effect of Remittances on Health-Care Access and Expenditures

Health-care access and expenditures can directly affect health outcomes. This section examines the effect of remittances on health-care access and expenditures. Table 18.2 builds on the systematic literature review on the impact of financial remittances on health-care utilization and expenditures in developing countries conducted by Nathaniel in 2019[27] and expands on this review with additional literature.

As in the previous section, the evidence in this field can be split into positive, mixed, and negative (although none of the review studies fall under this category). Again, the positive effects of remittances seem to vastly outweigh other/no impacts.

In studies that show mixed evidence, this was often because there was a positive effect in one area and no noticeable effect in another. For example, in Ecuador, Ponce, Olivié, and Onofa (2018)[28] found no effect of remittances on long-term child health variables, but remittances did have

TABLE 18.2 **The effect of remittances on health-care access**

Author	Effect	Country
Positive effect		
Amuedo-Dorantes, Sainz, and Pozo (2007)[1]	Health-care expenditures increased with the receipt of remittances, with hospital expenditures being the most responsive. This remittance income effect was higher than other sources of increased income.	Mexico
Frank et al. (2009)[2]	Remittances were found to be complementary to formal access to health care. Individuals who lacked insurance coverage or who were covered by the *Seguro Popular* program were significantly more likely to reside in households that spent remittances on health care than individuals covered by an employer-based insurance program.	Mexico
Drabo and Ebeke (2011)[3]	Remittances were an important determinant of access to health-care services. Remittance receivers were more likely to switch to private-sector access for the richest recipients.	Developing countries
Piette et al. (2012)[4]	Access to health care of chronically ill family members was highly dependent on receipt of remittances, as the majority of respondents reported to have reduced health-care visits and medication purchases due to a loss or reduction of remittance income during the 2009 economic downturn in the United States.	Honduras
López-Cevallos and Chi (2012)[5]	Migration was associated with use of antiparasitic medicines and health-care visits among low-income Ecuadorians (quintiles 1 and 2).	Ecuador
Salinas (2008)[6]	Found that the elderly with family members abroad were able to better manage their diabetes due to the economic assistance through remittances compared to their peers with no migrant family members.	Mexico
Nguyen and Nguyen (2015)[7]	Found that remittances increased both inpatient and outpatient health-care visits of children. The effect was higher for adolescents than for children.	Vietnam
Farooq and Iqbal (2015)[8]	Concerning health-seeking behavior, they found that remittance-receiving households were more likely to consult a private doctor/hospital when sick. Moreover, overseas receivers were more likely to consult "official" (more expensive) practitioners than non-receivers, who tended to rely on informal practitioners. Concerning vaccination, they did not find significant differences among the three groups (non-receivers, receivers in country, receivers from abroad). Regarding maternal care, the data showed higher utilization of prenatal and postnatal care among the overseas migrants but no distinctive difference between within-country migrant and nonmigrant households. This suggests that the households preferred better quality services if they had enough resources, as in the case of migrant households due to remittances.	Pakistan
Pellet and Jusot (2018)[9]	Remittances increased health-care expenditures and reduced the likelihood of abandoning or postponing care. Outpatient ambulatory expenditure was more likely affected by remittances.	Tajikistan

TABLE 18.2 *(continued)*

Author	Effect	Country
Negative effect	None	
Mixed effects		
Ponce, Olivié, and Onofa (2018)[10]	There was no effect of remittances on long-term child health variables, but remittances did have a positive effect on health expenditures, deworming, and vaccinations and medical expenditure when illness occurred.	Ecuador
Murrugarra (2002)[11]	Remittances did not seem to increase demand for health care, but they did provide a safety net in the case of adverse shocks.	Armenia

Sources: [1] Catalina Amuedo-Dorantes, Tania Sainz, and Susan Pozo, "Remittances and Healthcare Expenditure Patterns of Populations in Origin Communities: Evidence from Mexico" (Buenos Aires: Inter-American Development Bank, 2007).
[2] Reanne Frank et al., "The Relationship Between Remittances and Health Care Provision in Mexico," *American Journal of Public Health* 99, no. 7 (July 1, 2009): 1227–31, https://doi.org/10.2105/AJPH.2008.144980.
[3] Alassane Drabo and Christian Ebeke, "Remittances, Public Health Spending and Foreign Aid in the Access to Health Care Services in Developing Countries," Etudes et Documents Du CERDI (1 Centre d'Etudes et de Recherches sur le Développement International, 2011).
[4] John D. Piette et al., "Report on Honduras: Ripples in the Pond—The Financial Crisis and Remittances to Chronically ILL Patients in Honduras," *International Journal of Health Services* 42, no. 2 (April 1, 2012): 197–212, https://doi.org/10.2190/HS.42.2.c.
[5] Daniel F. López-Cevallos and Chunhuei Chi, "Migration, Remittances, and Health Care Utilization in Ecuador," *Revista Panamericana de Salud Pública* 31 (January 2012): 9–16, https://doi.org/10.1590/S1020-49892012000100002.
[6] Jennifer J. Salinas, "Tapping Healthcare Resource by Older Mexicans with Diabetes: How Migration to the United States Facilitates Access," *Journal of Cross-Cultural Gerontology* 23, no. 3 (September 1, 2008): 301–12, https://doi.org/10.1007/s10823-008-9076-4.
[7] Cuong Viet Nguyen and Hoa Quynh Nguyen, "Do Internal and International Remittances Matter to Health, Education and Labor of Children and Adolescents? The Case of Vietnam," *Children and Youth Services Review* 58 (November 1, 2015): 28–34, https://doi.org/10.1016/j.childyouth.2015.09.002.
[8] Shujaat Farooq and Nasir Iqbal, "Migration and Health Outcomes: The Case of a High Migration District in South Punjab" (Islamabad: Pakistan Institute of Development Economics, 2015).
[9] Sandra Pellet and Florence Jusot, "Barriers to Health Care: The Relief Effect of Remittances in Tajikistan," 2018, 30.
[10] Juan Ponce, Iliana Olivié, and Mercedes Onofa, "The Role of International Remittances in Health Outcomes in Ecuador: Prevention and Response to Shocks," *International Migration Review* (July 19, 2018), http://journals.sagepub.com/doi/10.1111/j.1747-7379.2011.00864.x.
[11] Edmundo Murrugarra, "Public Transfers and Migrants' Remittances: Evidence from the Recent Armenian Experience," vol. 2, World Bank Economists' Forum working paper, 2002.

a positive effect on health expenditures, deworming, and vaccinations, as well as on medical expenditure when illness occurred. In Armenia, Murrugarra (2002)[29] found that remittances did not seem to increase demand for health care, but they provided a safety net in the case of adverse shocks.

Most other studies found positive effects of remittances on health-care access (Drabo and Ebeke 2011[30]; Piette et al. 2012[31]; Nguyen and Nguyen 2015[32]; Farooq and Iqbal 2015[33]), expenditure (Amuedo-Dorantes et al. 2007[34]; Frank et al. 2009[35]), and utilization (López-Cevallos and Chi 2012[36]; Salinas 2008[37]; Farooq and Iqbal 2015).[38] Again, many of these studies were conducted in the Mexican or other Latin American country contexts but did cover other geographical areas.

4.0 Concluding Remarks

While this chapter reviewed the literature on the effects of remittances on health-care outcomes and access, it is clear that there is still more work to be done in different contexts and under different conditions. Most studies were cross-sectional and did not follow households or individuals over time. More time-varying studies would help to understand the difference between short-, medium-, and long-term effects. Additionally, studies were not always able to disentangle the effects of migration (the absence of a person or the transfer of norms and values) with the effects of the financial remittances. While some studies did cover a large swath of low- and middle-income countries, the majority of country case studies are still dominated by the Mexican and more general Latin American context. Much could be gained by understanding the relationship between remittances and health in more varied contexts around the world.

While some of the findings are mixed in different contexts, the overall picture shows that remittances are important for improving health outcomes, particularly related to children as well as health-care access. From a health policy perspective, that means that encouraging governments to make it cheaper, easier, and safer to send remittances can go a long way in increasing health outcomes and access. Additionally, making sure that there are more "safe, orderly, and regular" ways to migrate as discussed in both the Sustainable Development Goals and the Global Compact on Migration could help to increase remittances in a meaningful way, among all of the other positive benefits of migration on health.

CHAPTER NINETEEN

Technology and Migrants' Health

Access, Opportunity, and Ethical Challenges

Ebiowei Samuel F. Orubu, Carly Ching, Ahsan M. Fuzail, and Muhammad H. Zaman

1.0 The Importance of Technology for Migrants' Health

Technology, defined as "a capability given by the practical application of knowledge,"[1] is now ubiquitous in the twenty-first century and influences how we live, learn, interact, travel, and work. Increasingly, its role in managing and accessing health care has also grown. Technology in all forms—applications, point-of-care diagnostics, equipment—is in use today globally.

Migration—the movement of people within or away from their home countries because of conflict or economic reasons—is a global phenomenon. With an ever-increasing number of people being displaced forcibly from home due to conflict or climate change and remaining vulnerable, we focus our attention on this group of migrants, broadly defined as those who are forcibly displaced and living as refugees outside their home countries, asylum seekers, or those who are legally classified as stateless. The "temporariness" of forced displacement exposes migrants to many socio-economic determinants that predispose them to negative health outcomes.

Access to technology—defined here as the ability and capacity to use technology—presents an opportunity to improve the quality of and access to health care itself for migrants and host populations alike. The United Nations, as an example, aims to harness this opportunity to leverage attainment of the Sustainable Development Goals (SDGs)—specifically through

SDG-9c, which aims to "significantly increase access to information and communications technology and strive to provide universal and affordable access to the Internet in least developed countries by 2020."[2] Collectively, Least Developed Countries (LDCs) host one-third (33%, 6.7 million) of the global refugee population.[3] The hosting of such numbers places an additional burden on these countries and their health systems.

Equitable access to technology, while important for all — as technology facilitates progress and creates agency — remains a challenge. In 2019, according to the SDG 2020 Report, only 19 percent of the population in LDCs used the internet, compared to 87 percent in high-income countries, despite a mobile-broadband coverage of about 79 percent, with key barriers being cost and poor digital skills.[4]

In this chapter, we highlight some uses of technology, examine recent examples and initiatives, and address migrant health challenges both in low-resource countries/refugee settlements and in high-resource countries. We also discuss gaps and ethical considerations and provide some recommendations on how to address these gaps.

2.0 Developments in Technology Addressing Migrants' Health: An Overview

To highlight the ongoing efforts to implement solutions to health-care access and issues using technology, we provide a survey of areas in which technology is being used in humanitarian contexts. These technologies are sponsored by host governments, United Nations agencies, nongovernmental agencies, technology companies (both well-established and start-ups), and academic institutions. Some of these technologies are *generic* (widely available), while others are *customized* (specifically designed for humanitarian contexts).

In the following sections, we provide an overview of some selected applications of digital technology in the health sector addressing the need of migrants. These applications include communication, health records, mental health services, clean water, and diagnostics.

2.1 Communication and Access to Care

Language and communication barriers can exist for migrants.[5] While interpreters have been considered the gold standard, there are many limitations, including cost, trust, time, and availability. Thus, digital translation and communication tools are being incorporated and developed to address this barrier. The incorporation of a digital communication assistance tool (DCAT) prior to consultation and mobile health facilities with live translation services, both piloted in Germany, are two examples of the use of technology to provide better care to refugees in places where they do not speak the native language.[6] Other examples include Tarjimly, a mobile application that connects migrants with volunteer translators,[7] and HeRAMS (Health Resources Availability Mapping System), which is an electronic tool sponsored by the World Health Organization (WHO) and used for assessing availability of medical resources for emergency responses in Syria, Sudan, Yemen, Bangladesh, Lebanon, and sixteen other locations. This tool relies on individual contributors on the ground to provide an accurate and cohesive description of a project site's resource availability.[8]

2.2 Electronic Health Records

The limited availability of migrant's health records is another barrier to continuity of care. To address this issue, electronic health record (EHR) systems have been adopted. One example is the United Nations Relief and Works Agency for Palestine Refugees in the Near East (UNRWA) e-Health system for Palestinian refugees in UNRWA operations; deployed in 2010, it is a web-based application that supports the provision of its field-based primary health-care services. In addition to maintaining patient records, the e-Health system has a built-in appointment system, medicine lists and analysis tools, auto-populated forms for prescriptions based on clinical guidelines, and more.[9]

2.3 Clean Water

Access to safe, clean water is essential to avoid outbreaks of infectious diseases. The United Nations High Commissioner for Refugees (UNHCR) is using gateway technology to monitor water truck deliveries in Uganda and other countries using a series of networked ultrasonic water-level sensors. This helps ensure the supply of clean water.[10] In Cox's Bazar refugee settlements in Bangladesh, the UNHCR has implemented solar-powered safe water systems that have already provided clean water to forty thousand refugees. In this, the use of green technologies is highlighted.[11]

2.4 Mental Health

Premigration trauma and post-migration stress increase the burden and risk of mental health disorders in displaced populations.[12] Numerous electronic or mobile mental health technologies have been developed to address this health issue.

One such example is Step-by-Step (SbS), an e–mental health application developed by the WHO.[13] SbS assists in training users in behavioral activation and psychoeducation. Guided by an illustrated story of an individual suffering from depression, users obtain the necessary therapeutic information over five sessions. Following that, the users go through an interactive component to practice the skills they have learned, such as activity scheduling, stress management, positive self-talk, and/or relapse prevention. The SbS was piloted in Lebanon and further tested with Syrian refugees in Germany, Sweden, and Egypt.[14]

Two other examples are the University of Zurich/University Hospital of Zurich's Multi-Adaptive Psychological Screening Software (MAPSS-2015)[15] and the Open Data Toolkit (ODK) by Palestine Children's Relief,[16] both of which provide options for self-reporting (former) or collection and assessment (latter) of mental health symptoms via mobile applications.

One further example is the HADStress screening tool combined with telepsychiatry, which allows for post-traumatic stress disorder (PTSD) screening based on four symptoms: headaches, appetite changes, sleep changes, and dizziness.[17]

2.5 Diagnostics and Devices

Technological advances in low-cost diagnostics can improve health outcomes. An Artificial Intelligence (AI) diagnostic application, Tibot, was implemented in refugee camps in Bangladesh. With the application, users upload skin conditions and answer questions. The application then uses AI to go through a database of images and sends back matches that health providers can use. Using the application, health providers can see 25 percent more patients a day.[18]

3.0 Key Gaps: Opportunities and Challenges

While the use of technology in improving migrant health has shown encouraging outcomes, gaps remain. Though there has been an increase in the development of digital and information communication technology, there has been less focus on point-of-care (POC) innovation. New advancements in manufacturing, 3D printing, imaging, and paper-based rapid diagnostic tests (RTDs) provide many opportunities for innovation for customized solutions beyond the application of routine POC and RDTs implementation for refugee populations.[19] However, these types of innovations require increased awareness, investment, and multi-sectoral approaches.[20]

Concerning POC innovation, progress suffers due to the prevailing trend of improving the performance of devices—particularly medical devices—as compared to improving the cost of development or implementation. Global health communities and international organizations should redirect focus to increasing the influence of disruptive innovation in the refugee health space.

Similarly, with digital and information communication technology, a gap remains in widespread implementation, scalability, and uptake, with issues such as internet connectivity, user training and support, and the involvement of multiple agencies serving as barriers. Another recurring barrier for uptake of these technologies is lack of trust.[21] While numerous digital and information technologies are being conceptualized or developed, far less get widespread implementation. Greater coordination and communication through each phase of innovation is needed to avoid duplication of applications and efforts and ensure feasibility. Additionally, the quality, accuracy, and timeliness of the information provided by digital technology remain concerns.[22]

Further user-side and situational barriers to the deployment of technology remain for the use of technology as a means of providing agency to refugees and the forcibly displaced. Issues that need to be considered include digital literacy, affordability, power, the need for identification, network coverage, and technical support.[23]

4.0 Ethical Challenges and Considerations

Despite the ability of technology to leverage or promote health outcomes, ethical considerations built on an operating principle of "do no harm" are necessary.[24]

Bangladesh currently hosts over a million Rohingyas at the world's largest refugee camps in Cox's Bazar District, which borders Myanmar.[25] In September 2019, Bangladesh shut off access to internet and telephone services in Cox's Bazar, affecting both the refugee camps—the Rohingya are not allowed to own SIM cards—and host Bangladeshi communities on grounds of security.[26] Bangladesh had in the past restricted access to social media platforms and call services across the country for the same reason.[27]

The ethical implications of this mobile telephone and internet ban are complex. Bangladesh requires a national registration number, or a passport by non-locals, for obtaining a phone number. This, coupled with the government's concern about rising crime, are the basis for restricting access in the camps. However, this has led to concerns about access to healthcare services and information concerning Covid-19, creating a dilemma between policy, security, and access to health services by displaced persons in Bangladesh.[28] This restriction was lifted in August 2020, following international pressure.[29]

This restriction contrasts somewhat with the situation in Uganda, which hosts Africa's largest refugee population of about 1.3 million people. In 2019, the government extended access to mobile telephony in allowing the use of several forms of identification, outside of the usual national ID cards, to enable refugees in its settlement camps to obtain SIM cards.[30]

Harm can also come in the form of privacy concerns with big data.[31] Technology should not be deployed to surveil forcibly displaced populations or to promote access to services based on their vulnerability (conditional consenting).

For forcibly displaced people, there is a lack of clarity and information regarding data privacy and how the data is or will be used, and this may compromise the development and implementation of digital technology in response to the global refugee crisis. Often, the willful and consensual submission of biometric or personal data by refugees is later used for surveillance, detention, and deportation. This was primarily the case with data submitted as part of the application process for the Deferred Action for Childhood Arrivals (DACA) in the United States and the deportation of migrants from France in 2006 as part of a host government data-collection scheme.[32] Ethical considerations in the use of data have led to the Signal Code, a set of five considerations for ensuring the fundamental human rights of the forcibly displaced in the development and deployment of technology.[33]

5.0 Recommendations

Addressing gaps in access to digital technology in migrants would require a collaborative approach between governments, donors, and service providers. Funding, increased network coverage among migrants (and their host communities), including incentives for doing so, and the institution of protocols/conventions to monitor ethical issues would be necessary. Some of these solutions are discussed in Devika Nadkarni et al. (2017).[34] Generally, solutions encompassing both the host communities and their guests are more likely to be sustainable.[35]

CHAPTER TWENTY

Intersectionality

From Migrant Health Care to Migrant Health Equity

Denise L. Spitzer

1.0 Migrant Health

The World Health Organization's 2008 World Health Assembly outlined an agenda for migrant health that included, among other issues,
the promotion of health policies attentive to migrant populations, more
extensive training of medical professionals to enhance culturally safe and
gender-sensitive care, bilateral and multilateral agreements to ensure access
to health-care services throughout their journeys, and the implementation
of best practices to support and improve their well-being.[1] Subsequently,
the First Global Consultation on Migrant Health in 2010 promoted intersectoral collaboration and work on legal mechanisms to facilitate the
expansion of migrant-responsive health services.[2] Seven years later, the
Second Global Consultation acknowledged that migrant health had not
uniformly advanced as hoped.[3] This chapter briefly outlines how migrants'
encounters with health-care services and systems are differently experienced. Furthermore, it argues that intersectionality can help to critically
nuance our understanding of the complexities of migrant health, which
can contribute to the development of medical-care systems and services
that are not only accessible and responsive, but that also truly engender
migrant health equity.

1.1 Defining Intersectionality

Rooted in Black, Indigenous, queer, and postcolonial feminisms, the term *intersectionality* was brought into the lexicon by Kimberlé Crenshaw in 1989 to illuminate the multiplicity of interacting categories of social differentiation that inform lived experience.[4,5] "Intersectionality is an approach which draws our attention to the ways that social locations interact to produce advantage and disadvantage for groups and for individuals. It also helps us to consider how these positions interact with, and are constituted by, social policy and social structures."[6] Intersectionality draws attention to the mutually constituted and fluid constellation of social markers, including socioeconomic, racialized, and migrant status, gender, sexuality, ethnicity, Indigeneity, ability, geography, and so on—and their attendant power relations—contextualized by historical and contemporary systems of (neo)colonialism and globalization that situate individuals and communities within the social landscape.[7,8] Importantly, intersectionality does not automatically privilege particular axes of difference (e.g., gender, class), but instead highlights the totality of these interacting categories, which is how we are presented (and respond) to the world where we experience, depending on context, varying degrees of both oppression and privilege.[9,10]

1.2 Categorizing Migrants

Leaving one's homeland to migrate to another locale involves a complex set of decisions, rationales, and strategies. Yet the messiness of these contexts and realities are subsumed under the boundaries of common juridical categories—immigrant, migrant, refugee, asylum seeker, or internally displaced person—that are further differentiated as documented or undocumented. Each of these labels is situated on a continuum marked by two major dimensions—one that turns on the degree of voluntary (economic immigrant, migrant worker, family-class migrant) and involuntary (refugee, asylum seeker, internally displaced person) departure and the other that is focused on temporality, from intended permanent resettlement (immigrant, refugee) to temporary stay (migrant[1]). In reality, these categorizations are slippery. For example, documented and migration status may fluctuate. Moreover, some immigrants may be best regarded as

---

1. Given the slipperiness of these terms, when not explicitly specified, the term *migrant* is used throughout this chapter as a shorthand to refer to the diversity of mobile foreign-born populations.

"involuntary voluntary" migrants if the decision to move, perhaps to accompany or join family, was not wholly endorsed. Additionally, intentions
about—or regulations pertaining to—the permanence of resettlement
may shift over time.[11,12]

The acquisition or imposition of these labels by state actors in concert
with agreements laid out in international conventions structures migrants'
mobility across sites of departure, transit, and destination. Importantly,
gendered and racialized divisions of labor are strongly intertwined with
these assignations. Racialized persons from the Global South are more
likely to be recruited into temporary migrant categories, while permanent
resettlement is increasingly reserved for select global knowledge workers
and immigrants from the North.[13,14] Migration status, particularly upon entry to a destination country, places the newcomer on a trajectory that will
contour their access to determinants of health, yet even within categories,
migrants are not uniformly treated. In Canada, for example, the female
partners of heterosexual couples migrating as family class immigrants are
often designated the dependent of male principal applicants. This distinction enshrines their dependency on their male companions and shapes
their access to, *inter alia*, language training—critical to health literacy and
employment.[15]

Despite international bodies declaring health care a basic human right,
migration status—informed by notions of deservingness—generally structures access to medical services.[16,17] Considerations about migrants' potential economic contributions to the host society influence the ease with
which individuals may settle, the location and duration of their stay, and
which rights they are granted.[18,19] Underpinned by racism and xenophobia, refugees and asylum seekers are often perceived as uneducated and
unskilled, while migrant workers are suspected of stealing local jobs even
when migrants are undergoing a process of de-skilling as their own education and work experience are uncredited in the host environment.

1.3 Encounters with Health-Care Services

The organization and content of health-care services are influenced by a
host of factors, ranging from the political-economic context, historical legacy, government policies, professional interests, values, and gender ideolo-
gies to the training, attitudes, and modalities offered by health professionals and the composition and expectations of the community.[20] Migrants
must navigate their way between often dissimilar systems. For example,

some newcomers may be frustrated by the need to seek a primary care practitioner for referrals to specialists.[21] Moreover, encountering disparate health systems along migratory journeys creates difficulties. Refugees may receive health care from a patchwork of nongovernmental organizations, volunteers, and, when necessary, emergency services. The absence of personal medical files complicates treatment plans and follow-up in transit and at the destination country.[22]

Although the right to health care includes universal health coverage (UHC), undocumented migrants, migrant workers, asylum seekers, and other noncitizens may not be eligible despite the long-term economic and social benefits, such as enhanced social cohesion, of an inclusive system.[23,24,25,26,27] In the United States, one of the few high-income countries without UHC,[28] migrants are less likely than native-born residents to have medical insurance and a committed provider, with women reporting the greatest barriers to care.[29] A European Union study found that some private medical institutions hesitated to treat refugees and asylum seekers because of required administrative efforts or because their fees exceeded the amount reimbursed by national health insurance schemes.[30] Even when available, migrants may not be aware of their ability to access health-care services—particularly if their status changes. Additionally, they may be concerned about required documentation or financial outlay and avoid seeking treatment.[31,32,33,34] Furthermore, health-care professionals uncertain about the eligibility of migrants to access services may be placed in the role as gatekeepers to the system; in some instances, they are required to report undocumented migrants to the authorities.[35,36,37,38]

Despite the prevalent discourse that raises concerns about the deservingness of migrants' access to medical care and the perception that they overburden local health-care resources (influenced in part by some migrants' exclusion from all but emergency services), they generally underutilize formal services.[39,40,41] As noted, structural aspects of health services may constrain migrants' use of needed care, which may contribute to greater health, social, and economic costs if infectious and chronic diseases are untreated.[42] As migrants, racialized women in particular occupy the lowest echelons of local labor markets and may be engaged in multiple low-wage positions that offer little flexibility and few supplementary benefits. Resultantly, both financial costs of visits (where levied) and treatments and taking time for medical appointments during working hours may be problematic. Transportation barriers and childcare responsibilities may further complicate making appointments, and women, in particular, may prioritize the health of family members and forgo their own care.[43,44,45] Even where migrants are entitled to health services, they may not be adapted to their needs.[46] Moreover, migrants may face challenges or prolonged waits finding preferred culturally, linguistically, and gender-matched health-care providers, which may be critical for some women seeking sexual and reproductive health services.[47,48,49]

Fear and experiences of exclusion, stigma, and racism further affect utilization of health services.[50,51,52] Health-care reforms have been propelled by neoliberalism that supports the hollowing out of government support for public services generally in the health, education, and social services sectors. These reforms have contributed to staff shortages and the enhanced rationalization of time as a commodity to be spent with patients, disproportionately affecting racialized patients who are sometimes bypassed by time-stressed staff as they are *presumed* to present demanding language and cultural challenges—interactions that can be experienced as racism by those patients.[53]

2.0 Complicating Migrant Health

2.1 Intersectionality and Migrant Health

The complexity and fluidity of migrants' status structuring their interactions with health-care systems and services requires a more nuanced understanding. Highlighting intersectionality may reframe our thinking and action to promote migrant health. Intersectionality allows us to unpack the tangled relationships among social location and social structures that underpin health disparities.[54,55] An intersectional lens allows for greater scope of inquiry, accounts for fluidity and complexity, and acknowledges the limitations to what can be uncovered and/or understood, which more accurately reflects the messiness of lived experience. Highlighting migrant status surfaces an individual's backstory, including home country and familial context, migratory journey, reception of host society, shifting gender and other social roles, mobility in socioeconomic and employment status, and changing sources and conditions of social support, which can impact access to determinants of health and health outcomes. Moreover, it illuminates the influence of policies, programs, discourses, and values that are implicated in an individual's and community's placement in the social landscape.[56]

Despite the complexity of these issues, biomedicine focuses attention on the individual and proximate causes of the current complaint, potentially erasing the patient's life trajectory and the broader social context in which they are situated.[57] Resultantly, migrant health programs and policies often target specific health conditions and outcomes rather than upstream factors that could change the shape of the system.[58] An intersectional approach attends to issues of power and the dynamic interactions among macro- and meso-level forces and institutions and the bodies of individuals in their historic and current context.[59,60] Deploying intersectionality is therefore critical to uncovering and subsequently remedying health disparities to work toward to goal of migrant health equity.

3.0 Minding the Gaps

3.1 Health Care

Efforts to address disparities in migrant health and the diversity among migrant populations are generally focused on encounters with health-care practitioners. Filler et al. (2020) found that clinicians felt both ill-equipped to provide culturally responsive care and inadequately remunerated for providing care to migrant patients.[61] For decades, cultural sensitivity and cultural competency, where service providers gain an understanding of the dominant health beliefs and practices of their client base, have been promoted as a means of offering more effective migrant health care.[62,63,64] This approach, however, has been critiqued for its tendency to rely on and reinforce cultural stereotypes and for identifying culture as a decontextualized and singular barrier that needs to be breached in order to assimilate migrant patients, who may hold disparate ideas about health, illness, and treatments, into the local biomedical system.[65,66] Patient-centered care has been forwarded as a more holistic approach wherein the health-care practitioner offers more individualized attention and interchange with the patient. Linguistic issues, time constraints, and focus on culture as the most salient social marker in patient-healer interactions, however, may remain.[67,68] Bourgois et al. (2017) suggest clinicians focus on structural vulnerability, which is "produced by one's locale in a hierarchical social order that is embedded in diverse networks of power relationships and effects";[69] to this end, they propose a focus on *structural* rather than cultural competency, which would allow health-care providers to refer patients to other nonmedical supports they may require.

Another approach to addressing migrant health disparities—the introduction of cultural brokers and community health workers who can mediate between professional and patient worldviews—has been regarded as beneficial across sectors.[70,71] As members of migrant communities who have

experienced many of the same challenges as the client population, community health workers can not only help patients navigate the system, they
can, where their work is meaningfully included, facilitate system change by
insisting on recognition of intersectionality and unequal power relations.[72]

3.2 Beyond Health Care

Improving the access to and the development and uptake of structurally
competent medical services for migrant populations is vital; however, improving their overall well-being requires us to move beyond health care.
Migration policies that limit the possibilities of settlement and family
reunification and/or that tie migrants to a particular employer, especially
in workplaces such as private households, maritime, or agricultural settings
where their movements are further constrained, contribute to precarity,
which is associated with worsening health status. Moreover, studies have
identified a gradient in health inequities between native-born and migrant
populations linked to the immigration policy, with more restrictive policies
engendering worse health outcomes.[73] Reception in the host country further
influences health and well-being such that a European study asserted that
problems with migrant integration could be regarded as a determinant of
health inequity.[74] Most migrants arrive in their destination countries in better health than the resident population; however, many lose that advantage
over time. This loss of health status is not uniform, with racialized women
reporting the most precipitous decline.[75] Overrepresented in low-wage employment and often subject to de-skilling, even well-educated professionals are vulnerable to downward mobility, which is associated with delete-
rious health effects.[76,77] Depending on migrant status (and often economic
wherewithal), family reunification may be delayed or denied, resulting in a
paucity of social support, a well-documented determinant of health, and the
intensification of worries about the well-being of family in their home country, which contributes to stress-related disorders.[78] More inclusive immigration policies and programs that facilitate migrants' integration into their host
society are essential to improve the health and well-being of migrants.[79,80]

4.0 Conclusion: Toward Migrant Health Equity

The movement of people across and within borders is a prominent feature
of our globalized world. Migrant health equity supports a more produc-

tive population and enhances social cohesion, both of which are critical to local projects of nation-building. Actualizing the calls for health care as a right for migrants, regardless of migration status, requires international cooperation to ensure access to migrant-sensitive health care and social protections in transit and in destination countries.[81] UHC is both an economically and socially sound investment.[82] To be optimally effective, health-care services, however, must be responsive to the migrant communities in all of their diversity. An inclusive workforce that incorporates community-health workers as respected (and adequately remunerated) members and that truly engages (and listens to) local communities for their input can enhance uptake of services and reduce some of the communication and other challenges health-care providers report.[83,84,85] Implementing structural competency in health education and practice is critical to patient care and to enhancing their longer-term health and well-being. Both cross-sector and cross-border collaboration is essential to this practice, creating potential for helpful synergies to emerge.[86]

Adopting these practices and policies that attend to the diversity of migrants and illuminate the dynamic interactions of forces that produce their differentiated social locations is consonant with intersectionality as patients are regarded as persons situated in the social world. Working toward the reduction of health disparities and the enhancement of health equity, however, requires a broader focus that directs action more decidedly on the upstream processes that engender inequality and that operates to break down policy, practice, and institutional silos to support intersectoral participatory, evidence-informed policy-, program-, and decision-making.[87] These efforts could well inform migration policies that would address precarity, mobility, social protections, labor, and political rights, which have salient health impacts. Thinking intersectionally calls for treating migrants as individuals and as members of both global and local communities with both singular and shared histories, identities, strengths, hopes, and disadvantages. Collaboration across multiple borders and fields is required to realize migrant health equity.

CHAPTER TWENTY-ONE

The Ethics and Justice of Recognizing Migrants' Right to Health

Wendy E. Parmet

1.0 Introduction

In the late winter and early spring of 2020, as Covid-19 spread around the globe, then President Donald Trump used his immigration authority to bar non-US nationals from China, Europe, and Iran from entering the United States.[1] Other nations responded to the pandemic similarly, denying entry on the basis of citizenship or passport status, rather than exposure to the virus.[2]

The decision to shutter borders to non-nationals during a pandemic reflects the common perception that national health policies should privilege citizens over others, including noncitizen residents. Whether the policy relates to the distribution of vaccines or the implementation of travel bans and quarantines, many assume that nations should favor their own when it comes to health.

This chapter challenges the ethics and justice of that assumption. In so doing, it does not ask whether states have the right to control their borders, nor what rights, if any, they owe to those beyond their borders. It also does not examine in detail the rights provided to noncitizens under international law, a topic more fully covered in chapter 8.[3] Rather, the focus here is on the ethics and justice of the common practice of favoring citizens over noncitizen immigrants with respect to health.

2.0 Citizenship and Solidarity

Even before Covid-19, nationalism was ascendant across much of the world, as evidenced by Trump's "America First" approach to immigration and foreign affairs and the United Kingdom's decision to exit the European Union.[4] Although Trump lost his bid for reelection and President Joe Biden promised a new approach, nationalism remains a potent force that speaks to the widely held view that nations "do not have any obligations to non-citizens, including immigrants."[5]

This view aligns with the positivist claim that rights are simply entitlements that come from states.[6] Citizens, in turn, are those to whom states choose to give rights.[7] True, the class of rights-bearing citizens has grown over time to include women, racial and religious minorities, and non–property owners, as has the list of rights granted to citizens.[8] Nevertheless, to the positivist, rights belong only to citizens.

In his influential discussion of citizenship, Michael Walzer analogizes states to membership organizations that can limit benefits to their members.[9] Just as a book club can decide not to distribute books to nonmembers, states can deny *some* rights to noncitizens. For Walzer, this limitation is closely connected to the goal of having citizens actively engage in the political life of their state.[10] Yet, precisely because only citizens have the right to make critical decisions, Walzer argues that citizenship must be open to newcomers, so that they can have a say in important decisions that affect them.[11]

Other arguments for preferencing citizens rely on the claim that the conferral of positive, social welfare rights requires a closed community with whom individuals share a sense of solidarity.[12] In effect, in the modern world, citizenship replaces family, tribe, and clan as the community of concern to whom citizens are willing to provide aid and support.[13]

The argument that citizenship is critical for solidarity presupposes exclusion; citizenship ties people together precisely because it leaves some outside its bounty.[14] This view gains support by the observation of a rough correlation between the generosity of a state's social benefits and its homogeneity.[15] Further, many states have responded to increases in migration by reducing health benefits.[16] This implicates what Peter B. West-Oram calls the "progressive dilemma,"[17] the danger that by seeking social benefits for migrants, progressives risk undermining support for social programs.[18]

Whether the progressive dilemma is inevitable, however, is questionable. Although the rise of nationalism in the wake of increases in global migration hints at ties between citizenship, solidarity, and exclusion (often covering for racism and religious bigotry), the relationships may be more complex than those who would limit health rights to citizens presuppose. First, there is little empirical evidence supporting the claim that the recognition of rights to health for migrants would bankrupt wealthy nations. To the contrary, pre-Covid-19, migrants to high-income countries were healthier than native-born citizens and in many instances contributed significantly more to national health systems than they took out.[19] Moreover, the claim that an exclusive version of citizenship is required to support rights to health overlooks the complexities of immigration law.[20] Notably, the assumption that residents can be neatly divided into three camps — citizens, documented migrants, and undocumented immigrants — ignores the nuanced and dynamic nature of those categories. Further, many citizens and noncitizens live in mixed status households. For example, in the United States, over 13 percent of children have a noncitizen parent.[21] In countries that have as many migrants and mixed-status families as the United States and many other Western countries, the assumption that a willingness to support others depends on citizenship seems facile.

The claim for the necessity of exclusion also ignores the fact that solidarity can arise from shared interests and experiences.[22] These can relate to health, as was evident in New York and many other hard-hit cities in the early days of the Covid-19 pandemic. Every evening, people thanked health-care workers as they changed shift.[23] At that moment, the immigration status of medical personnel, their patients, and those thanking the workers seemed irrelevant. Everyone was in it together.

The moment did not last. During the weeks and months that followed, partisan division in the United States shattered the unity.[24] Yet, rather than confirming that solidarity requires exclusion, its dissolution over Covid-19 highlights that the existence of solidarity and a nation's willingness to support health is contingent on a host of political and social factors other than citizenship. With divisive leadership and intense polarization, even the exclusion of noncitizens from a nation's public health agenda cannot ensure support for the health of citizens.

2.1 Should Citizenship Matter for Health?

Despite the arguments for exclusion, every country grants noncitizen residents, including those who are unauthorized, some rights and access to many services. For example, nations provide basic police and fire protection to all residents, regardless of citizenship status. Further, most countries grant all noncitizens (including those who are unauthorized) access to emergency medical care.[25] Thus, rather than asking why noncitizens should have rights to health, we might ask if there is any justification for denying rights to health while granting other rights to noncitizens.

One way to answer that question would be to consider if there is something special about health that merits its exclusion from the rights and services granted to noncitizens. It is hard to think of such a characteristic. In contrast to voting or holding political office, rights to health do not depend on the type of close connection to a nation's governance that we associate with citizenship. Nor is there any empirical evidence to support the common claim that granting noncitizens rights to health serves as a magnet for migration. Rather, migration is spurred by civil unrest or persecution in the country of origin, lack of economic opportunity, and the desire for family unification.[26] The exclusion also cannot be justified by the claim that health is simply a private matter. To the contrary, as discussed further below, health has many features of a public good in that individual health is influenced by and can affect the health of others. In this sense, health is quite similar to fire and police protection, the type of services that are generally afforded to noncitizens.

Health's moral weight further suggests that rights to health belong in the bucket of rights granted to noncitizens.[27] The Universal Declaration of Human Rights proclaims that everyone "has the right to a standard of living adequate for the health and well-being of himself and of his family, including food, clothing, housing and medical care."[28] Article 12 of the International Covenant on Economic, Social and Cultural Rights requires states to respect "the right of everyone to the enjoyment of the highest attainable standard of physical and mental health."[29] Multilateral and regional declarations, such as the American Convention on Human Rights in the Area of Economic, Social and Cultural Rights and the Bratislava Declaration on Health, Human Rights and Migration issued by the ministers of the European Union, provide further support for the recognition of some health rights for migrants.[30] Although there is ambiguity under international law as to whether rights to health apply fully to all (especially undocumented) noncitizens,[31] these global and regional agreements attest that health matters more than most other goods and services.

Many scholars agree and argue that a just society must provide at least some level of support for health. Drawing upon John Rawls's *Theory of Justice*,[32] Norman Daniels explains that "health is of special moral importance because it contributes to the range of opportunities open to us."[33] Importantly for Daniels, the moral importance of health is not limited to individual health care; it reaches the wider array of goods and services that protect health at an individual and population level.[34] Martha Nussbaum likewise includes "bodily health" among the capabilities that are critical to well-being.[35] Amartya Sen writes that "in any discussion of social equity and justice, illness and health must figure as a major concern. . . . Health equity cannot but be a central feature of the justice of social arrangements in general."[36]

These theories elucidate why a just society must provide some level of health protection to all. However, even if they fail to convince that health should be regarded as a right, they support the claim that health is central enough to justice that it should not be within the class of rights that are denied to noncitizens. Thus, once a state recognizes some type of right to health, justice demands that that right, however broad or narrow, be among those rights that are granted to noncitizen residents.

2.2 Health Owed

Principles of responsibility and reciprocity offer further support for the recognition of health rights for noncitizens.[37] This is most obvious when states directly harm the health of migrants, as when the United States separated young children from their parents and put them in cages.[38] In such cases, because the state caused the harm, it is ethically responsible for the children's care. Likewise, if a state detains migrants in conditions that expose them to a communicable disease, as has happened in the United States during the pandemic, the state would seem to have a clear obligation to reduce exposure or, if illness occurs, provide treatment.[39]

This responsibility extends far beyond these simple examples. In the last several years, scholars have recognized that immigration status is itself a negative determinant of health.[40] The myriad vulnerabilities created by immigration law, from the fear of deportation, to legal barriers to accessing health care, endanger the health of migrants and their families. Even beyond immigration law, a wide array of social factors—the so-called social determinants of health—can increase the health risks experienced by migrants and their communities.[41] Because the state can influence many of these factors—for example, by establishing or eroding labor standards—the state is significantly responsible for enhancing or reducing the health risks faced by migrants (and others).

Reciprocity offers an additional reason for respecting the health rights of migrants. In many wealthy nations, newcomers account for a large percentage of the health-care workforce. For example, in the United States, 29 percent of physicians and 17 percent of nurses are foreign-born.[42,43] Migrants, especially immigrant women of color, also make up a significant share of home health-care and nursing home workers.[44] Other wealthy nations benefit similarly from the labor of migrants. In the United Kingdom, 28 percent of the physicians are immigrants.[45] Because nations rely so heavily on migrant workers for their health, reciprocity demands that they provide care to those workers.

2.3 The Public Nature of Health

The *public* nature of health offers a final, compelling reason why health belongs within the bucket of rights afforded to noncitizens.[46] Although we often think of health as a personal good, our health is frequently dependent on the health of others. This is most apparent with communicable diseases. High rates of Covid-19 among migrants cannot be contained within immigrant communities, nor are migrants spared high rates of disease among citizens.[47] The risk of contagion, however, is not limited to infectious diseases. Lack of prenatal care for migrants impacts the health of citizens (in countries that recognize birthright citizenship). Untreated mental-health and substance-use disorders among migrants can also affect citizens, and vice versa. Further, as Covid-19 shows, preexisting disparities related to noncommunicable diseases (such as diabetes) can magnify the dangers of communicable diseases and increase the strain on health-care systems. Thus, the realization of the right to health for citizens depends significantly on its extension to noncitizen residents.

3.0 The Nondiscrimination Principle

The argument that justice requires states to grant noncitizens the same right to health that they grant to citizens does not compel states to recognize a right to health, nor does it demand that states interpret the right to health in any particular way. It only requires that states treat noncitizen residents equally to citizens with respect to health.

So narrowed, the claim avoids two criticisms often aimed at the right to health. The first relates to the capaciousness of the term *health*, which is amenable to broad and contested interpretations. Indeed, given the role of social determinants, we need to accept that a right to health may implicate a broad array of services, benefits, and structures. Thus, determining what is required by a right to health is an infamously difficult task. By limiting noncitizens' rights to health to those benefits and protections the state already recognizes, the claim for noncitizens' rights avoids the definitional problem.

Second, rights to health, like other positive rights, are often criticized as implicating policy choices that are not well-suited for judicial enforcement.[48] But by limiting the claim for noncitizens' right to health to those rights already recognized for citizens, these problems are avoided. No specific policy determinations need to be made by judges; all they must do is reject discrimination, a task that is quite familiar to them.

4.0 Closing Borders

What about shuttering borders to noncitizens during the pandemic? Because the nondiscrimination principle applies to noncitizen residents, it would not condemn either all bans on travel or those limited to nonresidents. However, responding to the pandemic with border closings that are predicated on passport status rather than exposure to the virus sends the misleading signal that noncitizens pose a greater danger than citizens.[49] This age-old identification of noncitizens with disease and risk can blind nations to the need to look within and do the hard work required to control disease within their own borders. Thus, by discriminating against others with respect to the right to health, nations endanger their own citizens.

PART IV

Approaches to Understanding the Relationship between Migration and Health

CHAPTER TWENTY-TWO

The Relevance of Culture for Migrant Health

Tilman Lanz

1.0 Introduction

This chapter discusses the role of culture and social attachments in the context of health and migration. Culture's influence on complex migration processes is significant but often underestimated. In each culture, specific norms mediate how illness is expressed, received, discussed, and addressed in the social domain. Health and illness themselves are defined through cultural norms and conventions. Culture heavily influences notions of health and illness by creating culture-specific categories and mediating appropriate articulations of health and illness. While culture's influence in health matters is significant, it is also, most often, subtle. It surfaces in a myriad of small occurrences in migrants' everyday lives, in the enactment of cultural norms. Because of the subtle and intrinsic character of these notions, difficulties and problems can emerge during migration. When people move from one cultural context to another, the presence of two or more cultural systems and their attendant norms frequently leads to misunderstandings, false readings of interpersonal signals, or generally failed communication. Migrants frequently suffer because of failed communication with health providers. This suffering can be minimized through an improved understanding of the important and specific role that culture plays here. Raising awareness for the relevance of culture frequently involves making subtle and implicit categories and conventions explicit—especially when they conflict across cultures and impede cross-cultural communication.

In what follows, a selection of contexts in which cultural issues relate to migrant health will be discussed. This chapter first gives a brief account on the various disciplines dealing with the role that culture plays in conjunction with health and migration and how they are grouped around the subfield of medical anthropology. Then it engages in three important debates on health and illness and shows the importance for understanding the cultural input in each of these debates.

2.0 Culture, Health, and Migration — Emergence of an Interdisciplinary Field

Today, the famous statement about migrants coined by Swiss writer Max Frisch in light of migration to Central Europe in the 1950s and 1960s no longer holds true. With his adage "workers were called for and people came," Frisch put the spotlight on how Europe treated migrants at that time. It was important to Central European societies to cover their labor needs, but how the people providing this labor were faring was considered quite unimportant.[1] During the 1970s and 1980s, a gradual interest in the lives of migrants emerged.[2] This meant that subsequently, the health of migrants was also considered important as a worthwhile area of study and as part of the larger field of migration studies. It was understood over the following decades that studying the lives of migrants was important to understanding them and assisting them in becoming, over time, full-fledged members of their new home societies.[3,4] Migrant communal and individual health became an integral part of these studies.

About the same time, medical anthropology emerged as a new subfield in anthropology, particularly in the anglophone world. Rooted in Rivers's early, pioneering work, medical anthropology concerned itself with the relations between culture and human conceptions of body, health, and illness.[5,6,7,8] In this context, medical anthropologists also became interested in how migration, here understood as changing cultures, influenced perceptions of health and sickness as well as the medical syncretisms emerging from such change.[9,10] Medical anthropology became, over time, the principal field through which migrant health and its cultural implications would be studied. Its specific value lies in a biocultural approach, which understands human behavior and *physis* as dialectically connected throughout the lifespan.[11] Yet, studies on culture and migrant health remain quite interdisciplinary in character, frequently borrowing from fields as diverse as linguistics,[12,13] political science,[14] anthropology,[15] or history.[16] The research object's three-pronged complexity makes for the open character of the field. Medical anthropology, with its willingness to weave interdisciplinary connections, has today emerged as a hub for the study of how culture impacts migrants' health. Over the past few decades, medical anthropology and migration studies have successfully merged to provide a viable platform for the culturally sensitive research of migrant health.

3.0 The Role of Culture in Health and Migration

3.1 Field Surveys and Reference Works

A relatively small number of researchers work in the highly specialized field of culture, health, and migration. As a consequence, literature reviews, overviews of the field, or surveys are relatively sparse. Yet, there are comprehensive surveys affording orientation. Helman's narrative text provides a thorough introduction to the field, explaining the development of scientific discourses around migration and health and with a particular eye for the relevance of culture.[17] Kumar and Diaz report directly from health practitioners' positive and negative experiences.[18] The volume uses these narratives of cross-cultural communication to provide concrete advice for those very practitioners. Sargent and Larchanché offer a comprehensive account of the field, focusing on its development over the past half century but also detailing the specific areas of research that have emerged until today.[19] Hadley provides a similar but shorter introduction to the same topic.[20] A recently published policy brief by the World Health Organization (WHO) indicates that culture has been significantly underrepresented in research on migrant health and that this needs to be remedied in future studies.[21,22] Providing an overview of the field, the text also makes suggestions on how culture can be better integrated in medical studies with migrants. The journal *Ethnicity and Health* is a specialist journal covering a wide range of topics, many of which are related to the issue of health and culture in migration. There are finally a number of glossaries that help to further orient newcomers in this subdiscipline.[23]

3.2 Global Health: Universal and Particular Aspects

The notion of global health aims to implement the universal equity principle, upon which the UN was founded, within the domains of collective and individual health. With the founding of the WHO in 1948, global efforts started to be made, especially in the field of epidemiology, to eradicate or contain the spread of a large number of infectious diseases. Over the past twenty years, efforts to establish medical standards across the globe have complemented the earlier struggle against infectious diseases. Over this period, it has also become more evident that cultural considerations had been neglected for quite some time. It was realized that issues of culture contact especially needed to be considered to a greater extent. In global health, the antagonism between universal and particular views of health and illness plays a significant role. This antagonism cannot simply be resolved by choosing sides. Rather, global health strategies need to reconcile particular local interests of patients, health professionals, and other stakeholders with universal interests of various kinds.[24] The consequences of ignoring cultural particularities and the need for intercultural communication in contexts of global health practices can be severe. In a sensitive way, Fadiman shows this in her ethnography about a Hmong migrant woman in California struggling with epilepsy.[25] The woman's own cultural beliefs and those of California's medical system are at odds in reading her illness, with the former reading it as a rare spiritual gift and the latter as a neurological disorder. She suffers immensely in the experience of the culture gap and her inability to reconcile both interpretations. Instead of a medical pluralism fusing her own cultural and Western medical beliefs, she encounters the dominance of the latter. Though this is still a problem, awareness of issues related to cultural contact is growing.

Universal demands for global health standards as well as particular understandings and interpretations of health and illness are in need of reconciliation in each given case. Such reconciliation efforts are frequently difficult because they involve the questioning of much-loved personal certainties, derived from one set of social and cultural norms.[26] But although this process takes time, it is well worth the effort.[27] As global health practitioners move forward, they will need to find ways to reconcile universal and particular aspects in their work, as also required in other domains facing global processes today.[28] Recent proposals to further develop global health practices demand much more local aspect inclusion than so far.[29]

3.3 Mental Health and Cultural Competence

The mental health of migrants relies heavily on their cultural competence (i.e., on their ability to learn and use the norms and values of their new host society).[30] It is now widely recognized that cultural competence plays a significant role in migrant well-being and especially in migrant mental health, whether collective or individual. Mental health, in turn, is a necessary requirement for successful migrant integration, which crucially rests on cultural competence.[31] However, it is a matter of debate how cultural competence is to be achieved and what it entails. Some argue that cultural competence means primarily a competence in the culture of the new home society, largely ignoring the importance of the culture of the heritage society. This has been pointed out as a severe shortcoming, since the culture of the heritage society often acts as a crucial stabilizer in times of insecurity in the new homeland.[32] Further, cultural competence models need to consider that cultures are not hermetic systems, offering ready-made value packages to their adherents; rather, they are open systems, able to adjust to changes of needs or circumstance as well as individual agency.[33]

At the same time, the cultural competence of migrants also crucially includes their ability to maintain meaningful ties with their former homeland.[34] It is important to maintain essential support from family and friend networks in the former homeland.[35] To maintain such ties, it is highly useful to speak the language, for example.[36] Thus, for migrants, it is often a difficult balancing act to make choices on which cultural norms to follow—those of the old or of the new homeland.[37] The difficulty of this is sadly a frequent source for mental problems, as it often becomes impossible to maintain equal ties with the culture in the new and the old homeland, whether due to practical issues (access) or ideological conflicts between both cultures.

It is, in this instance, particularly important to understand migration and the integration of migrants as a long-term process, fraught with uncertainties and possibilities for failure. The upheaval, often perceived as a crisis, of switching from one (set of) culture(s) to another in the context of migration usually requires years, decades, and sometimes generations to overcome.[38] This is so especially when contemporary forms of communication have made it much easier to stay in touch with a former homeland, hence delaying the process of integration in the new homeland.[39] The uncertainties of this process make migrants susceptible to mental problems, particularly when they are not able to successfully negotiate their former and present cultural affiliations. In such instances, health professionals have frequently used the lifecourse approach when aiming to assist migrants in improving their mental health. These lifecourse approaches are embedded within a robust understanding that two cultures are important for migrants—that of the present and the former homeland.[40] Successful approaches to improving the mental health of migrants take this dual view of cultural competence into consideration.

3.4 Sunset Migration: Elderly Migrant Care and Health Issues

Contemporary images of migration are dominated by pictures of hapless refugees, economic migrants, and youth seeking a better future. In recent decades, these conventional images of migrants have been complemented by those who migrate in old age to improve their living conditions. This phenomenon has aptly been labeled "sunset migration" in the past.[41] The seemingly innocent term suggests a rather care-free, affluent existence, perhaps almost paradisical bliss. But migration in old age comes with its own specific problems, especially in terms of health care. Two such issues resurface time and again.

First, elderly migrants are distrustful of the health providers in their place of migration, sometimes with reason, sometimes out of distrust toward an unknown, alien health system. Since sunset migration often happens more to less developed places in order to get more house for the buck, elderly migrants frequently move to contexts where health care is not provided at the same standards without realizing this. Only after some time living in the new home do elderly migrants realize that their health care is not the same as in their former homeland.[42] Sometimes this leads to unusual solutions, as evidenced by the case of an elderly German retiree to the Cevennes in France. She takes a high-speed train from Lyons to Frankfurt once a month to visit her German dentist because she does not trust the French health-care system. It is a six-hour train ride.

Second, deteriorating health of these migrants over time raises the issue of more substantial daily care, where, again, quality is an issue. To this are added language and cultural customs to which elderly migrants often adapt only with difficulty.[43] These issues are more pronounced when national borders are involved. The situation in the United States, for instance, with many elderly migrants moving to its sunny south, is more manageable because, in principle, the health-care system does not change. In the European Union, with its myriad of different health-care systems, a move from the Netherlands to southern France might already be more difficult to master. If, say, a German elderly couple moves to Turkey, the situation is difficult in terms of their assured care to the standards they were used to in Germany. This is, sadly, also true for Turkish citizens who have worked for decades in Western Europe and returned to Turkey upon retirement. Frequently, they are successful in reintegrating into Turkish society, but over time, their health forces them to return to Western Europe because of the quality of the health-care system.

In these instances, the culture-specific quality of the system is, apart from objective standards, a central issue. Switching between different (national) health-care cultures is, as sunset migration shows, also problematic, since they differ from each other quite significantly. Here, it is not individual or collective migrant cultures causing difficulties, but rather health-care system cultures. This is just one more reason inducing us to create systems that are more open to ethnic, cultural, gendered, and religious diversity.

CHAPTER TWENTY-THREE

The Sociology of Migration and Health

The Decline in Migrants' Health Due to Adverse Environments and Limited Options for Care

Steven J. Gold

1.0 Introduction

The number of international migrants globally reached an estimated 272 million in 2019, an increase of 51 million since 2010.[1] International migrants now comprise 3.5 percent of the world's population, up from 2.8 percent in the year 2000. Given this large and growing number, the investigation of migration and health will continue to be an enterprise of significant importance.[2] This chapter draws on the discipline of sociology — the analysis of human group life, social change, and social inequalities — to consider why persons migrating from relatively poor to more affluent locations frequently experience declining health and well-being.[3]

Historically and during the present era as well, societies that are the destinations of numerous international migrants have commonly considered some fraction of newcomers to be threatening. They often assume that migrants are of low character and lacking in positive physical and mental attributes. In many points of settlement, migrants' health, resilience, intelligence, and way of life are viewed as inferior to that of natives.[4,5] As a consequence, migrants, especially the impoverished and those with unfamiliar cultural, linguistic, and religious orientations, are seen as vectors through which diseases are transmitted.

The following quote from an historical study about migration and health describes how, during the nineteenth century, Americans attributed the prevalence of disease to migrants from Ireland:

> In 1832, a severe cholera epidemic swept across the Atlantic and devastated New York and several other cities. . . . Along the east coast, large numbers of immigrants got sick and perished. Especially hard hit were the poorest newcomers which included the Irish. In an era well before germ theory, some Americans saw a link between two unwelcome arrivals—cholera and the Irish. . . . Anti-Irish nativists were only too willing to believe that bars and political clubhouses that were frequented by the Irish were breeding grounds for cholera and that the disease was disproportionately visited upon the Irish as divine punishment for their sinful ways.[6]

As suggested by the following, the same form of reasoning attributes contemporary diseases like HIV/AIDS and Covid-19 to migrants' presence: "By referring to COVID-19 as a 'Chinese' disease, Trump appears to be blaming the disease and its transmission on people with Chinese and East Asian ancestry. When that attitude comes from the presidential bully pulpit, it easily spreads. For instance, a Kansas county commissioner claimed his county didn't need stringent public health measures because it had so few Chinese people, making it safe. Such rhetoric mistakenly suggests China and Chinese people are medically or pathologically diseased. Referring to the virus as 'Chinese' also encourages people to assume perceived race or cultural practices are health risks."[7]

In a related manner, residents of host societies worry that immigrants' bodily processes, racial characteristics, and patterns of fertility, sexuality, and reproduction threaten the survival and dominance of natives.[8] As a consequence of such denunciations, immigrants have been attacked, quarantined, and subject to deportation in misguided efforts to protect the health, well-being, and way of life of the host population.[9,10]

2.0 The Healthy Migrant Phenomenon

Despite the prevalence of assumptions about the superior health and vitality of local populations and the threats of contagion presented by immigrants, a considerable body of contemporary cross-national research has found that immigrants are in fact healthier than the local citizenry of societies where they have settled. This finding is unanticipated, since immigrants tend to come from locations characterized by higher rates of poverty and lower standards of living than in points of settlement.[11] Because of the counterintuitive nature of this discourse, the *healthy migrant phenomenon* has become one of the most well-studied and conceptually significant topics of research in the study of migration and health.

Migrants' well-being is found to be superior to that of natives over a wide range of health measures. This has been observed in the United States, Canada, Australia, and several countries in Western Europe.[12] Immigrants have better infant, child, and adult health outcomes than the native-born in general, as well as native-born members of their own ethno-racial group in host societies.[13] Immigrants are less likely to die from cardiovascular disease and have a lower incidence of all cancers, fewer chronic health conditions, lower infant mortality rates, lower rates of obesity, fewer functional disabilities, and fewer learning disabilities.[14] Immigrants also have lower rates of depression and alcohol abuse than the native-born.[15] What is more, migrants' health advantages over natives are most visible among demographic categories typified by less education and lower earnings.[16] In addition to maintaining better health than the native-born, immigrants also have a longer life expectancy. "This pattern does not suggest that immigrants are free from diseases" and other health problems, "but rather [that] they show a general health advantage when compared to the native-born."[17] It should be noted that voluntary labor migrants are the border-crossing population that reveals the greatest health advantages. In contrast, refugees, forced migrants, and undocumented immigrants often experience higher levels of premigration and post-migration stress and trauma. Moreover, because refugees and forced migrants are often escaping wars and may spend extended periods in crowded and poorly organized refugee camps before being resettled, their levels of physical and mental health are often negatively impacted.[18]

2.1 Accounting for Migrants' Better Health

Scholars of migration and health point to a variety of causes to account for healthy migrants. First, as a self-selected group, migrants tend to be healthier than the average member of their country of origin. Individuals lacking good health, energy, and ambition are unlikely to migrate. And if the less healthy do migrate, they are more likely to return to the country of origin than are those experiencing good health.[19] Accordingly, the remigration of those who are sicker or less fit enhances levels of health among the migrant population as compared to nonmigrants.

A considerable body of research reveals that migrants more often practice habits and lifestyles associated with good health—such as consuming a nutritious and low-fat diet and engaging in regular exercise.[20,21,22] They also refrain from injurious behaviors like smoking, substance abuse and other detrimental habits that are prevalent among the native-born.

It is true that migrants sometimes benefit from improvements in points of destination, such as educational and occupational mobility, a cleaner and safer environment, better health-care services, and improved housing.[23] Nevertheless, such benefits are disproportionately accrued by college-educated and highly skilled migrants, rather than the less skilled and less educated.[24]

2.2 Migrants' Long-Term Loss of Health

While migrants are initially healthier than local residents, the healthy migrant phenomenon tends to decline over time. Migrants who have lived in the host society over an extended period, as well as their descendants, tend to have poorer health than the recently arrived. Reductions in migrants' health are generally attributed to the social, economic, residential, and occupational locations and conditions in which migrants find themselves.[25]

Despite their entry into societies that are more affluent and technologically advanced than their countries of origin, unskilled migrants generally remain in environments and occupations that, while economically essential, are difficult, debilitating, and poorly compensated. "Migrants tend to be overrepresented in low-qualified, temporary, and high-risk jobs with resulting higher rates of occupational injuries and sickness presenteeism (the tendency to carry on working despite being ill). Occupational health is a particular challenge for labor migrants working in irregular employment.[26]

Accordingly, migrants' decline in health is the consequence of poverty, environmental pollution, employment in dangerous and unsanitary jobs, precarious living conditions, and being subjected to social stressors like discrimination and social isolation.[27,28] In the midst of the Covid-19 pandemic—whose impacts tend to be most serious and widespread among those living in crowded and impoverished conditions—the destructive effects of such circumstances on health and well-being have been obvious.[29]

3.0 Critiques of the Healthy Migrant Phenomenon

The ability of impoverished migrants to maintain good health despite their being subjected to difficult circumstances shows their resilience. However,

immigrant advocates generally discourage excessive emphasis on the healthy
migrant phenomenon because its celebration is likely to foster indiffer-
ence to migrants' health problems and may absolve the host society for
its reluctance to provide care.[30] The authors of a major study on migration
and health contend that while the desire for improved health may drive
migration, conditions in the host society often preclude immigrants from
achieving that goal.[31]

4.0 The Pursuit of Low-Cost Labor and
the Rationing of Health Services for Migrants

Beyond environmental and occupational causes, an additional source of
migrants' difficulty is the trouble they confront when obtaining health
care. Research and planning that focus on the improvement of migrants'
health conclude that programs need to be affordable and compatible with
the needs, expectations, ways of life, and language competence of the populations being served.[32,33,34] Moreover, while a number of international
organizations like the United Nations (UN) and the World Health Organization (WHO) espouse the belief that "the highest attainable standard
of health [is a] fundamental right of every human being,"[35] few nations are
willing to allocate the resources required to meet this high-minded goal.

Because of cost-cutting policies as well as practical contingencies that
limit migrants' health access, major migrant destinations tend to provide
deficient health services. "Since the 1990s, many European countries have
witnessed political backlash over immigration, with a particularly hostile
reception for asylum seekers and a rise in anti-Muslim rhetoric."[36] Such
countries seek to discourage migrants' presence by limiting or altogether
denying access to health care.[37] Indicative of this trend, several countries
have recently cut funding for migrants' medical services even as they have
upped allocations for dependent natives.[38]

In addition to documenting the impact of policies that have the effect
of reducing migrants' health, the health and migration literature offers
numerous examples of practical and logistical problems that make it hard
for migrants to obtain health care. As the authors of an article on migrants and health published in the *Annual Review of Anthropology* note,
in order to address their health needs, migrants must learn how the host
society health system works, both in terms of demonstrating eligibility and
obtaining care.[39] Because immigrants are often unfamiliar with the orga-

nization of host society health-care systems, lack native language fluency, and may be employed in unconventional work routines, communication between them and medical personnel is often fraught with confusion. Faced with such difficulties, health-care providers develop biases against immigrant clients. In reaction, immigrants learn to avoid accessing health care from public sources.[40,41,42,43]

Acquiring health care is especially difficult for undocumented immigrants, who account for a sizable fraction of the global migrant population. As of 2017, there were 10.7 million undocumented migrants in the United States and 4.8 million undocumented migrants in Europe.[44] In many locations, neither employer nor host society offers more than emergency care. Moreover, undocumented migrants are known to avoid interaction with health-care providers out of fear that such exchanges will reveal their lack of legal residency and ultimately result in their being punished or deported.[45] Finally, because of their marginal status, undocumented immigrants are understudied, leading to a dearth of knowledge about their health needs and the strategies that they rely on to obtain health care when access to it is limited.

The fact that immigrants' health status declines as a consequence of their migration to and work within affluent host societies reveals a significant impediment to fulfilling the long-standing immigrant bargain between immigrants and the nation of settlement, whereby parents' sacrifices are redeemed through their children's advancement.[46] Instead, the benefits of migrants' efforts accrue to employers, consumers, and other well-situated members of the host society who profit from their low-cost labor.

4.0 Conclusion

This chapter directs attention to the irony of the healthy migrant phenomenon as it shapes human experience. Migrants arrive in the host society with a level of health exceeding that of locals. They perform necessary but difficult, dangerous, often irregular, and poorly paid jobs while living in squalid conditions. Despite being subjected to working and living circumstances that are detrimental to their health, they find that their access to health services is limited by restrictive funding and delivery systems that are unfamiliar and difficult to utilize. While these challenges affect all migrants, accessing health services is especially demanding for undocumented workers, who account for a sizable fraction of employees in many national settings.

Even more striking is the fact that, due to their generally good health, immigrants' health care costs only a fraction of the amount required per capita for meeting the needs of the native-born.[47]

While the healthy migrant phenomenon may bring to mind a reassuring appearance of resilience, the consequences of unwholesome conditions and the less-than-adequate health care extended to migrants in many nations are a human tragedy. The significant disadvantages that migrants face indicate that nations and employers have rejected NGO's assertions about making available and high-quality health a human right.

The denial of health services leads to the growth of unmet physical and mental health issues and feelings of alienation among migrant populations on a global level. Such problems will only worsen over time, demanding ever more costly and time-consuming treatment. Limiting migrant workers' basic health care will leave them unable to perform the socially and economically significant tasks they were recruited to accomplish. Finally, recent governmental efforts to establish new means of payment for the health care of low-income persons, such as the US Affordable Care Act, are directed toward citizens and consequently are incapable of providing for the needs of undocumented immigrants.[48] While the provision of health care for undocumented immigrants is somewhat more flexible in the United Kingdom and Germany, accessing medical services is described as restrictive and hard to understand for both physicians and health consumers in the European Community.[49] Given the importance of the sectors that undocumented workers serve in the economy (e.g., service and agriculture), providing affordable health coverage for undocumented workers is the right thing to do and makes good sense.[50]

CHAPTER TWENTY-FOUR

Economics in Migrant Health

Migrant-Sensitive Service Improvement as a Driver for Cost Savings in Health Care?

Ursula Trummer, Lika Nusbaum, and Sonja Novak-Zezula

1.0 Introduction

Data from the Organisation for Economic Co-operation and Development (OECD) show that for high-income countries, migration is good for the economy, as it positively contributes to the labor market, the public purse, and economic growth.[1] The health-care labor market is among those heavily relying on a migrant workforce. Nowadays, migrants are at the forefront of the essential workers supporting the economy of hosting societies heavily affected by the Covid-19 pandemic.[2] From an ethical perspective, the human right to health is enshrined in various global and European documents, and equity in health service provision is a set goal in global and European normative frameworks.[3] This entails paying attention also to the needs of disadvantaged and marginalized populations like asylum seekers and undocumented migrants who find themselves in a difficult position of entering labor markets for various reasons.[4]

Researchers in the field of health and migration, collaborating in the framework of the European Public Health Association / Section Migrant and Ethnic Minority Health have started to integrate economic arguments in their work and developed a research agenda accordingly in 2020 after holding workshops on the issue at the annual EUPHA conferences in 2016 (Vienna) and 2019 (Marseille).[5] This starts from the increasing evidence on the cost-saving potential of decent access to quality health-care services for migrant populations, including vulnerable migrants. Socio-logical and service utilization studies that look at economic costs with different methods come to similar results, namely that besides the ethical obligation to safeguard the human right to health, it is also economically reasonable to aim at universal access to health care.[6,7,8] It also can be argued that healthy migrants do make better contributions to the economy, and even through a pure economic lens, early access to health care for migrants should be a rational choice for societies and policy development.

1.1 Good Communication as a Central Quality Factor in Health Care

Existing knowledge on key factors in effective health care highlights the importance of good communication between caregivers and patients. Experts in communication strategies accentuate the importance of provider-patient interaction.[9] They acknowledge the challenges faced by clinicians in their efforts to find the right way and right words to get the health message across in a way that is simple, clear, and acceptable to patients and that is tailored to meet their personal needs and health concerns.[10] Good oral communication, complemented by easy-to-understand written material when appropriate, is key to ensuring that patients succeed in expressing their concerns to clinicians who are able to understand the complaints and plan appropriate diagnostic, treatment, and instructional steps. It is also essential to convey health information back to the patient verifying they understand their health and how to deal with it in order to achieve better health outcomes.[11] Good communication considerably influences care processes and has shown to speed up recovery after surgery.[12]

Communication gets more difficult and demanding when different languages come into play. Language barriers lead to more unnecessary diagnostic procedures and specialty referrals.[13] They also cause medical mistakes, irreversible damage to migrant health, and even death.[14,15] A Swedish study showed that immigrant women, compared to women of Swedish origin, had several cases of infant deaths during labor or in the first month of their lives. In these cases, infant deaths were attributed to the flawed communication between mother and clinicians and could have been avoided.[16] A study conducted in six US hospitals demonstrated that patients with low proficiency in English suffered from physical harms and death almost twice as much as the group of English-speaking patients.[17] Findings from these and other studies explicitly demonstrate how the language people speak may negatively affect their experiences within the health-care system and determine their family health and well-being.

1.2 Professional Interpreting Services Are Crucial for Migrant-Sensitive Health-Care Provision

Health-care structures sensitive to migrant health therefore should include professional interpreting services (PIS). PIS have been described as a distinctive factor for migrant health, especially for those migrant groups that are socially disadvantaged (having low command of local language, low education level, and scarce economic resources). The use of PIS to communicate in medical settings is now increasingly recognized as essential for good care for patients who do not speak or understand a local language well. It ensures greater satisfaction of the migrant patients[18,19] and providers,[20] responding to their needs and expectations. Further, the use of PIS facilitates access to care, reduces medical errors and delays in clinical processes, and improves health-care outcomes among migrants.[21,22] For example, the provision of PIS in primary care settings has been shown to improve understanding of the clinical picture by physicians and to increase the trust in medical diagnosis by migrants in the Netherlands.[23] Patient trust in their diagnosis is crucial for their involvement in medical consultations, treatments, and continuing care. Using PIS in the palliative setting improves understanding by patients of their health and treatment goals and supports better symptom management.[24]

1.3 Professional Interpreting Services Are Not Established as Routine Services

The evidence described above suggests an integration of PIS to facilitate proper communication as a decisive factor of good quality health care. Still, and despite this evidence, such services do not seem to be part of the established public health structures in a majority of high-income public health systems. An analysis of eight medical codes of conduct (global: World Medical Association; national: Australia, Canada, Germany, New Zealand, Switzerland, United Kingdom, United States) shows that only one, the Australian, explicitly addresses the responsibility of doctors to ensure good communication with migrant patients by using PIS.[25] It defines the doctor's duty as "familiarising yourself with, and using whenever necessary, qualified language interpreters or cultural interpreters to help you to meet patients' communication needs" and informs about the availability of government-funded interpreter services.[26] In health-care organizations, language barriers were identified as the most prominent area of concern in providing care for migrant patients in a needs assessment among twelve European hospitals, with PIS rarely implemented.[27] A look at the availability of PIS in the Migrant Integration Policy Index (MIPEX) Health reveals twenty out of thirty-four countries where PIS is, in principle, available. Interpreting methods include in-person, telephone, video interpretation, credentialed volunteers, and employment of "cultural mediators" and competent bilingual or multilingual staff. However, this does not give information about the level of implementation of such services in practice.[28]

In everyday professional work, results from interviews and focus groups in ten EU countries show language barriers as one of the main challenges for health-care personnel, with translation often provided by unqualified individuals. As a consequence, care is provided on the basis of poor understanding.[29] A survey in four outpatients departments in Austria reports that the majority of staff experienced high levels of strain through lack of easy-to-access interpreting services and uncertainties concerning responsibilities and procedures for proper communication with migrant patients.[30]

A prominent argument for not establishing PIS is their economic recurring costs.[31,32] The Netherlands in 2012 stopped already-established national financing of interpreting in the public health system. This is in line with the 2010 Coalition Agreement of the minority government of Christian Democrats and Liberals, with the support of the anti-immigrant Party for Freedom, which includes a paragraph saying that participation in society requires sufficient educational and language qualifications and that society is entitled to expect this of newcomers. Up to this point of time, the Netherlands had covered the cost of interpreting by the state and therefore had been the forerunner in terms of interpreter provision in Europe in the early twenty-first century. Saving €19 million was the goal of the Dutch Ministry of Health when deciding to abolish all subsidies for translation and interpreting from January 2012 onward.[33]

However, such arguments do not take into account the potential costs of not providing interpreting services or the potential cost savings associated with their provision. What evidence is available on these points?

2.0 A Rapid Review on Available Evidence on Cost Savings or Economic Costs of Not Providing Interpreting Service

To provide an answer to this question, a rapid review on original research reports published in English between January 2000 and October 2020 was conducted. A total of 212 articles were identified by search in EBSCOhost and PubMed databases, using keywords *interpreter/ing*, *health care*, *costs*, *savings*, *economic*, and *financial*. After analysis of the abstract, 188 articles that did not examine the economic effects of PIS on the health-care system were excluded from the review. Twenty publications (fifteen US studies; two Switzerland studies; one each in Canada, Australia, and Germany) were included in the final analysis. Seven of these studies reported only direct costs of PIS. Among the remaining thirteen, several studies examined the effect of PIS through the assessment of length of stay (LOS) in the medical facility, return visits, and admissions and readmissions to the hospital. These studies showed mixed results.

Regarding hospital LOS, two studies did not find any impact, one showed an increase in LOS, and two others demonstrated shorter LOS in hospitals that provided PIS at admission. Three additional studies showed longer visits in the emergency department (ED) and in the primary care for patients with PIS. Only one study evaluated the effects of PIS on chances for admission to the hospital from pediatric EDs. The group with the highest odds for admission was the group for whom the PIS was unavailable during their visit. Researchers assumed that not all admissions were clinically justified for this patient group and that the physicians were simply trying to ensure that families would not leave the ED with misunderstandings about the condition of and recommended treatment for their child.[34]

There are also several studies providing information about the effect of PIS on return visits to the ED and primary care clinics. Only one study (US) demonstrated a reduction in visits to the ED along with the increase in clinic visits during the subsequent thirty days after the interpreted encounter. Fewer ED visits could indicate a decrease in urgent medical conditions, reflecting better health mediated by improved patient-provider communication enhanced by PIS.[35] A similar increase in clinic visits, following the provision of PIS in four primary care centers (United States), was suggested to reflect an improvement in access and delivery of primary health care and reduction in disparities in health.[36]

Regarding hospital readmissions (all US studies), two studies found no effect of PIS on readmissions; two others reported positive effects of PIS in preventing readmissions. One large study demonstrated a statistically significant decrease, from 17.8 percent to 13.4 percent, in the thirty-day readmission rate for a patient who utilized telephone PIS, compared to the period before this intervention was delivered. This research estimated cost savings of $161,404 per month, stemming from 119 avoided readmissions during the eight-month intervention period.[37]

Six studies (five in the United States; one in Switzerland) discussed additional factors behind the potential financial benefit of PIS. Most of the studies that performed estimates of the financial impact of PIS on the utilization of diagnostic tests and treatment showed a lack of effect or higher uses and costs for patients with interpreters. A retrospective analysis of five hundred cases treated in the ED of a US teaching hospital demonstrated that PIS was linked to a modest increase in charges and in the number of tests, intravenous fluids, and medications given, compared to patients with language barriers without the interpreter. Yet, these numbers have been lower compared to English-speaking patients, who also had the longest stay in the ED and highest total charges for the thirty-day follow-up period.[38] The findings of higher costs attributed to increased use of health-care services and materials were also observed in asylum seekers who received PIS in a health clinic in Switzerland, compared to asylum seekers without language barriers.[39] Only one study conducted in the ED demonstrated the highest cost and number of tests for patients with language barriers without the PIS.[40]

The unavailability of timely and quality PIS may result in disastrous diagnostic and treatment errors, health complications, and higher medical costs. In the research study by the University of California, Berkeley School of Public Health and National Health Law Program, Quan and Lynch[41] analyzed the costs of 1,373 medical malpractice claims in the US health-care system. Based on their report, thirty-five medical malpractice claims were related to language barriers. Financial analysis of these claims demonstrated avoidable charges of $5,082,000 paid by institutions due to poor health outcomes following the failure to provide PIS. Among these malpractice cases, one patient became comatose as a result of flawed communication, one had a leg amputated, and another one experienced major organ injury.

3.0 Discussion and Conclusion

Studies that integrate economic indicators into considerations on pros and cons of interpreting services are scarce. Those that are in place show mixed and inconsistent results concerning the patterns of effect of PIS. So far, there is no unequivocal evidence to economically justify the use of interpreters. Although there is considerable evidence supporting the argument that PIS can curb expenses due to a decrease in medical mistakes and the prevention of costly admission, readmission, and returns to the ER, an economic price tag is rarely put on these findings. This may be caused by the limited interdisciplinary composition of research groups, where having economists in the team seems to be an exemption.

The available body of evidence, with its uncertainties considered, suggests that the economic benefits of introducing interpreting services may be considerably higher than the economic costs of such services. It would strengthen the impact of research findings on policy development if such economic analysis would be integrated more often. Available studies also suggest that research designs need to be improved to answer these types of questions.[42]

Good communication is an essential part of good health care and has a demonstrable impact on economic costs of care. Discussions on migrant health need to include discussions about professional services facilitating communication and bridging language barriers. They bring considerations on patient-provider communication closer to the center of attention of quality development in health-care provisions. These discussions can contribute to interdisciplinary quality development of health care for all patients and providers, including those with migrant backgrounds.

CHAPTER TWENTY-FIVE

Multilevel and Mixed-Methods Studies of Migration and Health

Joshua Breslau and Lilian G. Perez

1.0 Introduction

S tudies of migration and health face a number of distinct methodological challenges that stem from the social and cultural conditions that shape migration. Migrant populations, including intra- and international migrants and refugees, commonly maintain connections that can influence their health in at least two geographic settings, and these settings are likely to differ dramatically in social, cultural, environmental, and economic conditions. Moreover, in the United States and other high-income countries, the majority of migrants originate in regions that lack public health information infrastructures that collect data that can provide a foundation for population-based health research. A different set of challenges arise in destination settings. Large portions of migrant populations may lack legal documentation of their residency status, go uncounted in official statistics, and be unwilling to participate in research. Migrants are culturally distinct and often marginalized populations within their host societies, and their concerns about health and health care can go unnoticed or be stigmatized.

In this chapter, we discuss two research approaches that address some of these theoretical and practical challenges: multilevel and mixed-methods studies. Multilevel studies aim to understand multiple levels of social organization or environmental exposure that influence population health. In the context of migration, a multilevel study might aim to account for individual level factors, such as gender, age, and acculturation (e.g., age at migration), as well as community level factors, such as neighborhood characteristics (e.g., immigrant composition), to understand social conditions affecting the entire community. Studies that are informed by such multilevel models often use a set of statistical methods, sometimes called multilevel models, to test hypotheses at one level while accounting for simultaneous processes at other levels. These statistical methods are particularly valuable for informing policy strategies that address contextual factors, such as neighborhood conditions.

Mixed-methods studies integrate a combination of qualitative and quantitative methods into a coordinated project. The qualitative components of these studies tend to be exploratory and collaborative, taking advantage of the open-ended nature of qualitative data collection. The quantitative components, which include probability-based sample designs and structured survey instruments, provide for generalization of findings to the broader population and testing of hypotheses that are not possible using qualitative methods. In the context of research on migrant communities, in sending or receiving contexts, the combination of qualitative and quantitative methods enables researchers to identify factors that are significant to migrant communities, build trust between researchers and those communities, and communicate findings in ways that reflect migrant community perspectives.

The goal of this chapter is to introduce multilevel and mixed-methods research methods and their contributions to understanding the relationship between migration and health. Each method is illustrated through an examination of exemplar studies in which they were applied. In presenting examples, we focus on landmark studies and a selection of other studies that illustrate the breadth of application of these methods in the literature, but we do not attempt a comprehensive review of methodologies or results. We focus on studies that address mental health and substance use outcomes, though the same methods can be applied to other health outcomes. For each study, we discuss the theoretical model motivating the research, the study design, the analytic methods, and the novel findings that were produced.

2.0 Multilevel Studies

The Project on Human Development in Chicago Neighborhoods (PHDCN) is a landmark multilevel study initiated during the 1990s that has made important contributions to understanding the relationship between migration and health in the United States.[1] The primary goal of the study was to understand how characteristics of local environments within an urban area (e.g., neighborhoods) influence a range of developmental outcomes including health. The city of Chicago, with its diversity of neighborhoods, including large immigrant neighborhoods, provides a setting where variation in neighborhood characteristics, such as average educational attainment or proportion of native-born, can be distinguished from variation in individual characteristics, such as the sex, age, and race/ethnicity of individual respondents living in those neighborhoods. Multilevel theoretical models have a long history in sociological research, going back to the work of the Chicago School sociologists of the early twentieth century and including some important early psychiatric epidemiological research.[2]

Distinguishing the effects of contextual factors, which influence all the inhabitants of an area, from the effects of individual factors is particularly important for policy research, since many social policies related to housing or infrastructure affect area characteristics most directly. For example, previous studies from the United States, Spain, and Germany show that tobacco or alcohol outlets are more concentrated in disadvantaged neighborhoods, including those largely comprised of low-socioeconomic status (SES), racial/ethnic minority, and immigrant residents, and this may be contributing to inequities in substance use behaviors and related outcomes (e.g., violence).[3,4,5] Thus, reducing the availability of such outlets in these neighborhoods would be an important policy target. Multilevel studies have been used to investigate the health effects of policies that address neighborhood conditions with respect to access to food,[6] greenspace,[7] and housing.[8]

Multilevel theoretical models are relevant to migration and health in urban settings because of the ways in which residential patterns are shaped by immigration, as new immigrants commonly relocate to areas with residents of the same ethnicity or immigrant background and that provide cultural familiarity. In the United States, immigration has contributed to the creation of structural residential patterns that include immigrant enclaves (neighborhoods with high concentrations of immigrants) and co-ethnic neighborhoods (defined by the proportion of people of the same ethnicity).[9,10] These patterns may help facilitate immigrant adaptation to the host community by providing immigrants with opportunities to develop social networks, access cultural goods, and access housing and employment opportunities, among other pathways.[11,12] However, such residential patterns can also be a source of vulnerability, as they are often characterized by disadvantage in terms of their low access to resources that support health, such as physical activity facilities and culturally and linguistically appropriate health care,[13,14] and are disproportionately targeted by discriminatory policies (e.g., immigration, labor, and education) that reduce opportunities for social and economic mobility.[15]

2.1 Multilevel Study Design and Statistical Analysis

To investigate how immigrant concentration and other neighborhood factors are related to health in Chicago, the PHDCN was designed with a multilevel framework.[16] Specifically, researchers used a two-stage sampling design in which neighborhoods were identified first and then persons were sampled within each neighborhood. This created a multilevel data structure (level 1 = individuals and level 2 = neighborhoods) with two key sources of random variation: individual variation within neighborhoods and variation between neighborhoods. Survey data were collected at the community and household levels and subsequently linked to census-based structural neighborhood measures (e.g., immigrant concentration). The PHDCN also collected multilevel data from three main sources: a community survey of adult residents in 343 neighborhood "clusters" (derived from census tracts) that focused on perceptions of neighborhood social processes (e.g., collective efficacy); household surveys with children and their primary caregivers; and census-based structural neighborhood variables (e.g., immigrant concentration) linked to the neighborhood clusters.

The multilevel theoretical model and design of the PHDCN were matched with statistical models, known as multilevel or hierarchical linear models (HLM). Multilevel statistical models take account of the correlations between observations that arise from the design (e.g., correlations between individuals within neighborhoods).[17] Ignoring these correlations can lead to the misestimation of standard errors and inflate type 1 error (false positives, i.e., when a significant association is found when there is not one). Multilevel methods adjust for correlated errors to properly estimate associations between variables at two or more levels. Using these models enables studies like the PHDCN to identify associations between neighborhood characteristics, such as the proportion of the neighborhood's population that are immigrants, and health outcomes while accounting for the characteristics of the individuals in that neighborhood (e.g., country of birth).

Multilevel models can be challenging to interpret.[18] Methodologists point out two incorrect interpretations to which they are prone: the ecological and the individualistic fallacies.[19,20] The former occurs when group-level relationships are interpreted as individual-level phenomena. For example, an association between neighborhood immigrant concentration and prevalence of depression does not imply that individuals exposed to more immigrant neighbors are more likely to be depressed. The latter occurs when inferences about group-level phenomena are made from aggregated data collected at the individual level. An example of the atomistic or individualistic fallacy is when a study makes inferences about the relationship between neighborhood immigrant concentration and area-level depression when data about depression were collected among only a few individuals and aggregated to the group level.

Another criticism about multilevel research is that contextual effects may be the result of confounding by individual-level variables. In neighborhood research, this can result from selection bias, which would occur if characteristics that lead people to live in similar neighborhoods may also make them likely to have similar outcomes.[21,22] For example, if new immigrants with similar characteristics (e.g., low-SES, non-English speakers) reside together in the same neighborhood, then these individual characteristics may better account for their health or behavioral outcomes than the neighborhood environmental characteristics to which they are exposed. The issue of selection bias is critical because multilevel studies tend to focus on causal effects of neighborhood characteristics on individual outcomes, but, if selection bias plays a role, causation may in fact run in the opposite direction.

2.3 Three Examples of Multilevel Studies of Migration and Mental Health

Two examples of health-related research projects from the PHDCN can help illustrate the advantages of this study design for understanding relationships between migration and health. In a PHDCN publication on mental health among children (aged three to nine years), two-level hierarchical regression models were used to examine associations between the census-based structural neighborhood measures and child internalizing problems, adjusting for child and family characteristics.[23] A subsequent model included the perceived neighborhood social process measures to test for potential mediating effects. Findings showed that children residing in neighborhoods with higher concentrations of disadvantaged populations had more internalizing problems than those residing in more advantaged neighborhoods. However, this effect became nonsignificant when the neighborhood social process measures (collective efficacy and organizational participation) were added to the model, suggesting that social processes may buffer children from the negative effects of neighborhood disadvantage.

In a different PHDCN publication on substance use among adolescents (aged nine to fifteen years), two-level hierarchical Bernoulli regression models (analogous to logistic regression) were used to examine associations between the census-based structural neighborhood measures and three dichotomous substance use outcomes (cigarette, alcohol, and marijuana use), adjusting for adolescent sociodemographic and psychosocial factors (e.g., self-control).[24] A subsequent model included the perceived neighborhood social process measures to test for potential mediating effects. Findings showed that census-based neighborhood immigrant concentration, but not concentrated disadvantage nor residential stability, was associated with alcohol use, even after adjusting for the neighborhood social process measures. That is, adolescents residing in neighborhoods with a higher percentage of residents from immigrant backgrounds were less likely to report drinking alcohol than those residing in neighborhoods with fewer immigrants. No neighborhood correlates were found for marijuana or cigarette use.

A third example applying multilevel methods used data from the Smoking Inequalities—Learning from Natural Experiments (SILNE) study,[25] which involved surveys of adolescents with immigrant backgrounds (first-generation or higher) across six European cities.[26] This publication examined the association between social networks and substance use among immigrant youth.[27] Similar to the PHDCN, the SILNE study used a two-stage sampling design. In this case, schools within each city were identified first, and then students were sampled within each school. This created a multilevel data structure where the first level units were adolescents and second level units were the schools. Adolescents' social networks were measured using a name generator approach in which adolescents nominated up to five best friends from their school. The social networks were characterized based on different metrics, such as homophily (e.g., similarity in terms of immigrant background). Multilevel logistic regression models were used to examine the associations of the different social network metrics with three dichotomous substance use outcomes (smoking, alcohol, and cannabis use), controlling for sociodemographics. The models included random effects for each school to account for differences between the schools in terms of immigrant composition and other characteristics. Findings showed that among adolescents with immigrant backgrounds, higher social ties with nonmigrants were associated with increased use of cannabis and alcohol, but not smoking.

3.0 Mixed-Methods Studies

All social and epidemiological studies are informed by both qualitative and quantitative research findings. The term *mixed-methods studies* describes studies where these different types of methods are integrated into a single study design.[28] These studies aim to use the distinctive strengths of each research modality. Qualitative methods, such as participant observation, key informant interviews, and focus groups, are less structured in advance by the researcher than quantitative methods, and they are usually, though not always, used for exploratory purposes. They enable researchers to discover locally salient features of a social environment that may shape health and health behavior. Qualitative methods are also important for describing institutional structures and highlighting divergent perspectives, particularly among underrepresented groups.[29] Critically, because of their open-ended nature, qualitative methods are more amenable to collaborative research processes, in which researchers and members of communities being studied jointly shape the content and process of research. Given the power differentials between researchers and migrant communities, the qualitative component of mixed-methods research projects have been particularly important in migration and health research.[30]

The qualitative components of mixed-methods studies can be integrated with quantitative components in a wide variety of ways.[31] In many cases, qualitative components are conducted to help identify key constructs and measurement strategies, and these results are used to inform the design of instruments for collecting quantitative data. In other cases, quantitative research may precede the qualitative research. For example, a mixed-methods study might use quantitative methods to identify variation across individuals or communities and use that information to guide selection of cases for in-depth qualitative studies. In both cases, these designs enable studies to combine the in-depth, open-ended, and often collaborative aspects of qualitative methods with the ability to generalize to target populations and test hypotheses using formal statistical methods provided by quantitative methods.

3.1 Mixed-Methods Studies, Migration, and Mental Health: The Mexican Migration Project

Mixed-methods studies have played important roles in migration studies because of their ability to address gaps in existing administrative or survey data, link samples across national boundaries, and build trust between researchers and the often disadvantaged and vulnerable communities they study.[32,33] A landmark example that continues to influence migration studies around the world is the Mexican Migration Project (MMP), an ongoing collaborative effort between Mexican and American researchers that began in 1982 and has had an explicit focus on physical and mental health since 2007.[34] The MMP developed a mixed-methods approach called an ethnosurvey, in which a range of qualitative methods were conducted to inform the collection and analysis of survey data from representative community samples.[35,36] The ethnosurvey began with in-depth ethnographic fieldwork in migrant-sending communities in Mexico. Researchers spent time in the community building trust and interest in the study. Findings from the ethnographic fieldwork informed the development of a semi-structured interview guide, which was administered as an informal conversation rather than a fully structured survey interview yet allowed for systematic collection of information related to household composition, timing of trips to the United States, economic activity, and other areas related to migration. The qualitative work was also used to inform survey sample design.

A key goal of the MMP was to investigate the dynamics of migration between Mexico and the United States from both sides of the border, including both documented and undocumented migration. To achieve this goal, the MMP asked respondents in the sending communities in Mexico to provide contact information for people they knew who were living in the communities in the United States in which they themselves had lived as migrants. The study then contacted these individuals in the United States and, using snowball sampling methods, investigated migration from within the destination communities. The trust built up through the in-depth ethnographic research that had been conducted prior to the survey contributed to the study's success in collecting this sensitive information on both sides of the border.[37] Ethnosurvey methods, adapted from the MMP approach, continue to be widely used in migration studies around the world.[38,39]

Although health outcomes were not explicit foci of the MMP at the beginning, the foundation of the study in the mixed-methods ethnosurvey enabled robust studies of migration and health that were simply not possible in studies based within single countries. The health-related studies that were collected are generally quantitative in nature, but they build on the theoretical and methodological foundation of the ethnosurvey approach.

The study enabled innovative studies on three important aspects of the relationship between migration and health that had received little attention. First, the binational nature of the study allowed researchers to examine health impacts of migration as a transnational process, examining health predictors of migration (e.g., health selection), the health of migrants in the United States, and the health of return migrants in Mexico.[40,41] Second, the inclusion of undocumented migrants, both while they were in the United States and after they returned to Mexico, enable policy-relevant studies of how the conditions of life as an undocumented migrant impacts health.[42,43] Third, the ethnographically grounded theoretical understanding of the gendered nature of migration informed innovative studies of differential effects of migration between men and women.[44,45]

3.2 The Diversity of Mixed-Methods Study Designs

The MMP is a landmark study, and the ethnosurvey approach has now been used in many studies, but there are also a wide variety of mixed-methods approaches that have been developed and used to study migration and mental health in different settings around the world. Several examples can be used to illustrate the diversity and flexibility of mixed-methods approaches and the range of topics they have been used to address. A study of the mental health of the children of migrants in Southeast Asia used a mixed-methods design in which the order of qualitative and quantitative components was the reverse of the MMP.[46] In this study, a quantitative survey was conducted, and its results were used to strategically select research participants for more in-depth qualitative study. The quantitative survey assessed common mental disorders in a sample of 3,026 caregivers to children in families with and without a migrant head-of-household in Indonesia, the Philippines, and Vietnam. The survey was used to examine the relationship between having a migrant head-of-household and caregiver mental health. The survey data were then used to explore factors related to migration and caregiver mental health in a diverse group of respondents. Respondents for the qualitative interviews were selected to include individuals representing four types of caregiver and four categories of physical and mental health status.

Mixed-methods studies have played a particularly important role in understanding health and mental health needs among resettled refugee groups.[47,48] These studies tend to be smaller scale than those that address issues related to labor migration, since they tend to target specific refugee groups within a single city or country. However, this focus on a specific population enables researchers to identify needs and explore cultural and social factors influencing health in ways that can directly inform local practitioners and policy makers. The mixed-method design is particularly well suited for these situations, when there is a relatively small group of refugees who have distinct needs stemming from the often-traumatic experience prior to and during refugee resettlement. These groups often find themselves living as minorities within high-income countries and face cultural and social dislocation. For example, a mixed-methods study was conducted in Norway to examine cultural models of depression and their relationship to health and health-seeking behaviors among resettled Somali refugees.[49] Researchers first conducted a community survey (N=101) of cultural models of mental illness among the Somali refugee community using a standard narrative vignette to elicit judgements related to diagnosis and help-seeking behaviors for a mental health problem. Subsequently, the same vignette was used to structure open-ended discussions in focus groups comprised of members from the same community.

Another example of mixed-methods research on refugee mental health used a three-stage design to study economic hardship and psychological distress among Sudanese refugees resettled in Canada.[50] An initial phase of qualitative research, involving key informant interviews and community meetings, was held to identify key segments of the population that should be included in the sample and topics that should be covered in the interview. The sample design was important because of the diversity in geographic origin (e.g., North vs. South Sudan) and ethnicity (e.g., Nuer vs. Dinka) within the community. Reflecting the diversity of the refugee community, the survey was translated into five languages. The survey instrument included standardized assessments of mental health status along with assessments of pre- and post-migration experiences. Following the survey, a series of qualitative interviews were conducted to explore the survey results in greater depth and document special cases.

4.0 Conclusion

Multilevel and mixed-methods approaches provide valuable tools for conceptualizing and studying the complex relationships between migration experiences and health. As conceptual models underlying research projects, multilevel models are ubiquitous in migration health research. Most studies recognize that individual factors alone do not explain variations in health within migrant groups or between migrant groups and other populations in the countries of origin or destination. Multilevel conceptual models explicitly identify factors at higher levels of social organization (e.g., family and community characteristics) that influence migration and migrant health. As methodological tools for understanding these complex contextual influences, multilevel statistical models and the mixed-methods approach provide versatile research design strategies that address the many challenges facing research on migration and health. These challenges include the lack of robust administrative and survey data on migrant populations, difficulties conducting research with undocumented populations, and the need to conduct research that crosses national borders. Indeed, multilevel statistical models are one type of quantitative technique that can be incorporated into mixed-methods research projects. Both approaches have contributed to understanding the dynamics of health among migrant populations and potential policy responses to their needs.

CHAPTER TWENTY-SIX

Epidemiology and the Study of Migrant Health

Nadia N. Abuelezam

1.0 Introduction

This chapter aims to provide background on the field of epidemiology and the historical thinking behind epidemiologic studies of migrants. The chapter will discuss current research and the challenges to rigorous epidemiological work among migrants. It will conclude with a discussion of future goals of this work.

2.0 Epidemiology

Epidemiology is a field concerned with understanding the ways in which disease is distributed and experienced in a population.[1] Epidemiologists find themselves conducting interdisciplinary work that allows them to understand the determinants of health and the ways in which health can be improved through intervention.[2] Epidemiologists are concerned with an exposure, sometimes called a treatment, that precedes the health outcomes of interest. There are many different study designs that epidemiologists use to understand the relationship between a particular exposure and outcome. The gold standard study design in epidemiology is the randomized controlled trial in which participants are randomized to one of two exposures and are followed over time to observe the outcome.[3] Randomized trials allow epidemiologists to control the study environment and ensure that outside influences do not affect the outcome. These experiments are not always possible and often can be unethical.[4] Epidemiology therefore relies on observational studies in which behaviors and exposures are observed over time but are never assigned. Some observational studies are considered natural experiments that allow epidemiologists to observe changes to individuals' lives that may influence their health without intervention. One natural experiment that has fascinated epidemiologists for decades is immigration.[5] During migration, migrant populations leave their native environments and arrive in a host environment. The host environment may result in different exposures than were present in the native environment. The migration process can be considered an exposure because it may have consequences for an individual's health.[6] Epidemiologists recognize that no research design is capable of accounting for all possible changes to the environment that result from migration.[7]

The process of migration provides an opportunity to understand the impact of changes in social, cultural, and environmental factors on health outcomes.[8] The relationship between migration and health is an interactive process that requires an examination of both temporal and environmental variables.[9] Epidemiology is well positioned to understand the impact of time- and context-dependent exposures on health outcomes.

2.1 Historical Perspectives

Epidemiologists have long been tasked with determining the best methods to understand migration's impact on health outcomes. Kasl and Berkman proposed an ideal epidemiological study[10] that would require epidemiologists to follow three groups of individuals before the migration process began: those who are migrating, native residents of the origin country, and native residents of the host country. Epidemiologists would then be able to characterize the health status and psychosocial status of all groups at repeated time points before, during, and after migration. This type of study would allow epidemiologists to account for all possible effects of migration, including potential environmental effects.

While this proposal would provide an opportunity to understand migration as a mechanism, the feasibility of this type of study is low due to prohibitive cost and time constraints. Epidemiological studies have therefore focused on examining the impact of migration on the migrating group or making distinct comparisons to individuals in their native environment or individuals in the arrival country.[11] A number of different outcomes can be considered when exploring the impact of migration on health, including categorizing the predeparture distribution of medical conditions, the health impact of migration, changes to health after arrival, and consequences of any potential return travel.[12] Many epidemiological studies occur at one time point after the migration process has occurred and do not account for follow-up. For example, some studies aiming to characterize the health of Latino immigrants to the United States only look at the outcomes of immigrants in the United States, and not immigrants who may have returned to their home countries or are thinking about migrating.[13] The challenge to epidemiological studies is therefore to account for the environmental and experiential differences of migrating individuals while maintaining scientific rigor and ensuring appropriate inference from the studies conducted.

Historically, the earliest explorations of the health of migrant populations utilized secondary data sources like life tables and census data.[14] Interest in immigrant populations existed among the epidemiological community primarily because of the potential impact migrant and immigrant populations would have on the host nation's health.[15] Immigrant populations have long been seen as vectors for disease and have been blamed for the health problems of the host country.[16] The majority of the early work on the health of immigrants and migrants focused on mortality[17] and infectious disease outcomes.[18] The past few decades of research have expanded the outcomes examined to include chronic disease[19] and mental health[20] and a wide variety of health behaviors.[21]

3.0 Current Epidemiological Research

Recently, due to big data initiatives and the unification of data collected in the European Union and other parts of the world, a large number of meta-analyses on migrant health have been conducted (although data on migrants in Africa and the Middle East still remains scant). A recent analysis found that migrants had lower mortality rates than individuals in their home countries across all disease categories (except for infectious diseases and injuries).[22] Ecological studies have examined how welfare eligibility and documentation policies increased the odds of mortality and poor self-rated health among migrant communities.[23]

Growing health concerns, like substance abuse, occupational health hazards, and antimicrobial resistance, have also been examined among migrant populations. Substance abuse among forced migrants was found to be higher in refugee camp settings than community settings.[24] International working migrants had a high prevalence of occupational health risks, including psychiatric and physical morbidities, although the prevalence of occupational health hazards was lower among domestic migrants.[25] Migrants in Europe had a higher prevalence of antimicrobial resistance than native Europeans, with the highest levels found in refugees, asylum seekers, and those living in high-migrant communities.[26] The latest research points to the potential for negative health outcomes among immigrant communities due to the Covid-19 crisis.[27]

3.1 Contributing Factors to Health Inequities for Migrants

There are a number of factors that have been shown to contribute to the health of migrants, including the stress of the migration process and acculturation status. Migrants' experiences with leaving their native countries may be different based on social and political circumstances. Differences have been observed in mental health, infectious disease, and mortality outcomes for forced migrants when compared to voluntary migrants. Acculturation is the process of acclimating or adjusting to the way of life in a new setting, including changes to diet, behaviors, or language choices. Acculturation leads to poorer health outcomes in immigrant groups,[28] although there is some controversy around this.[29] Acculturation status is often associated with length of residence in the host country, suggesting that as migrants spend longer periods of time in their new environments, their health may deteriorate. This does not always happen for all immigrant communities, as living in ethnic enclaves may delay the acculturation process and provide protection against adverse health outcomes.[30]

4.0 Challenges to Epidemiological Research on Migration

There are many challenges to assessing the epidemiological impact of the migration process on the health outcomes of migrants.

4.1 Identification of Population and Ability to Enroll Populations in Studies

Migrants are difficult to identify using standard health-related survey data.[31] In many countries, the only way to determine if someone is an immigrant is to ask for their country of birth. Other survey measures may ask for citizenship status. If data on citizenship or country of birth is not collected, other ways of determining immigration status may be to ask about racial and ethnic identifiers or primary language spoken—but each have issues associated with them (see section 4.5).

Migrants without legal status in their host countries may avoid accessing health care at hospital systems or may avoid accessing public benefits due to their fear of deportation in countries where immigration pathways are not easily accessible and attainable for all populations.[32] Recruiting immigrants to participate in epidemiological and public health research may be a challenge. Immigrants may be less likely to participate in research due to distrust, an inability to understand the research objectives, or a fear of deportation.[33]

4.2 Limited Data on Health Outcomes in Origin Countries

In order to understand the changes to the health status of migrants from their native country to their host country, comparisons must be made to individuals in the native country, often through existing data. Data may not always be available in origin countries.[34] When the country of origin's records are not high quality, there is the potential for characterization of only one part of the immigration process, and epidemiologists may not be able to get a full picture of the health impacts of the immigrant experience.

4.3 Loss to Follow-Up

By definition, migratory populations move around to multiple community settings and contexts. This means that immigrant and migrant populations may be difficult to follow and observe health outcomes for over time. The transitory nature of many of these groups impacts an epidemiologist's ability to follow individuals in longitudinal studies to better understand the temporal impact of immigration and to properly characterize all stages of the immigration process.

4.4 Selection Bias

Another methodological issue associated with the recruitment of immigrant groups into epidemiological research is selection bias. Selection bias occurs when the individuals being studied in the epidemiological study do not properly represent the larger group the epidemiologists are hoping to apply the conclusions to. One of the ways in which selection bias has impacted epidemiological studies of immigrant populations is called the healthy migrant paradox. This healthy migrant paradox emphasizes the notion that immigrants may not be representative of their countries of origin[35] and likely have advantages that allowed them to immigrate to a new context. This health advantage that first-generation immigrants have often deteriorates with further immigrant generations due to acculturation and other reasons.[36]

This selection bias has been given much attention in epidemiological literature. While the literature originally examined the healthy migrant paradox among Latin American migrants to the United States,[37] it has been documented in other immigrant groups, as well.[38] For immigrant groups that the paradox does not apply to, there have been other hypotheses made about the forces that have led to the health outcomes of these groups in the population.[39]

4.5 Inability to Properly Contextualize Immigrants' Lived Experiences

There is a need to contextualize an immigrant's lived experiences in order to better understand the positive or negative pressures on health. Some factors important to an immigrant's lived experiences include their social treatment in society. Racial and ethnic categorization is one way to understand how immigrants fit into the social hierarchy of their host country. Data collection on race and ethnicity may vary across different countries. The racial and ethnic reporting guidelines and standards, in the United States in particular, may not be representative of the ways in which immigrants think about their own racial and ethnic categories. It has been documented that immigrants to the United States from Brazil do not have the same racial categories as those imposed on standard surveys, which may cause a misclassification of the race and ethnicity of Brazilian immigrants.[40] Proper classification of immigrant status or race and ethnicity is important because health programs will receive funds based on compelling data. Without proper classification, these populations may continue to be underserved.[41]

The politicization of immigration in many countries, including in the European Union and the United States, may mean that collecting data may be politically motivated and may not ultimately improve the population's health. One group for which data are not available in the United States are Arab and Middle Eastern Americans, those with ethnic and linguistic heritage from the Middle East and North Africa (MENA).[42] This group's racial and ethnic classification has changed over time from non-White to White, depending on the political environment.[43] The White categorization of Arab and Middle Eastern Americans is not fully adopted because they often experience discrimination that makes them feel non-White.[44] Many studies have documented the health disparities between Arab and Middle Eastern Americans and Whites.[45] Evidence collected by the US Census Bureau shows that this population does identify with a MENA identifier.[46] Despite this evidence, the US federal government recently decided not to expand the racial and ethnic classifications to include an additional identifier for MENA.[47] These decisions affect the ability of researchers to understand the health needs of these populations and to advocate for the proper resources to assist these individuals.[48]

5.0 Future Directions in Epidemiology

The field of epidemiology has been evolving to meet the needs of the populations it is serving. Epidemiological research is focusing more on elucidating the structural and systemic mechanisms through which systems and societal forces influence health.[49] More emphasis has been placed on structural interventions that influence the physical and social environment in which individuals live in order to improve health. This work will be especially important to improving the lived experiences of immigrants and migrants in all contexts. With a better understanding of the ways in which the physical and social environment influence the health of migrating populations, preventive tools can be developed to ensure safe transitions for these vulnerable populations.

Additionally, epidemiological research in this field will need to focus on maintaining the safety and trust of immigrant populations in future research projects. This will require involving community members and advocates in conversations around how research should be done. It will also be necessary to ensure proper training pipelines to ensure a diverse epidemiological workforce interested in advancing immigrant and migrant health. By respecting the rights and prioritizing the safety and well-being of immigrant communities, epidemiologists can contribute to improving the health of this vulnerable population.

CHAPTER TWENTY-SEVEN

The Humanities of Migration and Health

Carrie J. Preston

1.0 Introduction

Humanity and the concern for human life are at the foundation of research and writing on migration and health. The title of this chapter, "The Humanities of Migration and Health," evokes two additional perspectives: (1) The humanities as a category of academic disciplines and intellectual pursuits; and (2) the humanities as a plural term appropriate to the fact that the experience of migration varies dramatically for different human beings based on their nation, race, class, gender, sexuality, ethnicity, and other identity categories. One of the promising contributions of humanistic disciplines to the study of migration and health is the development of a language and method for the critical study of identities.

This chapter introduces humanistic perspectives on the book's primary terms, *migration* and *health*, including the ideas that these terms are constructs or human inventions, they have histories, and the historical understanding of the terms affect official policies and the health of migrants. The humanities encourage critique of the fundamental premises of migration regimes in specific historical contexts and inspire us to imagine different, healthier futures. Ana Teresa Fernández's performance art, *Borrando la Frontera/Erasing the Border* (2011), reimagined a crucial symbol of contemporary migration, the border barrier, as Fernández, in a dress and heels, painted a section of the fence separating Tijuana, Mexico, and San Diego, California, a sky-blue color (see fig. 27.1).[1] She created a gap or pause in the fence that makes space for a world in which barriers and

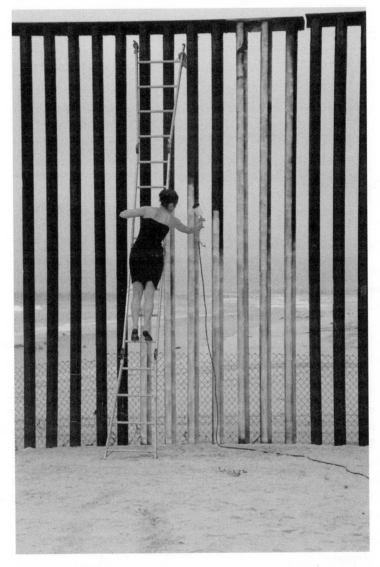

FIGURE 27.1. Ana Teresa Fernández, *Borrando la Frontera/Erasing the Border* (2011). Courtesy of the artist and Catharine Clark Gallery, San Francisco, CA.

guards, deportations and family separations, are not the only way of organizing migration. Closing with an analysis of Fernández's work, this chapter demonstrates how the humanities encourage the sustained analysis of cultural objects like *Borrando*, both to understand and reimagine, in this case, the cultures of migration.

2.0 Definitions and Concepts

2.1 The Humanities

The concept of the humanities as a category of learning emerged in the second half of the nineteenth century to encompass disciplines focused on human cultures and expressions.[2] Humanistic methods have a strong *historical grounding*; humanists often begin, as does this section, by offering the history of a concept or cultural object. Rather than experimental or quantitative methods, the humanities primarily use the critical interpretation and analysis of texts, objects, artworks, performances, and cultural practices. Many humanists are deeply committed to the value of free inquiry, critique of the operations of power and injustice, and creativity or artistic activity that is not necessarily or obviously instrumental. Humanists tend to be suspicious of the reductive nature of easy answers and direct their critique at solutions that accept the current dispensation of the world as a given. This tendency can be both a strength, when humanists identify underlying complicities or problematic assumptions and push for more comprehensive change, and a liability, when they are never satisfied with any intervention. A team working to solve problems of migration and health will benefit from the insights of a colleague trained in humanistic methods—particularly one who is aware (or can be made aware) of the limitations of seemingly unending critique and the likelihood that it will, at moments, frustrate more solution-oriented scholars.

2.2 Health

Disciplines in the humanities define *health* as a human construct with a history that is crucial, in part, because that historical category and its biases affect current understandings, policies, and health outcomes. While the field of *medical humanities* seeks to use humanistic knowledge for the goal of improving medical research and clinical practice, the more expansive interdisciplinary area called *health humanities* brings together insights from the humanities and arts to explore cultural, religious, ethical, and historical aspects of health.[3] Public health has long recognized the social and cultural determinants of health, particularly the impact of oppression rooted in race, gender, sexuality, class, ethnicity, and other identity categories for which the humanities provide a framework for analysis. The health humanities also consider how the category of health, itself, can become oppressive by establishing norms, demands, and prejudices that sometimes serve economic, political, and corporate goals.[4] Forms of biomedical surveillance and population control can be launched in the name of health, and so too can political platforms.

Take, for example, the pandemic of Covid-19 as it intersects with migration. In addition to being a deadly disease, Covid-19 is also a cultural event that is deeply intertwined with political and ethical aspects of human mobility. The spread of the disease outside China initially followed paths established by cultures of migration, global travel, and global capital, largely impacting urban centers.[5] Later, the virus reached the very different routes of irregular migration, including forced displacement, but Covid-19 was devastating even before migrants became ill due to political factors. States responded to the pandemic with travel bans, closed borders, and a refusal to process asylum applications, leaving asylum seekers stranded and pushing them into more dangerous journeys.[6]

In the United States, xenophobic rhetoric has long presented migrants as carriers of disease and additional burdens on the nation's health system.[7] On December 11, 2018, over a year before Covid-19 arrived, then US President Donald J. Trump tweeted that migrants bring "large scale crime and disease."[8] By January 25, 2019, the administration installed the Remain in Mexico program (Migrant Protection Protocols) to send non-Mexican asylum seekers back to Mexico to await judgement on their claims. In March 2020, the administration shut down asylum proceedings and began turning back all migrants at the southern border, citing a Title 42 ruling from the Centers for Disease Control and Prevention (CDC) designed to "mitigate the serious and increased danger of higher introduction of COVID-19 in the United States."[9] Brian Hastings, chief of the Border Patrol's Rio Grande Valley sector, claimed that without immediately turning back migrants, including unaccompanied non-Mexican children without family in Mexico, "we would have massive amounts of infections, massive amounts of commingling, and again, we would fill a hospital."[10] The Title 42 expulsions, which deported nearly 200,000 people during the first eight months of the pandemic (according to government data), alongside the Remain in Mexico program, resulted in undesignated, crowded camps across the border.[11] The humanities help to clarify how xenophobia, racism, and political interests can motivate responses to a pandemic that produce humanitarian disasters in the name of public health.

3.0 Migration

Humanities perspectives on *migration* work to reimagine the foundational frameworks for understanding human mobility, refusing to take for granted the division of the globe into nation-states and categories of people into migrants and natives. Humanities scholars regularly work with social science research that tracks and measures migration, and there is considerable overlap in approach, but humanists deploy the critical and analytical insights provided by transnational, border, postcolonial, diaspora, and critical refugee studies.[12] Humanists consistently emphasize that human mobility has a long history, and the modern definition of *migration* dates to the mid-nineteenth century. Before this moment, the word was used to describe conquest and colonization rather than movement of peoples to access economic opportunities or escape violence.[13] Humanists consider how the popular language used to describe groups of people, like *migrants*, provides a public definition for them, produces cultural assumptions about *who they are*, and constructs their self-understanding.

3.1 Migrants/Natives

Groups of people categorized as *migrants* are defined in opposition to those called *natives*, who are typically assumed to have the right to claim the privileges of citizenship assured by their nation. These claims rest on the accidents of birth and lack of subsequent migration beyond national borders — which, in turn, depend on the borders of a nation staying put. That is, the categories of migrant/immigrant and native/citizen rest on a series of rather arbitrary circumstances and do not describe enduring characteristics of the people who are labeled at any given moment. Yet, these categories are regularly understood as designating a coherent group. For an example of the presumption that migrants have a positive work ethic, take Lin-Manuel Miranda's standing-ovation-getting line in the smash hit musical *Hamilton* — "Immigrants: We get the job done!" — which is sung by Alexander Hamilton and the Marquis de Lafayette (neither of whom was technically an immigrant).[14] On the other hand, Trump regularly characterized migrants from South and Central America as "criminals," "rapists," and even "animals."[15] While Miranda's and Trump's comments would encourage very different policies on immigration, both share the logical flaw called *essentialism*—the tendency to attribute an essential, permanent characteristic to all people classified in a category that is fundamentally heterogenous and even incoherent.

A number of examples underscore the inconsistent, even imaginary, aspects of the constructs of the migrant and the native. The brutality of American racism affects the rights and privileges of Black Americans, who are rarely considered native to the United States because their ancestors are presumed to be forced migrants from Africa, brought to the United States as slaves as early as the 1500s. Yet, many Americans of European descent can trace the arrival of their ancestors in the United States to the nineteenth century or later, although they are generally categorized as natives with unquestioned rights. Ironically, indigenous or *Native Americans* are not afforded the full rights granted to those called *American natives* due to the ongoing policies of settler colonialism, histories of displacement and genocide, and American manifestations of *nativism*. Bearing the same root word as *native*, nativism is a set of attitudes expressed primarily by White Americans who claim the dominant race and ownership of the nation while denying citizenship rights to Native Americans and immigrants.

3.2 Borders

The changeable, even imaginary, status of national borders provides an additional example of the arbitrary nature of the categories of migrant and native. In *Borrando la Frontera/Erasing the Border*, Ana Teresa Fernández erased a fence marking a border between Mexico and the United States that has been disputed, renegotiated, and moved, partially in response to other shifting borders around the world and always in denial of the land claims of indigenous peoples.[16] When Mexico gained independence from Spain in 1821, the young nation held the land now called California (as well as the current states of Texas, Arizona, Nevada, New Mexico, Utah, and even parts of Kansas, Colorado, Wyoming, and Oklahoma).[17] The southern border of California did not take its current shape, from the Colorado River to the Pacific Ocean, until after the Mexican-American War (1846–1848), which was partially inflamed by competing claims over the borders of Texas—an independent nation, the Republic of Texas, from 1836 to 1845. In a twelve-year period, members of the Coahuiltecan tribe living between the Nueces and Rio Grande rivers who survived European aggression and battles with other displaced tribes could have been (mis) classified as Mexican, Texan, and then American—if citizenship rights had been granted to indigenous peoples. This violent history emphasizes the constructed and imaginary nature of the lines we have drawn to create our equally imagined nations.[18]

4.0 Analysis: *Borrando la Frontera/Erasing the Border*

Armed with sky-blue paint and dressed in a "costume" steeped in stereotypes of femininity, the ubiquitous little black dress and stiletto heels, Ana Teresa Fernández erased the border fence where it stretches into the ocean—as if it could even demarcate the nationality of the waves. Shortly after she began, border police threatened to arrest her, becoming unwitting collaborators in the performance. She managed to convince them to let her complete her project, suggesting that her dress and heels helped her avoid arrest because they popularly indicate both (passive) femininity and some wealth (see fig. 27.2).[19] This costume both emphasized her labor and made the work more difficult, as is clear in Fernández's series of paintings documenting the performance, *Foreign Bodies*. The same sub-

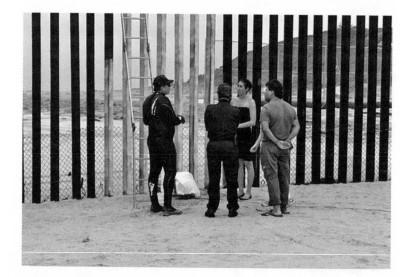

FIGURE 27.2. Ana Teresa Fernández, *Borrando la Frontera/Erasing the Border* (2011), with authorities. Courtesy of the artist and Catharine Clark Gallery, San Francisco, CA.

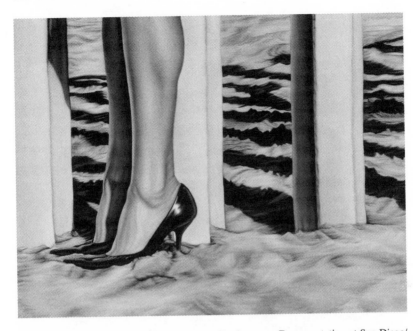

FIGURE 27.3. Ana Teresa Fernández, Entre #4 (Performance Documentation at San Diego/ Tijuana Border), oil on canvas, 10 × 40 inches, 2013. Courtesy of the artist and Catharine Clark Gallery, San Francisco, CA.

stance, *paint*, that signifies working-class labor in the context of painting a fence is high art when placed on a canvas by a person in a dress. Fernández's painted close-up on her own lower legs shows the skin around her ankles sagging against the brutal black heel; skin and tendons resemble the swirls of sand, while the stiletto heels puncture the beach in parallel to the posts of the fence (see fig. 27.3).[20] Fernández's border performances and documentary paintings suggest that the disastrous politics of migration are sunk deep in racism and misogyny.[21] Other paintings in the series feature Fernández in dress and heels mopping the waves or sweeping the sand near the border fence as if to clean up the political filth. The Mexican woman is considered a foreign body to the United States and consigned to specific forms of labor—certainly not art—although the truly foreign element is the border wall itself.

Born in Tampico, Mexico, Fernández immigrated with her family to San Diego at the age of eleven. She claims she was inspired to erase the border in 2011, when the Obama administration prohibited contact across the border wall at the Tijuana-San Diego Parque de la Amistad/Friendship

Park. Separated families had previously embraced through the barrier as they shared binational meals and holidays.[22] Fernández has repeated her performance whenever it is censored or painted over and has also adapted the piece for other border towns and community engagement. On April 9, 2016, Fernández coordinated a performance in the border cities of Mexicali, Agua Prieta, and Ciudad Juárez with volunteers and a livestream of the painting.[23] She performed the piece again at Las Playas, Tijuana, in December 2016, shortly after Trump won the US presidency with slogans like "Build the Wall." The annual binational Christmas party, La Posada Sin Fronteras, was taking place at the triply enforced barrier in Friendship Park, not far up Las Playas from where Fernández was painting.[24] The stunning visual effect she produced emphasizes the beauty of the beach, sea, and sky without the barrier scar and inspires a corresponding opening in the walls we erect in our minds.

CHAPTER TWENTY-EIGHT

Law, Migration, and Health in the US Context

Sondra S. Crosby, Michael R. Ulrich, and George J. Annas

1.0 Overview of US Immigration Law

America's identity is wrapped up in the mythology of its origins. The story is often told of the United States being a nation of immigrants who came to the United States (primarily from Western Europe) to find a better life. The story usually starts well after the genocide of the Native Americans and their forced relocation to reservations and the enslavement of Africans who were forcibly brought to the colonies and later to the states to be bought and sold for their labor. Slavery was officially ended in the United States by the victory of the North in the Civil War (Emancipation Proclamation and the Thirteenth Amendment), but its legacy has continued to this day in the form of discrimination, mass incarceration, and structural racism.

Prior to World War I, the United States was often described as a melting pot comprised of immigrants who came here to become Americans. The melting pot metaphor survived World War I, but only by becoming an anti-immigrant slogan relating to nationalism. As Teddy Roosevelt put it in 1915: "There is no room in this country for hyphenated Americans. . . . The one absolutely certain way of bringing this nation to ruin . . . would be to permit it to become a tangle of squabbling nationalities."[1] In Roosevelt's vision, to become a true American, one had to leave their culture behind and assimilate the pure American culture. The US eugenics movement in the first half of the twentieth century encouraged a view that the United States was for white people and that white people had an obligation to have as many healthy children as they could to prevent the country from being overrun by racial minorities. The United States Supreme Court also endorsed eugenic sterilization of the genetically unfit in its infamous 1928 *Buck v. Bell* opinion. During World War II, US citizens of Japanese origin were literally imprisoned in concentration camps because they were seen as disloyal to the United States. The US Supreme Court approved their imprisonment and did not find it unconstitutional (as being race-based) until 2018, in the same opinion in which the Court approved an anti-Muslim executive order.

Except for people from Asia, the US borders remained virtually open to immigrants prior to 1924. No immigration law had ever prohibited white people from entering the US. The Chinese Exclusion Act of 1882 was the first immigration law to discriminate based on race and class. Originally intended to block Chinese laborers from entering the United States, it later expanded to bans on immigrants from virtually all of Asia except Japan. The first modern immigration law was passed in the United States in 1924. It essentially excluded all Asians, including Japanese, and put strict quotas on immigrants from Europe. There were no quotas imposed on Western Hemisphere countries, and the border with Mexico continued to be essentially open to ensure a steady supply of farm workers.[2] Following World War II, the Convention Relating to the Status of Refugees (1951) was adopted. In the context of the Cold War, it was primarily designed to help people fleeing from oppression in the Soviet Union and Eastern Europe and seeking asylum. The 1967 Protocol expanded the scope of the 1951 Convention, making its provisions global and applying them to future crises. The treaty defined a refugee as someone who had "a well-founded fear of being persecuted for reasons of race, religion, nationality, membership of a particular social group or political opinion,"[3] is outside his or her country, and seeks to remain outside of the country because of this fear. The UN High Commissioner for Refugees (UNHCR) is responsible for the treaty but does not have the authority or resources to enforce it. The UNHCR estimates that at the end of 2020, there were 82.4 million forcibly displaced people in the world, which included 27 million refugees, 48 million internally displaced persons, and 4.1 million asylum seekers.[4] It is of note that while the treaty began with an almost exclusive concern with Europe, it has returned to that emphasis, with the large number of people displaced due to the Syrian War coming to Europe for sanctuary. The ten-year war in Syria has produced approximately seven million forcibly displaced people. Although most discussion is of Syrians coming to Europe, in fact most Syrian refugees are in Lebanon, Jordan, and Turkey.[5]

The contemporary refugee crisis in Europe has been well described by an official of UNHCR: "We've entered a desperate era, an extremely dangerous era, in which war is governing this massive displacement [of refugees]. We need political solutions to stop these horrible wars, and we need governments to support the smaller countries that are hosting large numbers of refugees. . . . The asylum and protection systems are uncoordinated and dysfunctional. Countries are taking unilateral action. We're seeing more restrictive policies. Xenophobia is becoming rampant, intolerance more frequent and mainstream."[6]

The most recent, major immigration law in the United States was passed under Lyndon Johnson in 1965, more than a half century ago. It continued the quota system and added Central and South America to the quota list. It also gave family members of US citizens and people with special skills the ability to apply for citizenship outside the quota system. The 1965 law had two major unanticipated results. First, it drove the United States to be much more racially diverse than it would otherwise have been. By one count, without the law, the United States in 2015 would have been 75 percent white, 14 percent Black, and 8 percent Hispanic; with it, it was 62 percent white, 12 percent Black, and 18 percent Hispanic. Second, because it imposed the first-ever quota on Western Hemisphere immigration, the law "laid the ground for our modern illegal immigration crisis."[7]

Immigration is a global phenomenon and continues to spark controversary both in the United States and around the world. In this chapter, we focus primarily on immigration's impact in the United States after the terrorist attacks of September 11, 2001, which has caused immigration to be seen through the lens of national security, with massive discrimination based on religion. This includes the contemporary politics of immigration that became so raw during the presidency of Donald Trump, who, as both presidential candidate and president, declared excluding South and Central American refugees and asylum seekers as his number one priority. The theme of the Trump presidency elevated the white nationalist values of those feeling threatened by immigrants, especially those from the Hispanic South, while continuing religious discrimination through the Muslim ban in 2017.[8]

Immigration is a complex subject with many moving parts, only a few of which are confined to the United States. Nonetheless, we think that by putting the US contemporary experience in the context of the Trump administration's blatantly anti-immigrant policies, we can identify at least some of the major determinants of health as they affect immigrants seeking to come to the United States primarily as refugees and asylum seekers.

These anti-immigrant policies were not born in the Trump administration and will not die with the Trump administration. Many anti-immigrant policies were exaggerated during Trump's time in office, but nonetheless represent policies supported by almost half of the country.[9]

2.0 Extreme Anti-Immigration Actions under Trump

The Trump administration made no pretense about their disdain for immigrants and was willing to cross boundaries unprecedented in civil society, some of which were shocking, to stop the flow of migrants into the United States. As a presidential candidate, Trump successfully built a strong political base on his campaign platform of building a wall at the southwest border of the United States to keep out the "murderers, rapists, and drug dealers." Indeed, "Build that Wall!" became a mantra at his rallies, and stoking a fear of immigrants as the enemy was a successful strategy that helped catapult Trump into the White House in 2016. No matter how logistically unrealistic the building of a three-thousand-mile fortress was, Trump was obsessed with following through on his campaign promise and started in full force immediately following his inauguration. According to Julie Hirschfeld Davis and Michael D. Shear, his overarching goal was to make the experience of crossing into the United States as perilous and terrifying as possible, and he wanted his wall to be dangerous enough that migrants would not even attempt to cross it. Trump's obsession was so great that the topic of the wall made it into almost every conversation he had with his secretary of Homeland Security, Kirstjen Nielsen.[10]

Refugees and asylum seekers are a vulnerable population. Many have been traumatized and even tortured in their home countries. Many have suffered atrocities that are impossible for most of us to comprehend — atrocities perpetrated either directly by the hands of government officials or by a lack of protection from harm by their governments because of race, religion, nationality, political party, or membership in a particular social group. Some have harrowing stories of escape and entry into the United States. One of us (Sondra S. Crosby) has listened to innumerable accounts of lives marked with atrocities and narratives of unspeakable suffering: the mother forcibly separated from her child after fleeing severe domestic violence; the man burned and mutilated with hot oil, rendering his hands unusable and his face disfigured; the woman who witnessed the rape and torture of her children and then watched her husband burn to death; the woman forced to witness the murder of a pregnant woman and the expulsion of the fetus; the man burned by necklacing, where a tire is placed around his neck, filled with gasoline, and lit on fire; the woman whose genitals were burned and mutilated after she was shackled to a tree. Asylum seekers are seeking safety and refuge, to which they are entitled under both domestic and international law.

The Trump administration promulgated more than four hundred executive actions on immigration, although this is the tip of the iceberg. Professor Lucas Guttentag, a law professor at Yale University and Stanford University, created the Immigration Policy Tracking Project to document each of these changes. In his words, "If we don't keep track it will take a new administration years just to unearth everything that has happened."[11] His group has fastidiously documented more than one thousand changes to the US immigration system during the Trump era. Some of these were established as formal rules that must be published in the Federal Register and opened to public comment. Many others flew under the radar through processes such as guidance memos and bulletins, which are subject to less scrutiny and are difficult to track and to reverse. The changes fell into broad categories of humanitarian protections, labor laws, immigrant visas, and citizenship, and include specifics such as border and interior enforcement, refugee resettlement and the asylum system, and Deferred Action for Childhood Arrivals (DACA), among many others.

On January 27, 2017, mere days after Trump was inaugurated as president, he signed new executive orders that were said to protect the country from terrorists entering the United States. These orders caused strife and chaos in refugee and immigrant communities, not only in the United States, but around the world. These orders (often referred to broadly as "the Muslim ban") banned immigrants from seven predominantly Muslim countries and suspended refugee arrivals to the United States for 120 days. Judges in New York and Massachusetts immediately blocked parts of the order. On March 6, 2017, Trump signed a second executive order. This new order was modified and less exclusionary—for example, Iraq was taken off the list of excluded countries' lawful permanent residents, refugees were allowed, and language was removed that gave religious priority to minorities—but it was also challenged, and another temporary restraining order was issued. In June 2017, the US Supreme Court partially lifted the suspension of the ban and agreed to hear the case in the fall of 2017.

Yet a third version of the travel ban was announced in September 2017, and this was the version ultimately approved by the US Supreme

Court in June 2018 by a five-to-four vote. The majority opinion, written by Chief Justice John Roberts, concluded that the ban was consistent with the president's national security powers and legitimately designed to prevent the entry of foreign nationals who could not be adequately vetted. Justice Sonia Sotomayor wrote a blistering dissent, arguing that the ban was a religious-based Muslim ban that violated the First Amendment. She joined with the Court's reversal of *Korematsu v. United States*, in which the Court had approved of the internment of Japanese Americans solely on the basis of race during World War II, but argued that the Court had just made the same constitutional error again and was "merely replac[ing] one 'gravely wrong' decision with another."[12]

3.0 Safety and Health Aspects of Immigration Laws

Perhaps the most significant impact on immigrant and refugee populations already in the United States resulted from executive orders designed to enhance public safety in the interior of the country. These measures included an increase in Immigration and Customs Enforcement (ICE) resources and discretion, threats to punish sanctuary jurisdictions, an increase in immigrant prosecutions, and a revival of the Secure Communities Program. The empowerment of ICE created and inflamed a toxic environment of fear, pain, and stress throughout immigrant communities. In 2019, the number of immigrants in detention in the United States hit a record-high daily average of over fifty thousand.[13]

Policies requiring individuals to provide evidence of immigration status limited access to resources, regardless of documentation status. For example, following the passage of Arizona Senate Bill 1070, which allowed law enforcement to detain persons who could not verify citizenship, Mexican mothers were less likely to use public assistance or take their infants to receive medical care.[14] Lower birth weights have been reported in Latina mothers affected by ICE raids,[15] and a spike in adverse mental-health symptoms has been reported in many immigrant communities.[16] A typical ICE raid is often experienced as a traumatic event. These raids frequently occurred in predawn hours, when agents, often with guns and body armor, stormed into homes in a militarized fashion, frequently in the presence of children. Fear of detention or deportation has resulted in a decrease in immigrants' willingness to report crimes, including domestic violence.

Aggressive ICE policies left families and communities in fear and reeling at the loss of loved ones. The downstream social impact of community and family insecurity is detrimental beyond those communities directly targeted. Indeed, this was the plan. ICE director Thomas Homan, in a 2017 House Appropriations Committee meeting, said that "if you're in this country illegally, and you committed a crime by entering this country, you should be uncomfortable, you should look over your shoulder, and you need to be worried."[17]

Several of the Trump administration immigration policies, including termination of Deferred Action for Childhood Arrivals (DACA), Temporary Protected Status (TPS), the Zero-Tolerance Policy directing forced separation of children from their parents, the Migrant Protection Protocol (MPP), Title 42, and Public Charge, deserve further comment and represent the major examples of the complex web of legal policies that impact the lives of and undermine the health of migrants. While the Joe Biden administration rolled back many of these policies shortly after taking office others still remain, and the impact of each policy will have long-lasting effects.

The Trump administration continuously attempted to rescind DACA, a program initiated by President Barack Obama and now preserved by the Biden administration. This was a landmark proposal, initiated with an executive order, to protect from deportation approximately 800,000 youth who arrived undocumented before age sixteen. The program required school attendance, completion of high school, or military service. It did not provide a pathway to citizenship (this would require an act of Congress) but provided economic opportunities and health care.

TPS is a humanitarian program that allows foreign nationals to remain in the United States if conditions in their country pose a danger to personal safety due to ongoing armed conflict or humanitarian disaster. The Trump administration took steps to end TPS for El Salvador, Haiti, Nicaragua, Sudan, Honduras, and Nepal. Many families who came to the United States with TPS have established roots and have children that are US citizens. President Biden pledged not to send TPS holders back to unsafe countries and extended TPS benefits into 2022 and beyond for eligible immigrants from nine nations, and expanded eligibility for immigrants from Haiti due to recent turmoil. Immigrants from Venezuela and Myanmar are newly eligible for TPS under the Biden administration and TPS currently covers approximately 700,000 immigrants from twelve countries.[18] But TPS is precarious and fluid, leaving many in fear of deportation and family separation. Currently, TPS does not provide a path to permanent residency.

In May 2018, former Attorney General Jeff Sessions announced the most controversial anti-immigrant policy of the Trump Administration: the Zero-Tolerance Policy, designed to prosecute parents who crossed into the United States illegally with children. Border agents forcibly separated children from their parents at the Mexican border to deter other parents from attempting to come to the United States with their children. The children separated from their parents were sent to government custody or foster care. Some of the children were warehoused in cages. The Biden administration announced it would try to reunite families and create programs to address the children's and families' mental-health needs, but due in part to lack of records, reunification of families remains incomplete as of the winter of 2022. Although the Biden administration announced that it would no longer separate families at the border, the administration ended negotiations over compensation to separated families in December 2021.

In December 2018, the MPP—often referred to as the Remain in Mexico program—was established. Under MPP, individuals who arrive at the southern border and request asylum are given notices to appear in immigration court and then are sent back to Mexico to wait for their court hearing. At least seventy thousand asylum seekers have been returned under this program. The decision to send a person or family back under MPP is discretionary and is made by individual CBP officers or Border Patrol agents and almost always puts the asylum seeker at significant risk of harm. Human Rights First previously tracked more than 1,544 reports of murder, rape, kidnapping, torture, and assault of people sent to Mexico under the MPP.[19] Multiple people, including at least one child, have died. The makeshift tent-city living conditions for people returned to Mexico under MPP (witnessed by Sondra S. Crosby) are inhuman: makeshift encampments, unsanitary conditions, a scarcity of food and potable water, limited medical care, and exposure to the elements. Families have also been separated under the MPP, which was discontinued but then reinstated under the Biden administration in December 2021 while litigation to abolish it continues.

4.0 Public Health and War Impacts on Immigration

As of the winter of 2022, asylum remained effectively prohibited at the southern border of the United States with an excuse first promulgated by Trump and then endorsed by Biden: the borders to Mexico and Canada were closed because of the Covid-19 pandemic. Section 361 of the Public Health Service Act, codified at § 264 of Title 42 of the US Code, granted the Secretary of Health and Human Services (HHS) extremely broad authority to prevent the introduction, transmission, or spread of communicable diseases from foreign countries into the United States. Both presidents relied on Title 42 authority to restrict asylum seekers from entering the United States, though many believed the use of Title 42 was illegal and speciously uses public health as a rationalization to keep asylum seekers from crossing the border.

For purposes of considering the US border with Mexico, it is important to note that the statute emphasizes that this authority "*shall not provide for apprehension, detention, or conditional release of individuals except for the purpose* of preventing the introduction, transmission or spread of such communicable diseases."[20] The statutory language gives the US discretionary authority to exclude individuals at the border only if there is credible evidence of a risk of spreading disease. The statute also clearly states that this authority is with respect to those individuals who are entering the country, as opposed to those already within the United States: "Regulations prescribed under this section, insofar as they provide for the apprehension, detention, examination, or conditional release of individuals, shall be *applicable only* to individuals *coming into* a State or possession from a foreign country."[21] This authority has been invoked to close the border to asylum seekers without the customary asylum screenings that would help ensure that the United States is not violating domestic and international law. The Trump-Biden Title 42 policy has no scientific base and instead undermines public health, all while damaging the public's trust and sacrificing the health and human rights of migrants and asylum seekers.[22] During Biden's first year in office, Human Rights First has tracked over 8,705 reports of violent attacks against migrant and asylum seekers blocked or expelled to Mexico through MPP and Title 42.[23] Another policy that directly affected health care access to immigrants living in the United States was expansion of an existing public charge rule. Public charge is a US government designation for an immigrant who is considered or is likely to become primarily dependent on government-funded benefits. Immigrants considered a public charge may be prevented from adjusting their legal status to lawful permanent resident or US citizen and may even be denied admission into the United States. Historically, noncash benefits were excluded from the original determination, however, the new Trump rule (rescinded by Biden in March 2021) included programs such as Medicaid, Supplemental Nutritional Assistance Program (SNAP), and public housing, all of which have a significant impact on health and wellbeing.[24] Even though the Trump public charge rule was reversed, the chilling effect persists, including throughout the Covid-19 pandemic. Immigrants have reported avoiding necessary medical services or other

TABLE 28.1 **Biden administration actions**

Biden actions as of January 2022
    Halting Trump's border wall construction.
    Ending travel ban on several Muslim-majority countries.
    Reversing plan to exclude undocumented immigrants from the census.
    Pausing deportations for certain noncitizens in the United States for one hundred days.
    Overturning executive order that pushed aggressive efforts to find and deport unauthorized
    immigrants.
    Instructing the Department of Homeland Security Secretary to take action to preserve and
    fortify DACA.
    Increase refugee admissions.
    Extended and expanded TPS.
    Rescinded Trump's Public Charge Rule.
    Stopped but then continued MPP after court refused to enjoin enforcement during litigation.
    Continued Title 42.
Legislative proposals: Biden's US Citizenship Act of 2021
    Create a pathway to citizenship for all undocumented individuals, including Dreamers, TPS
    holders, and immigrant farm workers.
    Reform family-based immigration system.
    Outlaw discrimination based on religion.
    New funding for immigration support programs.
    Increase employment-based visas.
    Improve immigration courts.

Source: https://crsreports.congress.gov/product/pdf/IN/IN11811

critical social services for fear that it might prevent their ability to adjust their status.[25,26,27]

Many of the most cruel immigration policies of the Trump administration had been revoked by mid-2021—but others, like Title 42, remained in place. A permanent solution would require majority agreement in Congress to revisit immigration policy for the first time since Lyndon Johnson. It is relatively easy to outline what not to do—such as separating children from their parents or denying immigrants health coverage—but getting agreement on a comprehensive immigration law, complete with a path to citizenship, is still a work in progress. Nonetheless, the inauguration of Biden has made the passage of new immigration laws at least plausible. As Biden put it shortly after being sworn in: "With the first action today, we're going to work to undo the moral and national shame of the previous administration that literally, not figuratively, ripped children from the arms of their families—their mothers and fathers at the border—and with no plan, none whatsoever, to reunify the children who are still in custody and their parents."[28]

Author and scholar Viet Thanh Nguyen emphasizes how US responsibility for creating refugee crises through its war machine repeated itself with the US withdrawal from Afghanistan in August 2021 after a twenty-year war. He noted that refugee stories are also war stories and compared the departure in Afghanistan in 2021 to the fall of Saigon in 1975. After the fall of Saigon, nearly a million Vietnamese fled by sea. Tens of thousands perished during escape, while others survived and lived in refugee camps, with some resettling in host countries. In April 1975, the United States evacuated about 130,000 vulnerable people from Vietnam and then admitted hundreds of thousands as refugees from Vietnam, Laos, and Cambodia over the next decades. Nguyen correctly opined that there would be a similar fate for many Afghans facing recrimination following the American retreat and takeover by the Taliban and, just as we saw following the Vietnam war, the new refugee crises will likely last for decades.[29] Biden committed to evacuating an unspecified number of Afghans to safety.

5.0 Conclusion

Immigration law and policies evolve over time and have profound health consequences for migrants and their family members still living under the threat of persecution or harm. Immigration law is inherently international law—but it is also under the jurisdiction of individual countries, virtually all of which offer waivers when major international crises and conflicts send people fleeing their countries looking for safety. We witnessed an extreme overreaction of fear and prejudice leading to horrific health consequences for immigrants during the Trump administration. Going back to the policies of the Obama and Bush administrations is necessary, but not sufficient. The challenge for the United States is to develop an immigration policy based on human rights and human dignity, with clear standards that are fairly and nondiscriminatorily applied.

CHAPTER TWENTY-NINE

Migration

A Health-Equity Lens

Felicity Thomas

1.0 Introduction

"The Universal Declaration of Human Rights reminds us that "all human beings are born free and equal in dignity and rights." Today, one of the single most fundamental determinants of the capacity of individuals to realise their full potential and rights is their place of birth. Some are born into opportunity and others into deprivation. Migration, properly managed, is a route for individuals to make the most of their lives and achieve the dignity that our predecessors enshrined in the Universal Declaration. Their quest for equality is a legitimate one. The global compact should ensure that they can pursue it in a safe, orderly and regular manner."
United Nations Secretary General at the United Nations General Assembly, 2017

Most governments recognize health as an essential human right. Promising developments in health policy in recent years have focused on the emergence of a global health equity movement concerned with understanding and addressing the social determinants of health.[1] Yet despite such developments, the global policy arena on migrant health remains largely uncoordinated and inconsistent, with major contradictions across migration and health-related policy agendas as well as discrepancies between policy and on-the-ground need.

Considerable variation in health-related entitlements and experiences exist across different types of migrants. Some countries, for example, allow wealthy foreigners to buy citizenship status with associated rights and entitlements attached or have bilateral or multilateral agreements that cover the portability of social protection benefits. However, such conditions predominantly apply to people moving between high-income countries.[2] For those migrants who are not deemed deserving, necessary, or useful to help meet wider economic ends within the host country, research (mainly from high-income countries) has shown that equity in health is often far more elusive.[3] Less is published on the situation within low- and middle-income countries, where high numbers of migrants may be hosted under already restricted conditions of health resourcing. However, research within such contexts has shown that while barriers to health care may be experienced by both migrants and native populations, migrants often face additional legal, economic, and language barriers[4] and that health equity may also be influenced by factors such as gender, ethnicity, residence within or outside of official refugee camps, and by political and/or religious affiliation.[5]

This chapter focuses on health equity as it relates to those defined as refugees and asylum seekers, undocumented migrants, trafficked people, and low-wage economic migrants. Here, the conditions in which migrants travel, live, and work can carry significant risks to their physical and mental health and well-being. Such risks are often linked to the social determinants of health and include restrictive legislation around immigration, employment and welfare, economic disadvantage and exploitation, poor housing and amenities, and discrimination. This chapter begins with an overview of the governance of migrant health. It then examines how a lack of health equity exacerbates vulnerability, the inequities that exist in health-care access and provision, and the health equity implications of migration for those who are left behind in home countries.

2.0 Governance and Access to Health Care

The right of everyone to enjoy the highest attainable standard of physical and mental health is established in the World Health Organization (WHO) Constitution of 1948. Ratified international human rights standards and conventions also exist to protect the rights of migrants and refugees, including their right to health. This includes the entitlement to preventive, curative, and palliative health care, as well as to the underlying social, political, economic, and cultural determinants of health, such as clean air and water and nondiscriminatory treatment.[6] The Sustainable Development Goals (SDGs) also identify migration as both a catalyst and a driver for sustainable development, with an aim to "leave no one behind," regardless of legal status, in order to achieve Universal Health Coverage for all.[7]

The 2016 New York Declaration for Refugees and Migrants was the highest-level UN meeting ever convened on global migration.[8] Within this, a new set of UN initiatives around managing movements of refugees and migrants in a "humane, sensitive, compassionate, and people-centred manner" requiring "international cooperation" was set out.[9] Other key developments promoting migrant health equity in the international governance arena in recent years include the World Health Assembly resolution Promoting the Health of Refugees and Migrants (2017) and the Global Compact for Safe, Orderly and Regular Migration (2018) initiated in line with target 10.7 of the 2030 Agenda for Sustainable Development to facilitate safe, orderly, and responsible migration.

While these developments assist in keeping migrant health on the broad radar of global governance agendas, in reality, a combination of political inertia, lack of clarity over how to implement multi-sectoral and universal health coverage to noncitizens,[10,11] contradictory migration-related interests,[12] concerns over national sovereignty, populist anti-migrant sentiment and state-endorsed discrimination, and the chasm between immigration and health agendas means that the rights enshrined within these conventions and standards do not always translate into entitlements in the form of national level policy.[13,14] Indeed, a recent Lancet Commission on Migration and Health affirmed that "when there is conjoining of the words health and migration, it is either focused on small subsets of society and policy, or negatively construed."[15]

For internally displaced persons and irregular migrants in particular, access to health care is often severely restricted.[16,17] Many states grant these people access only to emergency care, and even this is not guaranteed. At the same time, discrimination results in many, particularly those without secure residency status, avoiding health services or only attending health care at a late stage in their illness due to lack of resources or a fear of the potential repercussions of engaging with formal authorities.[18]

Benchmarking the equitability of migrant health-related policy is essential for monitoring progress and identifying positive and negative aspects of national level governance. While this kind of work poses considerable challenges, it has been made possible through initiatives such as the Migrant Integration Policy Index (MIPEX) in Europe, which includes a strand on health and clearly sets out how diverse policies play out to affect migrant health inequities across the European region.[19]

3.0 Vulnerable Groups

The health of migrants depends greatly on the structural and political factors that determine the impetus for migration and the conditions of their journey and their destination. Not all who move are especially vulnerable — indeed, many migrants are often initially healthier than native-born residents.[20] However, many groups of migrants face specific challenges and inequities, including punitive border policies, detention, physical and mental abuse, extortion, poor living conditions, restricted education and employment opportunities, and the denial of access to health care, all of which contribute to a deterioration in health status over time.

3.1 Gender

A wide range of evidence shows that population mobility and the health implications of migration are highly gendered. For women and sexual minorities in particular, gender-based violence and discrimination may be the cause of their departure. Women and children are also at particular risk when they migrate without the protection of social networks, as was seen in the widespread rape of Rohingya women forcibly displaced from Myanmar.[21] However, men, women, and sexual minorities all encounter different health risks and opportunities for exploitation and protection at different phases of their migration journey. Research with Syrian refugees in Jordan, for example, found that refugee men faced specific gender-related threats and circumstances that left them vulnerable, including forms of police harassment, forcible encampment, and greater likelihood for refoulement to Syria for alleged security reasons.[22]

3.2 Children and Young People

Children and, in particular, unaccompanied minors and irregular child migrants also face particular health challenges. For example, while it is known that education is a key determinant of future health and well-being, a study across twenty-eight high- and low-income countries found widespread challenges facing irregular child migrants in school access, such as cases of exclusion when children had not undergone health screenings and days missed due to poor access to health services to treat even simple illnesses.[23] Related to this, research in the United Kingdom and Italy has shown how prolonged and politically induced uncertainty over immigration status adversely affects the health and well-being of young people as they become legally adult while also stifling opportunities for them to pursue activities such as higher education and training that are critical in enabling them to improve their opportunities and life chances.[24]

3.3 Disabled Migrants

Relatively little is known about the health experiences and inequities experienced by disabled migrants, and there are few reliable statistics on their movements across borders. However, research suggests that people with physical or severe mental disabilities face significant structural barriers to migration, as well as negative assumptions that frame them as "unproductive."[25] Disabled people also tend to be ignored in migration policy and interventions yet have constrained rights to employment and welfare support because of their migration status. They are often unable to access the same level of health and social care support afforded to other disabled citizens, which further compounds experiences of disability and social exclusion.[26]

3.4 Impacts of Covid-19

While health inequities have long been a part of the migration landscape, they have been brought into even sharper relief during the global Covid-19 pandemic, as patterns of vulnerability and discrimination lie at the intersection of race, income, and status. Many countries have taken steps to reduce population movement, closing down migration corridors while also reducing or suspending humanitarian initiatives, such as search and rescue operations in the Mediterranean.[27] Those migrants and refugees living on the streets or in overcrowded conditions in camps often have little in the way of basic sanitation, meaning that the threat of contracting diseases is especially concerning.[28] A rise in xenophobia has also been reported, with an increased fear of abuse and violence likely to reduce migrants' willingness to come forward for screening, testing, and health care.[29]

Migrants make up a disproportionate share of the workforce in sectors that have remained active during the pandemic and often must work in risky environments with a lack of adequate protective equipment and hygiene facilities.[30] The poor living conditions of many migrants also make them particularly vulnerable to Covid-19 when they have inadequate access to health care and other essential rights. Insufficient inclusion of migrant workers in otherwise successful early containment efforts in Singapore, for example, saw a rise in new infections among migrants living in dormitories, which led to renewed closures, quarantines, and mobility restrictions.[31] Ensuring that all migrants, regardless of their status, are included in response programs and have access to health care is therefore a necessary condition for effective responses to Covid-19.

4.0 Inequities within Health Care

Legal barriers to accessing medical services constitute a major obstacle to enabling health equity for migrants. However, research has found that even among those with legal entitlement to such services, there may be relatively lower levels of engagement with public health facilities, screening and preventative programs, and prenatal and homecare visits than found among the general population.[32,33] Such findings suggest that even when migrants are entitled to access health care, the specific needs they face may be poorly understood and inadequately responded to.

Considerable attention has been given to the importance of health literacy in enabling migrants to make optimal use of health systems. Very often, however, programs of health education for migrants show little or no regard for migrants' own health beliefs and, as a result, do not succeed. It is important, therefore, that health services adapt in order to provide for diverse populations and needs and recognize that equity in health care involves offering care that is sensitive to needs of people from diverse backgrounds, rather than a one-size-fits-all approach to service provision that discriminates against those whose needs differ from the majority.[34]

Ensuring the provision of health care that is sensitive to the needs of people from diverse backgrounds is commonly referred to as *intercultural competence*.[35] In theory, intercultural competence is a two-sided process. First, it requires that health professionals are able to reflect on their own perspectives and biases, exercise cultural humility, and appreciate the existence of other perspectives and understandings.[36] Secondly, and central to this, is the need for health professionals to listen to their patients and to learn about their patients' beliefs and experiences relating to health and illness.[37]

The concept of intercultural competence has gained traction across many countries within the past two decades. In Europe, for example, the

Migrant Friendly Hospitals initiative played a key early role in improving hospital services for migrants and in raising awareness of the value of an interculturally competent approach to health-care provision.[38] Despite such advances, however, questions remain over the conceptualization of intercultural competence and how this plays out in practice. Particular concern is raised when static and often narrowly defined notions of culture become synonymous with race and ethnicity and when the fluid and constructed nature of culture and identity are overlooked.[39] Such challenges have led to the stereotyping and othering of patients and the inappropriate labeling of behaviors, responses, and conditions as cultural traits. This can be particularly problematic where culture is identified as an issue that is exclusive to migrants.[40]

Being understood and accepted is a key component of trust in the doctor-patient relationship and is highly associated with patient satisfaction.[41] Yet while guidelines and training initiatives relating to the use of professional interpreters are widely available,[42] and while language and cultural issues are commonly identified as a major problem for medical personnel, the use of professional, trained interpreters in routine practice is highly variable across settings. Research suggests that this is in large part due to resource constraints and to poor organizational practice and prioritization within health-care systems.[43] It is also known that many health professionals rely on informal interpreters (e.g., patients' family members) to support communication within consultations,[44] a strategy that risks compromising migrants' experience of health care when interpreting is of poor quality, when health issues are deemed sensitive, or when sociocultural norms negatively influence practices of care for particular household members. Using interpreters via video-conferencing technology can improve patient experience, yet this can be difficult to arrange in advance and may prove challenging when consultations are time constrained or undertaken in low-resource settings.[45]

Even when language is not a barrier, migrants will not necessarily be familiar with the diverse health systems and norms of practice that determine health seeking and health provision. Cultural mediators or navigators can therefore act as an important bridge between patients and health professionals, ensuring that migrants receive the support they require both within and beyond health-care systems. The use of such mediators is now well established in a number of countries, such as Spain, Italy, and Belgium, where research has suggested they constitute a positive element of work toward migrant health equity.[46,47] However, like professional interpreters, the use of cultural mediators is not yet widespread, a situation that is likely to remain unchanged in both high- and low-income countries without substantial reconsideration of resourcing and priorities.

5.0 Left-Behind Communities

Large numbers of migrants are separated from their family and core so-cial networks by distance and national borders. Understanding migration through a health-equity lens therefore encompasses not just the experi-ences of those who migrate, but also those who are left behind in home countries.

A key area where health inequities play out is the outward migration of highly skilled health workers. Health worker shortages remain a per-sistent and ongoing issue, with estimates of a global shortfall of eighteen million by 2030.[48] This affects all countries, but it is clear that the impacts are felt most harshly within low- and middle-income countries. While this is in part due to levels of resourcing and to the uneven distribution of health-care facilities within the country, it is also due to the migration of health professionals to higher-income countries, where health workers can secure higher wages and improved opportunities. Malawi, for exam-ple, trains around sixty new nurses each year. However, around a hundred nurses each year leave the country, with approximately half going to the United Kingdom, leaving a 75 percent vacancy rate.[49] In the past twenty years, ethical codes have been introduced to restrict active recruitment from particular low-income countries, and there is some evidence from the United Kingdom to suggest that this has led to a decline in health workers from some countries.[50] However, there is also evidence to suggest that such codes simply make migration more difficult and expensive for migrants from low-income countries, which may simply make them more vulnerable to exploitation and abuse.[51]

Evidence on the impacts of migration on the health of family members who are left behind is conflicting. Some evidence has demonstrated that remittances sent home by parents can facilitate access to health care and education for left-behind children. Evidence from Pakistan, for example, showed positive nutritional and growth impacts, with girls benefiting sub-stantially more than boys.[52] However, research from India, Peru, and Viet-nam has found that long-term parental migration reduced the health out-comes of children and reduced cognitive ability test scores in India and

Vietnam.[53] Most of the large volume of research on this issue stemming from China also shows that left-behind children of migrants have poorer nutritional and developmental outcomes than children of nonmigrant parents. A systematic review found evidence from China to show that parental migration can be especially detrimental to children's mental health, with children and adolescents having an increased risk of depression and higher levels of depression, anxiety, suicidal ideation, conduct disorder, substance use, wasting, and stunting.[54]

6.0 Conclusion

Population mobility is an asset to global health. However, this chapter has demonstrated that for many migrants, health equity remains far from a reality. Universal health care can only be achieved when everyone has the opportunity to access and make use of quality medical services and when population movement is considered core to the design of health interventions. This also means that the health of mobile populations must be fully considered across all of the Sustainable Development Goals and that governments should implement national programs of action that respond across multiple dimensions.

While current global governance arrangements aspire to the provision of health for all, profound gaps remain and are exacerbated by a lack of coordinated leadership around migrant health. It is clear, therefore, that achieving health care that is truly universal will require much more proactive and deliberative policy making to include and champion the needs of migrants.

PART V

Case Studies in Migration and Health

CHAPTER THIRTY

The United States as a Case Study

Policy, Access, and Outcomes

Sana Loue

1.0 Introduction

U S immigration law has long provided for the inadmissibility and consequent exclusion of individuals believed to be unhealthy in ways that would adversely impact the citizenry and/or economy of the country. *Inadmissibility* here refers to both physical inadmissibility to the United States, such as someone passing through immigration at an airport, and to the granting of an immigration status, such as to an individual seeking permanent resident status, whether applying at a consulate or at an immigration office in the United States. In addition to restricting those with specified health conditions from legally entering into or remaining in the country, US immigration and health laws also place restrictions on the ability of those physically present on its soil to access publicly funded health care.

Estimates suggest that there are currently 44.8 million foreign-born individuals living in the United States, accounting for 13.7 percent of the country's population. As of 2017, approximately 45 percent were naturalized citizens, 27 percent were permanent residents (green card holders), 5 percent were temporary residents (nonimmigrants), and 23 percent were undocumented.[1] Research has found that immigrants are generally healthier at the time of their arrival into the United States in comparison with native-born persons, an observation that has been termed *the healthy migrant effect*.[2] This is unsurprising in view of long-standing legislative and regulatory provisions that exclude from the United States intending immigrants and temporary visitors with specified health conditions.[3] However, this health advantage appears to diminish over time due to various factors, including changes in diet, lack of access to and knowledge about the medical-care system, anti-immigrant discrimination,[4,5] and challenges in communicating with health-care providers.[6] Immigrants' declining health status may also be attributable to existing policies, legislation, and practices that impact their ability, whether they are in the United States permanently or temporarily and whether they are documented or undocumented, to access care following their entry into the United States, potentially leading to worsened health status.[7]

2.0 Access to Publicly Funded Health Care Insurance Coverage

As of 2018, approximately 23 percent of nonelderly lawfully present immigrants and 45 percent of undocumented immigrants were uninsured.[8] Immigrants are significantly less likely than US citizens to be covered by employer-sponsored health-care insurance, often due to employment in low-wage positions that do not provide either health coverage[9] or wages sufficient to support the cost of private insurance. And, despite immigrants' disproportionately large contributions to the US economy through their payment of income tax and contributions to Social Security and Medicare,[10,11,12] numerous legal provisions limit their ability to access publicly funded health-care services. Table 30.1 provides a summary of these provisions, each of which is described below in greater detail.

2.1 Medicaid

Medicaid is a federal-state partnership program under Title IX of the Social Security Act that provides health-care services to low-income families with children, the elderly, and persons who are blind and disabled.[13] The statute specifically excludes from coverage individuals who are "not lawfully admitted for permanent residence or otherwise permanently residing in the United States under color of law."[14] Even those who are US permanent residents (green card holders) may be ineligible for Medicaid-funded health care under the terms of the Personal Responsibility and Work Opportunity Reconciliation Act of 1996 (PRWORA).[15] This legislation provides that most immigrants who were legally admitted after August 22, 1996, may not access publicly funded medical care, such as

TABLE 30.1 **Summary of legal provisions limiting immigrant access to publicly funded
health-care insurance**

Source	Impact
Medicaid (Title IX of the Social Security Act)	Excludes from coverage individuals who are "not lawfully admitted for permanent residence or otherwise permanently residing in the United States under color of law."
Personal Responsibility and Work Opportunity Reconciliation Act of 1996	Prohibits most immigrants who were legally admitted after August 22, 1996, from accessing publicly funded medical care for a period of five years after becoming "qualified" to receive "federal means-tested public benefits."
Patient Protection and Affordable Care Act	Some immigrants are eligible for marketplace tax credits under specified conditions; prohibits undocumented immigrants, individuals in the United States with a temporary status, and those with DACA status from participating in federally subsidized health exchanges or the Medicaid expansion.
Immigration and Nationality Act: "Likely to become a public charge"	Potentially renders inadmissible any non-US citizen who has received benefits for more than twelve months from specified programs within a rolling thirty-six-month period.

nonemergency Medicaid and Medicare, for a period of five years after becoming "qualified" to receive "federal means-tested public benefits." Individuals not legally in the United States are prohibited from accessing nonemergency Medicaid or Medicare regardless of their length of residence in the country. "Qualified" individuals include lawfully admitted permanent residents, individuals who have been granted refugee status or asylum, certain active military members and their dependents, battered and trafficked children and women, subject to specified conditions, and several other smaller categories of persons.

An exception to the prohibition against the use of Medicaid funding is made only in the case of emergency medical care, under the federal Emergency Medical Treatment and Active Labor Act (EMTALA).[16] Pursuant to this statute, hospitals that have an emergency department and that receive federal funds, such as reimbursement through the Medicaid or Medicare program, must provide appropriate medical screening to determine whether a medical emergency exists to individuals who present to the emergency department for examination and/or treatment of a medical condition.[17] Congress passed EMTALA in 1986 in response to hospitals' refusal to provide treatment to and their inappropriate discharge of patients who lacked adequate funds to pay for needed health-care services, a practice that became known as *patient dumping*.[18]

The scope of this emergency exception is narrow. The statute defines an emergency medical condition as one whose severity is such that the failure to provide immediate medical attention would reasonably lead to the serious impairment of bodily functions, the serious dysfunction of a bodily organ or part, or serious jeopardy to the individual's health. In the case of a woman experiencing contractions, the denial of medical attention constitutes an emergency medical condition if a transfer of the woman would pose a threat to the health or safety of the woman or the unborn child or if there is inadequate time to safely transfer the woman to another facility prior to delivery.[19]

Despite their potential eligibility for coverage for a medical emergency, many immigrants, whether in the United States legally or without authorization, may delay seeking medical care, potentially leading to adverse health consequences. Individuals have been reported to delay care for the treatment of gangrenous limbs resulting from severe diabetes and for severe hip injuries.[20] Many individuals live in mixed households that may include permanent residents, US citizens, and undocumented persons; as of 2018, almost nineteen million, or one-quarter, of all children living in the United States had at least one immigrant parent, and most of these children were US citizens.[21] Individuals may fear that presentation to medical personnel and/or reliance on publicly funded care may lead to adverse immigration consequences, such as the denial of their own or a family member's application for an immigration benefit or, in the worst-case scenario, to their own or a relative's deportation from the United States.[22]

Taken together, these provisions effectively bar many new permanent residents from accessing publicly funded health care for an extended period of time. States have the option to eliminate the five-year bar for children and pregnant women who do not have qualified status,[23] but more than one-half of the states have chosen not to do so for pregnant women and only slightly more than one-half have done so for children.[24] Even women who may be eligible for care have been found to delay prenatal care due to the fear of potential immigration consequences to themselves or their family members, leading to a higher risk of complications for both the mother and the child.[25,26]

2.2 The Patient Protection and Affordable Care Act

The Patient Protection and Affordable Care Act (ACA), intended to provide Americans with more affordable health care, included provisions to expand Medicaid and to establish health exchanges through which individuals could purchase coverage from private insurers.[27] Although the implementation of the ACA has gradually led to a decrease in the proportion of uninsured nonelderly persons in the United States, from 17.8 percent in 2010 to 10.4 percent in 2018,[28] immigrants' access to health care has generally seen little improvement. Immigrants who are lawfully present in the United States are potentially eligible for marketplace tax credits if their income is less than 400 percent of the federal poverty guideline. However, the ACA preserved the five-year bar instituted under PRWORA so that they are actually eligible only if five years have passed since becoming a qualified immigrant. Undocumented immigrants are explicitly prohibited from participating in either the federally subsidized health exchanges or the Medicaid expansion,[29,30,31] as are individuals in the United States with a temporary status, such as students and tourists, and those who entered as children and were granted status under Deferred Action for Childhood Arrivals (DACA).

2.3 Public Charge Provisions

The Immigration and Nationality Act of 1952 (INA)[32] provides for the inadmissibility of any alien applying for admission, adjustment to status of permanent residence (green card), or visa who is deemed to be "likely to become a public charge" (LPC). This provision, some form of which has been a part of US law for a century or more, is intended to identify those persons who are likely to rely on government resources as their primary source of support. Accordingly, an evaluation is to be conducted at the time of the individual's application to consider on a prospective basis whether the individual's age, health, family status, assets, resources, financial status, education, and skills are such that the individual is likely to become a public charge.

The Department of Homeland Security (DHS) had issued a final rule in 2019, effective February 24, 2020, that significantly changed the standard used by DHS in determining whether an individual would be LPC: any receipt of benefits for more than twelve months from specified programs within a rolling thirty-six-month period may now lead to a determination of LPC.[33] Additionally, the receipt of two benefits in one month was to be counted as two months, and the government officer was to consider, as well, the dollar amount of any benefit received. The rule would have exempted some categories of individuals from the rule's impact: US citizen children, members of the US armed forces and their family members, refugees, asylees, and certain visa applicants who have been trafficked and/or battered.[34,35]

This inclusion of both a specified duration and the dollar amount in the LPC evaluation significantly expanded the reach of the LPC provision, impacting not only those newly seeking legal status, but also those who are in the United States legally.[36] As an example, the receipt by a family of Supplemental Nutrition Assistance (formerly known as Food Stamps) for a US citizen child brings the noncitizen family members to the attention of the government agency. A family may decline to apply for this potential benefit out of fear that its receipt would lead to a denial of an immigration benefit, such as permanent residence, to noncitizen family members and, in the worst-case scenario, their deportation. This reticence to apply for the food assistance could lead to household food insecurity and poorer child health.[37]

However, on March 15, 2021, the US Citizenship and Immigration Service (USCIS) published a final rule that removed these regulations from the Federal Register and advised that it would not apply that standard to pending applications and petitions as of March 9, 2021. On March 9, a court order vacated the 2019 public charge rule after the federal government informed the Supreme Court that it would no longer defend the rule, which had been implemented under the Trump administration.[38]

Some individuals applying for permanent residence who cannot demonstrate on the basis of their own resources that they will not be a public charge may overcome their potential inadmissibility by presenting an affidavit from an individual who attests that they will provide the individual with the necessary support. These affidavits are most common in situations involving the immigration of a family member (e.g., when an adult citizen petitions for the immigration of his or her parents). Prior to the passage of the Illegal Immigration Reform and Immigrant Responsibility Act of 1996 (IIRAIRA),[39] affidavits of support provided by a sponsor on behalf of an individual seeking permanent residence were not generally enforceable legally. IIRAIRA provides for the enforceability of the affidavit and requires that the person signing an affidavit of support maintain the sponsored immigrant at an income level that is at least 125 percent of the federal poverty guidelines until the immigrant either becomes a US citizen or has been credited with forty qualifying quarters of work, whichever occurs first.[40] This sponsor support may be critical to individuals who have recently gained permanent residence and who develop health issues. If the individual does not have sufficient personal funds or privately funded or employer-sponsored insurance, he or she may have to rely on their sponsor's contribution to cover health-related expenses.[41] With very few exceptions, the sponsor's income will be deemed to the immigrant for a period of ten years or more, even if the sponsor's income is not actually available to the immigrant. It is unclear whether such affidavits will be sufficient to overcome a LPC determination in view of the more stringent standard that is now in place.

3.0 Implications of Restrictions

3.1 Health-Care Insurance Coverage and Access

It is clear that many immigrants who do not have employer-sponsored health insurance, coverage through a spouse or parent, or an individual health insurance plan will be unable to access health-care insurance at all due to these intersecting prohibitions in the health, immigration, and welfare laws. Even permanent residents are likely to experience difficulties accessing insurance if they have legally resided in the United States for ten years or less.[42] Those without insurance must pay out-of-pocket for their health-care expenses, self-treat, or seek care from a safety-net hospital or clinic.[43,44,45] Ongoing federal funding to safety-net facilities has recently been decreased based on the assumption that any such decreases would be offset by the numbers of newly insured individuals.[46] However, this diminution in funding raises questions as to the facilities' ongoing ability to meet the health-care needs of the uninsured population, including immigrants.[47] An inability to obtain insurance may lead to not only decreased access to needed care, but to adverse health outcomes, as well.

3.2 Case Example 1: Mental Illness and Substance Use Disorders

These measures impact particularly harshly on non-US citizens and their family members who are experiencing mental-health difficulties. Researchers utilizing a sample of 14,658 adults derived from consolidated data from the Medical Expenditure Panel Survey and the National Health Interview Survey from 2002 to 2006 found that immigrants were significantly less likely to use prescription drugs for mental illness compared to US-born citizens, a finding that was partly explainable by their lack of insurance.[48] A recent systematic review found that immigrants from Asia, Latin America, and Africa utilize mental-health services at a lower rate than nonimmi-grants, despite an equal or greater need.[49] Lack of insurance, the high cost of services, and fear of deportation were identified as major structural barriers to mental-health care.

Individuals detained by Immigration and Customs Enforcement (ICE), whether legally present in the United States or undocumented, may face not only a denial of needed treatment for an already-existing mental illness, but also exposure to conditions likely to exacerbate their illness. A study conducted by the Project on Government Oversight in 2017 that examined the records of the top fifteen immigrant detention facilities utilizing solitary confinement found that up to 82 percent of the records indicating solitary confinement at one detention facility pertained to mentally ill detainees.[50] Although placement in segregation may exacerbate preexisting mental ill-ness symptoms and increase the risk of suicide, mentally ill detainees in these facilities were often isolated for twenty-three hours per day, some for more than seventy-five consecutive days. An investigation of one detention facility by the US Office for Civil Rights and Civil Liberties concluded in 2018 that psychiatric leadership was inadequate, mental-health care was substandard, and detainees with serious mental disorders were routinely and inappropriately housed in administrative segregation.[51]

The potential impact of these various legislative provisions on eligi-bility for legal status and/or deportation and family separation has been found in various studies to be a deterrent not only to documented and undocumented immigrants' access to mental-health care, but to their US citizen family members, as well. Although children of immigrants who have been referred to the child welfare system have been found to have a similar level of clinical need compared with US-born children, those with undocumented parents are significantly less likely to receive needed mental-health services.[52] The inability to access these services is particu-larly troublesome in view of the violent and other traumatic experiences of many immigrants.[53] Even when they are eligible for services, individuals may avoid seeking care for fear that the providers will notify law enforce-ment personnel.[54]

Despite the removal of the 2019 regulations, the public charge provision likely continues to influence individuals' willingness to access even care for which they may be eligible. Because the provision relates to inadmissibility, it means that an individual's application for a particular immigrant status may be denied or that an individual may be denied entry to the country. Consequently, the provision may impact not only those seeking an immigration benefit, but their family members, as well. A parent applying for permanent resident status may delay seeking mental-health care for their US citizen child out of fear that their application for permanent residence will be delayed or ultimately denied, even though their child is eligible to receive publicly funded mental-health-care services. As yet another example, a permanent resident returning from a trip abroad may be questioned upon their return to a US airport by an immigration officer about their previous reliance on publicly funded services. An admission of their reliance on services for mental-health or substance-abuse care may lead to proceedings to find them inadmissible to the United States as likely to become a public charge[55] and, under a separate provision, as an individual with a mental or substance use disorder.[56] A false denial of such use could lead to proceedings to find them inadmissible on the basis of fraud or misrepresentation.[57] Even if the government's case against them were to prove unsuccessful, the individual and his or her family members would likely experience significant stress and expense to defend against the action.

3.3 Case Example 2: Trafficked, Abused, and Persecuted Noncitizens

There are no *health-focused* provisions in US immigration law or policy that are specifically directed to trafficked, abused, or persecuted noncitizens. However, individuals in such circumstances may be eligible for temporary or permanent legal status under various provisions of US immigration law. Eligibility for these immigration statuses may allow the individual to access publicly funded health care.

T visas, created by the 2000 Trafficking Victims Protection Act,[58] are potentially available to victims of severe labor or sex trafficking. A maximum of five thousand T visas may be granted annually.[59] The T visa grants individuals only temporary status in the United States. Successful applicants must present evidence proving that they:

- were forcibly transported for commercial sex or involuntary servitude;
- are physically present in the United States as a result of trafficking; and
- would experience "extreme hardship involving unusual and severe harm" if they were removed from the United States.

Additionally, a T visa applicant is required to comply with reasonable requests by law enforcement in their investigation and prosecution of their traffickers.

Later expansions of the statute provided access to this visa for children who have been kidnapped and enslaved by narco-traffickers along the southern US border.[60,61] Nevertheless, despite the 2016 loosening of the eligibility standard by the Department of Homeland Security, data suggest that a growing number of T visa applicants are being rejected due to an increasingly harsh interpretation of the definition of a victim of severe forms of trafficking.[62]

Individuals who successfully obtain a T visa are considered to be qualified for the purpose of receiving Medicaid, subject to meeting other eligibility requirements. They are also able to purchase private insurance through a marketplace plan established under the Affordable Care Act,[63] and, because they may obtain a work permit, they may potentially have access to employer-sponsored health insurance. T visa applicants are exempt from the public charge ground of admissibility and, as T visa holders, when applying for permanent residence.[64]

Permanent residence (a green card) is potentially available to T visa holders who can establish that they possess good moral character, have been continuously physically present in the United States for the lesser of three years or the duration of the investigation or prosecution, and would experience extreme hardship if they were removed from the United States.[65]

Like T visas, U visas are intended to protect noncitizen crime victims who assist or are willing to assist in the investigation and/or prosecution of a criminal offense. A U visa grants the holder temporary legal status for up to four years, which may be extended.[66] The statute provides for a maximum of ten thousand U visas annually.

In order to qualify for a U visa, the individual must demonstrate that:

- they experienced "substantial physical or mental abuse" as the result of being the victim of specified criminal activity, such as rape, trafficking, incest, being held hostage, false imprisonment, or sexual assault, among others;
- the criminal activity violated the laws of the United States or occurred in the United States or one of its territories or possessions;
- they hold information about the criminal activity;
- they have been helpful, are being helpful, or are likely to be helpful to the investigation or prosecution of the criminal activity;
- they have obtained certification from one of the specified authorities indicated in the statute to provide certification of their helpfulness; and
- they are not inadmissible.

Like recipients of the T visa, individuals who are granted a U visa are eligible to purchase private insurance through the marketplace established under the Affordable Care Act. They may also obtain a work permit and, depending upon their employment, may be able to obtain employer-sponsored insurance. However, they are not considered to be qualified for the purpose of Medicaid eligibility. They are not subject to the public charge ground of inadmissibility when applying for U visa status or when, as a U visa holder, they apply for permanent residence.[67] Permanent resident status is potentially available after they have been continuously physically present in the United States for three years, in addition to satisfying a number of other requirements.

Specified noncitizens who have been abused by a family member may be able to apply for permanent residence without having to rely on the abusive family member to sponsor them. The Violence Against Women Act,[68] originally passed by Congress in 1994 and amended since, permits the abused spouse or child of a US citizen or permanent resident or the abused parent of a US citizen son or daughter to seek permanent resident status through a self-petitioning process. With few exceptions, the abuser must be a US citizen or permanent resident. Additionally, the applicant must have been the victim of battery or extreme cruelty; must have resided with the abuser at some point in time; must reside in the United States or meet specified exceptions to this requirement; must be able to demonstrate good moral character; and, if it is a spouse petitioning for him- or herself, must demonstrate that they entered into the marriage in good faith. The applicant must be admissible, meaning that they are not ineligible for permanent residence on the basis of enumerated grounds of inadmissibility[69] or must qualify for a waiver of inadmissibility. In some situations, an abused spouse or child may include unmarried children under the age of twenty-one in their application. As noted in the previous discussion relating to Medicaid, individuals who receive permanent residence under this provision may be considered to be qualified for the purpose of determining Medicaid eligibility.

Asylum or refugee status is potentially available to individuals who are fleeing or who have fled their country on the basis of domestic violence, female genital mutilation, or LGBT status. Individuals who have been granted asylum or refugee status are also considered to be qualified for the purpose of receiving federally funded medical insurance and are not subject to the five-year waiting period.[70] A full discussion of the requirements for a successful application and process for either of these statuses is beyond the scope of this chapter. However, in brief, a successful asylum application requires that the applicant be physically present in the US; with limited exception, apply within one year of their last entry into the US; and demonstrate that they are unable or unwilling to return to their home country because:

- they have been persecuted in the past or have a well-founded fear of persecution in the future;
- by the government or a group that the government cannot control;
- because of their race, religion, nationality, membership in a particular social group, or political opinion.[71]

Courts have recognized that individuals who experience domestic violence,[72] who fear or have suffered female genital mutilation,[73,74] or who are persecuted on the basis of their sexual orientation or gender identity[75,76,77] may, depending upon the circumstances, be considered to be members of a particular social group that could form the basis of an asylum claim. Although individuals applying for asylum on these bases during the Trump administration had limited success, the Department of Justice has recently rescinded those Trump-era decisions.[78]

The importance of health-care access for these groups cannot be overemphasized. An analysis of 119 medical affidavits presented by asylum applicants in support of their applications found that 84 percent of the women had experienced some form of genital cutting. Almost three-quarters of the applicants experienced not only the acute effects of female genital cutting, but also suffered from chronic issues as a result, including post-traumatic stress disorder (72.4 percent), depression (65.9 percent), anxiety (51.1 percent), chronic difficulty with intercourse (81.7 percent), and chronic pain (42.4 percent).[79] The circumstances of battered immigrant women provide yet another example. Married immigrant women are at increased risk of physical and sexual abuse in comparison with unmarried immigrant women[80] and may have their immigration status used as a tool against them by their partners in an effort to keep them in the abusive relationship.[81] A New York City–based study found that 51 percent of victims of intimate partner homicide were foreign-born.[82]

4.0 Conclusion

Despite immigrants' sizable participation in and contributions to the US economy, the United States has implemented a complex, interwoven patchwork of laws designed to exclude, with few exceptions, non-US citizens from participation in publicly funded insurance programs. These provisions have been found to lead to decreased health-care access and adverse health-care outcomes for both immigrants and US citizens, raising questions as to whether they indeed fulfill their intended purpose of protecting the US economy and fostering self-sufficiency.

CHAPTER THIRTY-ONE

Eastern Mediterranean and Balkan Migration Route

Karl Philipp Puchner

1.0 Introduction

The Eastern Mediterranean and Balkan Migration Route (EMBMR) currently constitutes one of the most prominent channels of mixed migration worldwide.[1] Located in a fragile geopolitical context (as the western extension of the Middle East), the Eastern Mediterranean and the Balkans have repeatedly witnessed mass population movements in the past few decades.[2,3] Despite these historical precedents, continuous or even augmenting instability throughout the broader Middle East region for more than two decades has resulted in unprecedented numbers of refugees and migrants fleeing their home countries along the EMBMR since the beginning of 2015.[4] For most of the time in their recent history, host countries along the EMBMR have largely had a negative migration rate and thus lack experience in issues of the resource allocation and governance required with an influx of migrants.[5,6] Migration along the EMBMR is characterized by extremely dangerous border crossings, incomplete and often recurrent migration cycles, and volatile internal (i.e., between the states along the route) and external (i.e., toward central and northern European countries) flow dynamics—all heavily dependent on the geopolitical context of the region and the discrepant or often contradictory government approaches of the state actors involved.[7] This migration context can have a significant impact on the health status of those settling or in transit along the EMBMR. In this chapter, we will analyze the specific health risks, the burden of disease, and the access to health care of refugees and migrants in the region during different phases of the migratory process. We will also propose interventions for improvement of the well-being of this population.

2.0 Geopolitical Context and Forecast of Migration Flows

Sharing borders with various home countries of forcibly displaced people, like Syria or Iraq, Turkey constitutes the entry and first important junction point along this route. With almost four million refugees and asylum seekers residing within its national territory, Turkey has the highest refugee population worldwide and the fifth largest in relation to its national population (one in twenty-three residents in Turkey are refugees).[8] In addition, as an emerging economy with major airport hubs and booming metropolitan areas like Istanbul, Turkey has attracted large numbers of migrants from sub-Saharan Africa and Southeast Asia.[9] However, faced with prolonged political instability internally as well as at its borders and the emergence of serious economic challenges, Turkey is strained in its capacity to absorb migrant flows. With push factors for further migration multiplying, refugees and migrants residing for years in Turkey might re-enter the migratory process in the coming years to seek new destination countries.[10] On the other hand, Greece, as a member state of the European Union (EU) and often the second country along the EMBMR, and in 2020 hosted approximately 120,000 refugees and migrants. Greece attracts a substantial number of refugees and migrants seeking to apply for asylum in an EU country or be reunited with family members living in this or other EU countries.[11] However, despite significant political reforms, investments, and staff deployment in the past five years, the asylum process in Greece remains extremely lengthy and bureaucratic, often leaving refugees and migrants in a state of legal limbo for years.[12] Relocation and family reunification programs from Greece to other European countries, initially introduced in 2015, continue to exist, although output of these seems to be subject to changing political currents and priorities within the EU.[13] With its economy still recovering from a prolonged crisis of almost a decade, Greece, despite having attracted large numbers of economic migrants in the decades of 1990s and 2000s, currently has extremely low economic absorption capacities for refugees and migrants.[14] Further west in the EMBMR region, Balkan countries (Albania, Northern Macedonia, Bulgaria, Serbia, and Bosnia and Herzegovina) are less attractive to migrants and refugees. With the exception of Bulgaria, these countries are not members of the EU and have relatively weak economies and welfare states.[15] Thus, in the majority of cases, these are merely transit countries for refugees and migrants intending to reach their destination countries, mostly located in Central or Northern Europe, outside of regular migration channels.

Although movement along the EMBMR has decreased substantially since the beginning of 2020, it is still hard to foresee the long-term implications the Covid-19 pandemic might have on migration flows in the broader geographic area.[16] Toward the end of 2019, the total number of Syrian nationals in Turkish territory had stabilized, even as a significant influx of newly arrived refugees and migrants from Syria and other countries entering via land borders of the country kept the total numbers of refugees and migrants in the country at a record high.[17] Since the introduction of the EU-Turkey deal in 2016, which aspires to the return of refugees and migrants arriving outside the regular migration channels to the Greek Islands back to Turkey, the migratory influx to Greece has dropped substantially.[18] Nevertheless, with increasing securitization of its northern borders and swift changes in migration policies, including the temporary halt of family reunification programs of key European destination countries, Greece's refugee and migrant population has risen gradually to a record high of almost 120,000 in October 2020.[19]

Migratory movements occurring along the EMBMR are extremely volatile in terms of geography, speed, and intensity, although most movement patterns include some major junction points.[20] Although outflow through regular migration channels to other European countries has never ceased completely, a non-negligible proportion of refugees and migrants have been attempting to migrate further using border crossings and sea routes toward destination countries in Central or Northern Europe.[21] The majority of them travel through neighboring countries of the Balkans by following a constantly increasing number of different routes.[22] Serbia and Bosnia and Herzegovina are lately experiencing substantial increases of refugees and migrants stranded within their territories. In Bosnia and Herzegovina, the number of recorded new arrivals has skyrocketed from 755 in 2017 to 29,196 in 2019, as the country lies on a new route transiting Albania and Montenegro, two countries with still relatively porous borders.[23] Although absolute numbers of refugees and migrants in the Western Balkans are relatively small, the proper provision of humanitarian aid and protection is extremely challenging, as national governments and international agencies remain ill-prepared and often unwilling to improve migration governance in the region.[24] In addition, the extremely high mobility of refugees and migrants along the last part of the EMBMR and the not infrequently observed return to Greece—as none of the Western Balkan countries are seen as destination countries—make adequate planning and the implementation of proper humanitarian response and governance within the broader geographic area extremely difficult. Therefore, the EMBMR is characterized by an extremely fragmented geopolitical landscape, fluctuating push and pull factors, and volatile migration movement dynamics. This context significantly increases the vulnerability of those on the move and is likely to hinder the integration of refugees and migrants in the respective society and health system of the hosting countries.[25]

3.0 Demographics of Migrant Populations along the EMBMR

The migrant population moving along the EMBMR is extremely diverse and heterogeneous. The overwhelming majority of refugees and migrants residing in Turkey are Syrian nationals, who, in contrast to the other countries of the EMBMR, enjoy only temporary protection. It should be noted that the UN Protocol of 1967, which widened the definition of asylum seekers/refugees beyond the geographic scope of Europe as described in the initial Geneva Convention of Refugees in 1951, was never ratified by Turkey. Thus, Turkey does not recognize Syrian nationals as refugees but, through a Temporary Protection Regime, grants them the right to legally stay in Turkish territory and some level of access to very basic rights and services. Apart from this population group, there are a non-negligible number of Afghan, Maghrebi, sub-Saharan African, Iranian, and Pakistani refugees and migrants in the region.[26] While Syrian nationals used to be the most prevalent refugee and migrant group along the full length of EMBMR, the composition of the migrant population in each country of the region can vary substantially. Thus, while the majority of refugees and migrants arriving and residing currently in Greece are Afghans (followed by Syrians),[27] in the Western Balkans, people from Pakistan constitute the most prevalent migrant category.[28] Apart from the heterogeneity with respect to the country of origin, the migrant population reveals extreme demographic diversity; there are substantial numbers of unaccompanied minors, families, single male and female adults, pregnant women, people living with disabilities, and elders.[29] This demographic diversity adds complexity to the response and governance of the migratory process along the EMBMR, as distinct groups often exhibit quite different migration profiles, protection rights, integration potential, and heath needs.[30]

4.0 Health Status of Refugees and Migrants during Premigration Phase

As already discussed, refugees and migrants along the EMBMR originate from a range of different countries with diverse socioeconomic conditions, health systems, and epidemiological profiles. Refugees and migrants from conflict-torn countries like Syria or Afghanistan already have, in the pre-migration phase, poor mental health as a result of chronic exposure to stress, insecurity, and traumatic experiences.[31,32,33] In addition, some refugees and migrants from conflict-torn countries might have experienced war- or torture-related injuries with permanent musculoskeletal sequelae and disabilities.[34,35] Within the context of the epidemiological transition occurring in low- and middle-income countries (LMICs), the prevalence of noncommunicable diseases is increasing rapidly, particularly in countries of the Indian subcontinent and the Middle East,[36] while high levels of poverty and social exclusion, weak health-system performance, and ongoing conflict often hinder the provision of proper care for patients with chronic conditions in most of the countries of origin.[37] Major infectious diseases, like HIV or chronic viral hepatitis, might be already present in the premigration phase, particularly in refugees and migrants originating from high-endemic countries of sub-Saharan Africa and/or the Indian subcontinent. However, evidence from European destination countries suggests that refugees and migrants are highly likely to acquire these diseases during the migratory process due to increased vulnerability.[38,39] Latent tuberculosis (TB), for example, is highly prevalent among the general population in high-endemic TB countries of sub-Saharan Africa and the Indian subcontinent, might be present in the premigration phase, and may evolve to full-blown TB during the migratory process.[40] Finally, some refugees and migrants enter the migratory process along the EMBMR being pregnant or in the postnatal period. While these conditions do not constitute health problems, they can significantly increase the vulnerability of both the mother and the infant during the migratory process.[41]

5.0 Health Status during Movement Phase

During the movement phase of the migration cycle, refugees and migrants can be exposed to a range of health risks that can cause disease, aggravate already existing conditions, or even lead to death. Mode of travel, geography, level of militarization of borders crossed, migration governance and policies in transit countries, economic resources and travel documents of the individual refugees and migrants, and health status in the premigration phase influence the health risks people might encounter during the movement phase.[42] Within the context of the EMBMR, border crossing—often impossible via regular/legal migration channels—is extremely hazardous. The highly militarized southeastern land borders of Turkey constitute prominent entry points to the EMBMR. According to reports of the Turkish Armed Forces, in 2018 alone, a total of at least 224,358 people have been apprehended while trying to enter irregularly along the Syria-Turkey land borders in 2018.[43] With no option of applying for international protection directly at the border, refugees and migrants have to try to enter Turkish territory either by climbing a three-meter border wall, running the risk of being shot at by border troops, or paying smugglers or bribing border guards. Although exact numbers are unknown, numerous reports on fatal incidents and missing persons along this highly militarized border are suggestive of an extremely dangerous border crossing.[44] Borders to Iraq or Iran seem to be easier to cross; however, due to the mountainous nature of these border areas, exposure to extreme weather conditions for which refugees and migrants on the move are often ill-prepared frequently lead to frostbite, hypothermia, or even death.[45] Further border crossings toward Greece prove to be dangerous, as well. UNHCR statistics reveal a rate of dead and missing among new refugees and migrant arrivals to Greece, ranging from 0.01 percent to 0.06 percent since 2015 (table 31.1).[46] The majority of the fatalities are attributable to shipwreck and drowning—particularly of small children and infants—in the stretch of the Aegean Sea between the Turkish coast and the eastern Greek Islands. It is likely that total numbers of dead and missing along the Greek-Turkish borders are higher, as reports increasingly reveal dangerous pushback practices performed on the open sea by Greek coast guard authorities.[47] Resulting shipwrecks are likely to remain unregistered on both sides of the borders. Border crossings northward of Greece along the EMBMR are also associated with major health risks. There is growing evidence of extreme violence, brutal pushbacks, illegal forms of detention, and even torture practices by police forces and other non-state actors, particularly along the borders of Bosnia and Herzegovina to Croatia or Serbia to Hungary.[48,49] Sealing of the borders due to the Covid-19 pandemic has led to further aggravation of violence suffered by

TABLE 31.1 **New arrivals of refugees and migrants in Greek territory, 2015–2020**

Previous years	Sea arrivals	Land arrivals	Dead and missing (% of total N of arrivals)
2020	9,687	5,982	100 (0.06%)
2019	59,726	14,887	71 (0.01%)
2018	32,494	18,014	174 (0.03%)
2017	29,718	6,592	59 (0.02%)
2016	173,450	3,784	441 (0.02%)
2015	856,723	4,907	799 (0.01%)

refugees and migrants trying to move irregularly along the EMBMR.[50] However, it should not be forgotten that movement within the national territories proves to be hazardous, as well: there is increasing anecdotal evidence of refugees and migrants being involved in often deadly traffic accidents. This frequently happens within the context of refugees and migrants walking along unsafe roads like high-speed highways or railway tracks or being recklessly driven by smugglers.[51,52] High exposure to, and low protection from, violence, including sexual violence by non-state actors, is often reported by refugees and migrants on the move along the EMBMR.[53] Human trafficking and trafficking-related sexual and gender-based violence (SGBV) is a constant peril along the EMBMR, particularly for unaccompanied minors and women on the move.[54] States of temporary or prolonged homelessness, imprisonment, or detention are known to have an extremely negative impact on physical and mental health.[55] These conditions are experienced, often repeatedly, by a significant number of refugees and migrants along the EMBMR.[56,57] Finally, due to an unwillingness to delay transit and multiple barriers to health-care access, the use of health services by the refugees and migrants during this phase of the migratory process seems to be extremely low and almost limited to emergencies such as injuries or severe infections. This results in the aggravation of chronic conditions and inadequate prenatal and pediatric care and favors disease manifestation at a later stage.[58]

6.0 Health Status of Refugees and Migrants during Arrival and Integration Phase

The arrival phase follows a temporal or permanent conclusion of the movement phase and is usually reached by (provisional) settlement in a reception camp, registration facility, or junction point along the EMBMR. At this stage, the refugees and migrants might apply for asylum, seek a job, gather information and resources needed for further traveling, contact the existing migrant community, and start seeking health services for neglected and/or chronic health problems. Indeed, evidence from the EMBMR shows a clear shift in the pattern of conditions refugees and migrants present with when transiting from the movement to the arrival phase. The predominant causes for seeking health services during the movement phase are acute emergency-like conditions, such as trauma and infections. During the arrival phase, though, clear increases in chronic noncommunicable or reproductive health conditions can be observed among refugees and migrants,[59] and the impact of social determinants of health becomes gradually more evident.[60] Poor living and hygiene conditions and overcrowding characterize the majority of camps, reception, and registration facilities, resulting in the spread of infectious diseases — including those that are vaccine-preventable — and substantially increasing the burden of communicable conditions of this vulnerable population after arrival.[61] Camp-based syndromic approach surveillance data from both Turkey and Greece are indicative of periodical outbreaks, particularly of diarrheal and infectious skin diseases. Additionally, measles, hepatitis A, and varicella outbreaks among residents of refugee camps in both countries have been described in literature.[62,63,64] The extreme vulnerability of refugees and migrants to infectious diseases and their detrimental consequences is once again exemplified in the Covid-19 pandemic. Fast-spreading Covid-19 cluster outbreaks have been observed in many camps and reception centers along the EMBMR, while lockdown measures taken in order to respond to the pandemic — often involving the total quarantine of affected camps and treatment of cases found in situ — have aggravated the precarious socioeconomic and health conditions of refugees and migrants.[65,66] Settlement in camps and reception centers or urban junction points along the EMBMR can lead to further threats for those entering the arrival phase. Single women or unaccompanied minors are often lodged in overcrowded camps lacking safe zones, exposing them to the risk of sexual violence and exploitation. The failure to meet basic protection criteria is observed regularly among people settling in urban junction points. With less facilitated access to services and provisions than registered camp residents, refugees and migrants settling in urban centers find themselves in precarious socioeconomic conditions and may resort to survivor sex work or find themselves subject to forced labor and human trafficking in order cover their basic needs.[67,68] As temporary protection granted by the Turkish state is vaguely defined and subject to frequently changing practices and policies,[69] uncertainty about the exact nature and duration of their legal status, rights, and entitlements to services in Turkey exposes refugees and migrants settling in the country to toxic levels of chronic stress, which in turn may lead to mental-health disorders.[70] Prolonged stays in overcrowded substandard camps and reception centers and lengthy asylum procedures leave people in a state of legal limbo, which is typical of migration governance practices in Greece. These stays, together with arbitrary detention, are highly traumatizing experiences associated with mental distress and anxiety, further challenging the already poor mental health of many refugees and migrants.[71] It is during that phase or even later on, during the integration phase, that typical mental-health conditions begin to manifest and are diagnosed in the interactions of people with the health systems in both countries (Turkey and Greece). Indeed, evidence from these countries suggests that time elapsed since arrival in the host country may be an independent risk factor for major depressive disorders and other mental-health disorders.[72,73] However, it seems that migrant-friendly mental-health services, in particular, are at the moment insufficient in both these host countries. In conjunction with the scarcity of migrant-friendly rehabilitative and preventive services and the prevalence of multiple cultural and administrative barriers, access to health care for migrants and refugees settling in Turkey and Greece is poor, resulting in the overuse of emergency room (ER) services, low vaccination rates, inadequate primary and secondary health care, and poor health outcomes in this population.[74,75,76,77,78] These conditions not only fuel inequalities and overstretch the capacities of the respective health system; they also undermine social cohesion and obstruct integration of refugees and migrants in their host societies.[79] Access to health for refugees and migrants arriving in Western Balkan countries might be even more compromised. The medical systems of these countries, often hardly able to provide free services for the native population within,[80] run the risk of being completely overstretched by the influx of refugees and migrants, leaving this vulnerable population on the move without health coverage.[81] Finally, undocumented refugees and migrants, even in the case of successful integration in the socioeconomic life of the hosting countries along the EMBMR, find themselves excluded from the respective national or provisional health systems, and their access to health care is thus largely restricted to emergency services.[82,83]

7.0 Required Interventions and Recommendations

It is evident that the limited legal options offered to people seeking international protection and/or employment in countries of the EU fuel migration along the EMBMR. As long as the migration and asylum policy of the EU remains restrictive, movements along the EMBMR entailing hazardous borders will persist. Further militarization of borders along the EMBRM, as seen lately within the context of the Covid-19 pandemic, does not decrease and may actually increase exposure to health risks and the likelihood of injuries and fatal incidents among the people on the move.[84] Better documentation of reports and testimonies, the compilation of data from different national and international sources, and field studies are urgently needed. In parallel, rigorous advocacy at the national and international level for adoption of the Health in All Policies approach and a stronger commitment to the recently signed Global Compact for Safe, Orderly, and Regular Migration (which obliges signatory states to protect the safety, freedom, and fundamental rights of all refugees and migrants, regardless of legal status, and was signed by all EMBMR countries with the exception of Bulgaria and Kosovo), the health- and migration-related Sustainable Development Goals, and the WHO Constitution by state actors are key in order to protect the life and dignity of refugees and migrants moving along the EMBRM. In addition, the promotion of a regional and harmonized Migration Governance is urgently required in order to optimize humanitarian response to the observed migrant flows.[85] Targeted outreach health interventions along prominent transit routes,[86] the introduction of optional eHealth solutions, like the electronic personal health file,[87] and the scaling-up of refugee- and migrant-oriented primary health services in important junction points along the EMBMR could prevent health deterioration and secure some degree of continuity of care for people during the movement phase of their migration process.[88]

Multidisciplinary vulnerability assessments, improved protections, and the adequate coverage of basic needs are needed once the refugees and migrants arrive in order to address underlying social determinants of their health and reduce their vulnerability. Free voluntary primary health examinations provided within the context of the respective national health system and focusing on maternal and child well-being and both communicable and noncommunicable diseases should be made available to refugees and migrants soon after arrival. These health examinations might serve as the first step of educating them about the respective medical system and offer the opportunity of timely prevention, diagnosis, and treatment.[89,90]

Finally, unconditional access to health services and extending coverage so that it matches that of the native population at all phases of the migration process should be considered. There is growing evidence supporting the idea that unrestricted medical entitlements for all categories of refugees and migrants may drastically reduce expenditures on health systems and improve health outcomes in this very population.[91,92,93] Responsiveness of health systems to the special needs of refugees and migrants and tailored interventions in these communities should be fostered.[94] Finally, training medical professionals and students on transcultural health approaches, tackling institutional racism, and deploying cultural mediators at all levels of care would facilitate the integration of refugees and migrants in the respective health system.[95,96]

8.0 Conclusion

The EMBMR poses one of the most complex mixed-migration channels in current times. Exposure to risk factors specific to the geopolitical context, mode, and phase of migration can have major impacts on the health of refugees and migrants in the region. Multiple barriers to health-care access and the predominance of negative social determinants of health throughout the migration process along the EMBMR further threaten the well-being and increase the vulnerability of this population. Bold changes in migration and medical policies in the countries along the EMBMR and at the EU level are urgently needed in order to avoid rising health inequalities and excess mortality among the growing migrant population of the region.

CHAPTER THIRTY-TWO

Migration and Health in Nepal

Sabrina Hermosilla, Emily Treleaven, and Dirgha Ghimire

Migration directly affects almost half of Nepali households.[1] The Nepali migrant experience provides a unique opportunity to explore many of the key issues related to migration and health. This chapter examines the history of migration in Nepal, the drivers and demographics of migrants—both to and from Nepal—and the implications of these movements on population health.

1.0 Migration in Nepal: A Brief History

Tucked between China and India, Nepal—with a population of just under thirty million people—was historically a very isolated country, with limited nonregulated migration to India by the British Brigade of Gurkha soldiers starting in 1815.[2] With the Foreign Employment Act of 1985, transnational labor migration to destinations other than India first became a viable option. The act licensed nongovernmental institutions to mobilize the Nepali workforce abroad and legitimized labor contracting organizations, spurring streams of transnational migration, primarily to the Gulf Cooperation Council (GCC) countries and other East Asian Countries. Today, Nepali migrate to over 153 different countries.[3]

2.0 Nepali Migrants: At Home and Around the World

Understanding the complex relationship between migration and health requires an in-depth look into the unique geopolitical, cultural, and economic factors that shape the Nepali experience at home and abroad.

2.1 Nepali People Around the World: Who Is Migrating and Why

2.1.1 TRANSNATIONAL MIGRANTS.   Employment is the most common motivation for transnational migration from Nepal.[4] Similar to other migrant-sending settings where temporary transnational labor migration is a common livelihood strategy, a majority of transnational temporary labor migrants from Nepal have short contracts (two to three years), low levels of education, and are married men (most ages fifteen to forty-four) with children at home, though women are migrating in increasingly higher quantities.[5] While many migrants have family members who also migrate for work, most go on specific jobs and contracts alone.[6]

2.1.2 WHERE THEY GO AND WHAT THEY ARE DOING.   In 2018 and 2019, almost 85 percent of international labor permits from Nepal were issued for GCC destinations (Qatar, 31.8%; United Arab Emirates [UAE], 26.6%; Saudi Arabia, 19.6%; Kuwait, 6.8%);[7] however, this is a known underestimate, as many transnational migrants from Nepal travel informally via India to their final destinations.[8] Migrants to GCC countries must participate in the labor sponsorship system (*kafala* in Arabic) that requires permission from their sponsor before taking another position, making job mobility all but impossible. Migrants often go into debt to secure transnational labor permits, leaving them vulnerable to exploitation and trafficking, both at home from labor brokers and abroad.[9] Practices such as passport holding, salary withholding, and not registering with local governments for services such as health and education are common.[10] In addition to being geographically far from home, transnational labor migrants from Nepal to the GCC also live in a community with a different predominant religion, and very few speak local business languages, such as Arabic or English.[11]

India and Nepal share an open border, complicating the documentation of transnational migration.[12] Migrants to India are predominantly male, have little to no primary education, and are from the lowest-income families in Nepal.[13] They lack basic legal labor protections and experience delays in wages and unpaid overtime, live in overcrowded and unsafe settings, and lack meaningful access to health care.[14]

Transnational migrants from Nepal—regardless of destination country—often engage in work that is physically and emotionally taxing, such as construction and security. These jobs are often called the *three Ds* (dangerous, difficult, and dirty),[15] and employers frequently do not adhere to local health, safety, and labor laws.[16] In GCC countries, Nepali migrants typically live in (often overcrowded) camps organized by their employer and are segregated from local residents.[17] Beyond these harsh living conditions, at work, migrants have less access to protective clothing or equipment and thus have increased exposure to toxic agents, especially in agriculture, construction, manufacturing, and mining sectors.[18]

Although temporary labor migration is the most common motivation among Nepali people migrating transnationally, some Nepali migrate for education, family, or other reasons.[19] Women are more likely than men to report family reasons as the motive behind their migration.[20] These patterns reflect gender norms in Nepal, where men are expected to financially support their spouses, children, and parents as they age.[21] Given the lack of economic opportunities at home, migration, even with challenges, is a common way to meet these financial demands.

2.1.2 HEALTH PROFILE: TRANSNATIONAL MIGRANTS. Understanding the health profiles of migrants before, during, and after migration spells is essential to grasping the complex relationship between migration and health. In Nepal, as is common in transnational labor migration, migrants tend to be slightly healthier than those who stay behind.[22] However, migrants do not fare as well when they travel abroad.

Few studies have accurately documented the health profile of Nepali abroad. Nepali migrants suffer from occupational hazards. While data are scarce, Joshi and colleagues, who interviewed returned migrants in the Nepali International Airport and nearby hotels, found that Nepali migrants were more likely than local coworkers to suffer occupational injuries and disabilities, as 25 percent of migrants interviewed had experienced a jobsite accident and over half (56.6%) had experienced some health problem in the past twelve months abroad.[23]

Migrants' daily routines and access to services in their destination country also shape their health status. Many migrants return home early due to mental health problems arising from dangerous work and living conditions.[24] More than half do not have access to local health care, even when in the destination country on a legal work visa.[25] Official Nepal reports have documented 460 transnational labor migrant deaths by suicide while living abroad from 2010 to 2016.[26]

Given the temporary and cyclical nature of transnational labor migration originating and terminating in Nepal, the health profile of returnees is important to understand. While data around returned transnational labor migrants are limited, studies have found that among older adults (forty-five-plus years), people with a history of migration rate their overall current health worse and report higher functional difficulties compared to those without a history of migration. Migrants may also bring back adaptive habits meant to ameliorate the harsh working and living conditions while abroad. For example, studies have found that more than half of returned migrants are current smokers and alcohol users, substantially more than the local population.[27] While women make up a small proportion of the transnational labor force, returned women have high burdens of past-year depression and stress.[28] Migrants also appear to have increased rates of contraceptive use, as compared to nonmigrants.[29]

Given that health expenses are primarily the responsibility of migrants and their families,[30] migrants experience the negative effects of transnational migration across the social and economic gradient. They experience worse health outcomes if they are widowed/divorced, from a minority group (based on gender, caste, or religion), work in either a factory or security guard when abroad, are poorer, and are older.[31] The Nepali government has made efforts to support returnees; migrants are eligible for financial compensation should they become physically ill or die while abroad. However, this only applies to those on a work permit (thus none to India) and does not cover mental health conditions.[32]

2.2 Nepali Internal Migration

In Nepal, internal migration is primarily rural-origin individuals migrating to urban settings.[33] As compared to transnational labor migration, internal migrants are more likely to be female, young (over 75% are under twenty-nine years old), come from the high mountains and hills—areas with low agriculture productivity, difficult terrain, and harsh living conditions—and be somewhat more highly educated than transnational labor migrants, and they are just as likely to be married as unmarried.[34] Internal migrants move primarily for education and training (31.3% in 2011) and for family reasons (30.9%), while some are moving to look for work (13.0%) or work-related reasons (18.2%).[35] As with most processes in Nepal, this picture is highly gendered. For women, marriage (58.9%) and family reasons (20.1%) are the primary drivers of internal migration, with work coming in last at 6%. For men, however, almost half of internal migrants move for work (49.7%), and none list marriage as a reason (wives often move to a husband's household).[36] Internal migrants in Nepal are primarily employed in service (32.8%) industries.[37]

Few studies have explored the health conditions of these internal migrants within Nepal. While changing, Nepali culture has historically placed strong restrictions on women's and girls' movement and activities, and they have a higher chance of experiencing gender-based violence and exploitation, even while in their natal homes. Migrant female workers, away from traditional family and friend social networks, are at even greater risk of exploitation. A study among adolescent (fourteen- to nineteen-year-olds) garment factory workers in Kathmandu (capital of Nepal) reported a quarter (26.1%) of their first sexual experiences were the result of "force from partner."[38] The majority of adolescents also reported not using condoms during their first sexual encounter, even though education around condom use and availability is high.[39] Further studies around the impact of temporary and seasonal migration in Nepal are warranted to better understand the unique challenges and potential opportunities that such migration brings to the population.

2.3 Nepali Who Stay Behind

Migration affects the health and well-being of not only migrants themselves, but also the spouses, parents, and children left behind in households and villages of origin. Many of the young adult men who engage in transnational migration from Nepal are married with young children.[40] Given the nature of the formal labor contracts that allow these men to migrate, their family members typically remain at home.

Family members left behind must take up the labor and caregiving tasks previously performed by the migrant, which may have physical impacts. A spouse left behind with young children might be responsible for both maintaining the family farm and caring for children and elderly parents. Taking on this additional physical labor might cause physical stress for the left-behind parent, while the additional time demands might reduce their social participation outside the home, causing mental stress.

Health and financial security are interrelated in migrant-sending families. In addition to having direct effects on physical and mental health, migration can also affect access to health care among family members left behind, depending on how the family's financial situation changes after migration. For households whose economic status or security improves due to financial support from a migrant family member, migration may contribute toward improving the physical health status of those left behind if they have better access to health care. For young children, migrant remittances might allow them to enjoy a more diverse diet and enhanced food security, which can translate to improved health status and reduced undernutrition—especially important given Nepal's high rates of stunting, or chronic malnutrition.[41] However, for some families, migration represents a financial risk, leaving them more economically vulnerable compared to their position before migration.[42] If family members left behind experience food insecurity, children in these households may have a higher risk of undernutrition. These households may also be more likely to accrue health-related debts, which could make the family even more economically vulnerable over the long term. These types of financial stress and uncertainty can also negatively affect the mental health of left-behind family members.

2.3 Immigrants in Nepal

In addition to sending migrants around the world, Nepal is home to over 150,000 immigrants from three main countries of origin.[43] By population size, immigrants from India (87%) are the largest group; however, little is known about the health of Indian immigrants in Nepal. Nepal is also home to almost twenty thousand refugees; 64 percent of those are Tibetan refugees (who entered Nepal after the 1959 Tibetan uprising against neighboring China's rule in Lhasa, capital of the Tibet Autonomous Region),[44] and 32 percent are Bhutanese refugees (110,000 at their height in the 1990s, down to around 6,500 after third-country relocation efforts).[45] Having fled civil unrest in both cases, as with most forcibly displaced populations, these groups have higher levels of common types of responses to stress, including post-traumatic stress disorder, somatization of distress, and generalized anxiety disorder.[46]

3.0 Migration and Health in Nepal: Future Directions

What can the Nepali experience teach us about migration and health more broadly? As in many migrant-sending settings, understanding the connection between migration and health in Nepal is complex and hindered by insufficient information. Nepali migration is driven by economic opportunities, geopolitical affairs, and health on an individual, family, and community level. Individually, migrants make decisions, as all individuals do, to maximize their opportunities for themselves and their families. Given the current economic situation in Nepal, many of these opportunities lie outside the country. Families within Nepal recognize the importance and relative benefit that having a migrant abroad may bring; thus, they may come together to support both the migrant themselves and the family left behind. Communities and the Nepali government see an overall economic benefit from Nepali transnational labor migrants' financial remittances, but the health impact on migrants, their family members, and their communities is still poorly understood. Across the migration process, access to health care, including preventative measures and mental health services, is essential to ameliorate the stressors on migrants and their families. Labor protections at home and abroad shape migrant health and cannot be separated from the discussion of health and migration.

The Nepali migration experience will be better understood with complete longitudinal studies exploring the long-term consequences of both transnational labor and internal migration. To date, most studies have been cross-sectional and of limited sample size or nonrepresentative sampling techniques or qualitative designs. To guide responses to improve migrant health, rigorous, population-based, longitudinal studies are essential.

A better understanding of the Nepali experience will help us explore themes of inequality, gender-based exploitation, and social gradients of health that are salient in contexts far beyond Nepal.

Bibliography

Adhikary, Pratik, Steven Keen, and Edwin van Teijlingen. "Health Issues among Nepalese Migrant Workers in the Middle East." *Health Science Journal* 5, no. 3 (2011): 169–75.

Adhikary, Pratik, Steve Keen, and Edwin van Teijlingen. "Workplace Accidents among Nepali Male Workers in the Middle East and Malaysia: A Qualitative Study." *Journal of Immigrant and Minority Health* 21, no. 5 (October 1, 2019): 1115–22. https://doi.org/10.1007/s10903-018-0801-y.

Agudelo-Suárez, Andrés A., Diana Gil-González, Carmen Vives-Cases, John G. Love, Peter Wimpenny, and Elena Ronda-Pérez. "A Metasynthesis of Qualitative Studies Regarding Opinions and Perceptions about Barriers and Determinants of Health Services' Accessibility in Economic Migrants." *BMC Health*

Services Research 12, no. 1 (December 17, 2012): 461. https://doi.org/10.1186/1472
-6963-12-461.

Bennett, Lynn. "Sex and Motherhood among the Brahmins and Chhetris of East-
Central Nepal." *Contribution to Nepalese Studies* 3, no. Special Issue (June
1976): 1–52.

"Bhutan Refugees Rally for Help to Go Back Home." *Kathmandu Post*, December 11, 2018. Reliefweb.int. https://reliefweb.int/report/nepal/bhutan-refugees
-rally-help-go-back-home.

Cortes, Patricia. "The Feminization of International Migration and Its Effects on the
Children Left Behind: Evidence from the Philippines." *Migration and Development* 65 (January 1, 2015): 62–78. https://doi.org/10.1016/j.worlddev.2013.10.021.

Dhungana, Raja Ram, Nirmal Aryal, Pratik Adhikary, Radheshyam Krishna KC,
Pramod Raj Regmi, Bikash Devkota, Guna Nidhi Sharma, Kolitha Wickram-
age, Edwin van Teijlingen, and Padam Simkhada. "Psychological Morbidity in
Nepali Cross-Border Migrants in India: A Community Based Cross-Sectional
Study." *BMC Public Health* 19, no. 1 (November 15, 2019): 1534. https://doi
.org/10.1186/s12889-019-7881-z.

Gardner, Andrew M. "Labor Camps in the Gulf States." In *Viewpoints: Migration
and the Gulf*, 55–57. Washington, DC: The Middle East Institute, 2010.

Gardner, Andrew M, Silvia Pessoa, Abdoulaye Diop, Kaltham Al-Ghanim, Kien
Le Trung, and Laura Harkness. "A Portrait of Low-Income Migrants in Contemporary Qatar." *Journal of Arabian Studies* 3, no. 1 (June 1, 2013): 1–17.
https://doi.org/10.1080/21534764.2013.806076.

Global Focus UNHCR Operations Worldwide. "Nepal." Accessed October 20,
2020.. https://reporting.unhcr.org/node/10316.

Government of Nepal, Ministry of Labour and Employment. "Labour Migration
for Employment—A Status Report for Nepal: 2014/2015." Kathmandu, Nepal:
Government of Nepal, Ministry of Labour and Employment, 2016.

Government of Nepal, Ministry of Labour, Employment and Social Security. "Nepal Labour Migration Report 2020." Kathmandu, Nepal: Government of Nepal,
Ministry of Labour, Employment and Social Security, 2020. https://moless.gov
.np/wp-content/uploads/2020/03/Migration-Report-2020-English.pdf.

Graner, Elvira, and Ganesh Gurung. "Arab Ko Lahure: Looking at Nepali Labour
Migrants to Arabian Countries." *Contributions to Nepalese Studies* 30, no. 2
(2003): 295–325.

Gurung, Harka B. "Internal and International Migration in Nepal [in Nepali]."
Main Report. Kathmandu: HMG Population Commission, 1983.

Hull, Diana. "Migration, Adaptation, and Illness: A Review." *Social Science and
Medicine. Part A: Medical Psychology and Medical Sociology* 13 (January 1,
1979): 25–36. https://doi.org/10.1016/0271-7123(79)90005-1.

Joshi, Suresh, Padam Simkhada, and Gordon J. Prescott. "Health Problems of
Nepalese Migrants Working in Three Gulf Countries." *BMC International*

Health and Human Rights 11, no. 1 (March 28, 2011): 3. https://doi.org/10.1186
/1472-698X-11-3.

Kansakar, Vidhya Bir Singh. "International Migration and Citizenship in Nepal."
In *Population Monograph of Nepal*, 85–119. Kathmandu: Central Bureau of
Statistics, n.d.

Kollmair, M., S. Manandhar, B. Subedi, and S. Thieme. "New Figures for Old Sto-
ries: Migration and Remittances in Nepal." In *Migration and Remittances in
Developing Countries*, edited by N. Kumar and V. V. Ramani, 77–85. Hyderabad,
Pakistan: Icfai University Press, 2006.

Lu, Yao. "Test of the 'Healthy Migrant Hypothesis': A Longitudinal Analysis of
Health Selectivity of Internal Migration in Indonesia." *Social Science and Medicine* 67, no. 8 (October 1, 2008): 1331–39. https://doi.org/10.1016/j.socscimed
.2008.06.017.

Mills, Edward J., Sonal Singh, Timothy H. Holtz, Robert M. Chase, Sonam Dolma,
Joanna Santa-Barbara, and James J. Orbinski. "Prevalence of Mental Disorders and Torture among Tibetan Refugees: A Systematic Review." *BMC International Health and Human Rights* 5, no. 1 (November 9, 2005): 7. https://doi
.org/10.1186/1472-698X-5-7.

Nepal Ministry of Health, New Era, and ICF. *Nepal Demographic and Health Survey 2016.* Kathmandu: Nepal Ministry of Health, 2017.

Puri, Mahesh, and John Cleland. "Assessing the Factors Associated with Sexual
Harassment among Young Female Migrant Workers in Nepal." *Journal of
Interpersonal Violence* 22, no. 11 (November 1, 2007): 1363–81. https://doi
.org/10.1177/0886260507305524.

Puri, Mahesh, and John Cleland. "Sexual Behavior and Perceived Risk of HIV/
AIDS among Young Migrant Factory Workers in Nepal." *Journal of Adolescent
Health* 38, no. 3 (March 1, 2006): 237–46. https://doi.org/10.1016/j.jadohealth.2004
.10.001.

Rathaur, Kamal Raj Singh. "British Gurkha Recruitment: A Historical Perspective." *Voice of History* 16, no. 2 (2001): 19–24.

Seddon, David, Jagannath Adhikari, and Ganesh Gurung. "Foreign Labor Migration and the Remittance Economy of Nepal." *Critical Asian Studies* 34, no. 1
(2002): 19–40.

Sharma, Sanjay, Shibani Pandey, Dinesh Pathak, and Bimbika Sijapat-Basnett.
"State of Migration in Nepal." *Centre for the Study of Labour and Mobility*,
Research Paper VI, 2014.

Sharma, Vartika, Lopmudra Ray Saraswati, Ubaidur Rob, Mahesh Puri, and Avina
Sarna. "Life across the Border: Migrants in South Asia." New Delhi: Population
Council, 2015. https://assets.publishing.service.gov.uk/media/57a0897f40f0b649
740000e8/61263_Final-Migrant-Report_Life-across-the-border.pdf.

Shrestha, Maheshwor. "Push and Pull: A Study of International Migration from Nepal." *Social Protection and Labor Global Practice Group, World Bank Group*,

Policy Research Working Papers, February 8, 2017. https://doi.org/10.1596/1813 -9450-7965.

Shrestha, Shreejana. "Mental Cost of Migration." *Nepali Times*. July 15, 2016, sec. Nation.

Sijapati, Bandita, and Amrita Limbu. *Governing Labour Migration in Nepal: An Analysis of Existing Policies and Institutional Mechanisms*, 2017.

Singh, Chandni, and Ritwika Basu. "Moving in and out of Vulnerability: Inter-rogating Migration as an Adaptation Strategy along a Rural–Urban Contin-uum in India." *The Geographical Journal* 186, no. 1 (2020): 87–102. https://doi .org/10.1111/geoj.12328.

Thieme, Susan, and Simone Wyss. "Migration Patterns and Remittance Transfer in Nepal: A Case Study of Sainik Basti in Western Nepal." *International Migration* 43, no. 5 (2005): 59–98.

Van Ommeren, Mark, Joop T. V. M. de Jong, Bhogendra Sharma, Ivan Komproe, Suraj B. Thapa, and Etzel Cardena. "Psychiatric Disorders among Tortured Bhutanese Refugees in Nepal." *Archives of General Psychiatry* 58, no. 5 (2001): 475–82.

Williams, Nathalie E., Dirgha J. Ghimire, William G. Axinn, Elyse A. Jennings, and Meeta S. Pradhan. "A Micro-Level Event-Centered Approach to Investigat-ing Armed Conflict and Population Responses." *Demography* 49, no. 4 (2012): 1521–46.

Yabiku, Scott T., Victor Agadjanian, and Boaventura Cau. "Labor Migration and Child Mortality in Mozambique." *Social Science and Medicine*, special issue: *Place, Migration and Health*, 75, no. 12 (December 1, 2012): 2530–38. https://doi .org/10.1016/j.socscimed.2012.10.001.

"वैदेशिक रोजगार बोर्डको सचिवालय." Accessed November 5, 2020. http://fepb.gov.np/download #rules.

CHAPTER THIRTY-THREE

Persian Gulf Migrants

Maria Kristiansen

1.0 Introduction

Migration, health, and human rights are intrinsically linked, with migration being a key driver for population health and societal developments across the globe. There are substantial regional differences in migration patterns and in the living circumstances of migrants, their health status, and, not least, the recognition of human rights in relation to migrant populations.[1,2] This chapter puts the spotlight on the Arab countries located in the Persian Gulf region. This is a rapidly evolving and understudied region in Western Asia with a substantial and diverse migrant population representing an interesting case study of the intertwined forces of migration, health, human rights, and societal developments.

This chapter sets the stage by presenting the region and an outline of types of migrants and then focusing on the vast majority of low-income migrants. This is followed by an overview of living conditions, health status, and access to health-care services of migrants in the region, combined with a discussion of human rights concerns. The final part of the chapter suggests ways to improve the health and living circumstances of migrants of the region. The chapter concludes with summarized key points.

2.0 The Persian Gulf and Its Migration Patterns

The Persian Gulf is part of the Mediterranean Sea in Western Asia bordered by Iran and Iraq in addition to the six Arab nations that constitute the Gulf Cooperation Council (GCC) countries, namely Oman, the United Arab Emirates, Saudi Arabia, Qatar, Bahrain, and Kuwait. The GCC countries have become a central immigration hub over the past decades, since the discovery of oil that catalyzed considerable infrastructure development, rapid economic growth, and increased international engagement.[3] As the area moved rapidly toward modernization, the consequent need for expansion in the workforce led to an influx of migrant workers in particular over the past three decades.[4,5] The development has been swift, as exemplified by the State of Qatar, occupying a small part of the Arabian Peninsula. In the 1960s, Qatar had a small, homogenous Arab population of one hundred thousand. This population has since increased more than twentyfold to 2.2 million, primarily through immigration, with migrants making up 78 percent of the population and an estimated 94 percent of its workforce.[6] By 2019, migrants constitute between 38 and 87 percent of the total populations across the GCC countries, totaling approximately thirty million migrants.[7]

   This immigration pattern has turned the Persian Gulf region into one of the world's most ethnically diverse regions, and the number of migrants is expected to grow even further in the coming decades as the GCC countries continue their infrastructure developments and engagement in the international arena (e.g., in the fields of sports and cultural events). However, recent years have seen an increasing recognition of the vast inequalities emerging as part of the immigration patterns in the region, with conditions worsening by the ongoing Covid-19 pandemic.[8,9,10,11] One need only spend a few hours in the bustling capital cities of GCC countries, many of which are increasingly used as stopovers during long-haul flights or hot spots for financial and cultural events, before the inequalities in living circumstances and wealth between different types of migrants and between migrants and native populations become apparent. The complexity is significant. On the one hand, immigration has helped GCC countries accelerate development, and the resulting remittance flows have unquestionably had a positive effect on the economic conditions of certain economically developing regions in the countries of origin of main migrant groups, including in parts of India, Nepal, and the Philippines.[12,13] On the other hand, inequalities are significant, as migrant workers in the GCC come from a range of countries and represent different migration backgrounds that expose them to varying health risks and provide them with very different living circumstances in the receiving countries.[14,15] A very small minority among migrant populations in the GCC have their origins in North America, Western Europe, and other economically developed regions. Due to a lack of systematically collected and detailed data on country of birth of migrants in the region, the exact proportion of these migrants is unknown. These workers, called *expats* in public discourse, typically spend relatively short periods of time in well-rewarded professional positions with few health risks, decent housing, and comprehensive health insurance. This is in contrast to the experiences of the overwhelming majority, mainly unskilled low-income workers — predominantly male — from Bangladesh, India, Indonesia, Pakistan, the Philippines, and Sri Lanka.[16] These migrants tend to be employed in the construction sector or in services jobs, which expose them to health risks and are associated with substandard access to health-care services and higher risks of suffering from human rights violations (see table 33.1).[17]

3.0 Living Conditions, Health, and Human Rights

A limited, albeit growing, number of studies have explored living conditions, health status, and access to health-care services among migrants in the GCC countries. A more substantial body of work focuses on human rights concerns and has gained media attention in recent years, partially fueled by large-scale sporting and cultural events, such as the 2022 FIFA World Cup to be hosted by Qatar and the Expo 2020 in Dubai. In this brief overview, the focus will be on the overwhelming majority of low-income migrants. As indicated above, these migrants are often short-term employees working in construction or as domestic helpers in private homes, cleaners, and drivers. Overall, these jobs are characterized by low payment, long working hours, and, at times, physically and mentally hazardous working conditions, which may negatively affect the health of migrant workers.[18,19] Variations in working conditions both within and across countries exist, as reflected in a survey conducted among migrants in the GCC showing that workers in Saudi Arabia reported the lowest wages, lowest levels of workplace satisfaction, and highest exposure to verbal abuse in the region.[20] Further, many low-income migrants experience

TABLE 33.1 **Overview of migrant populations, September 2019**

Country	Number of migrants	Percentage of total population
Bahrain	741,200	45.2%
Kuwait	3,000,000	72.1%
Oman	2,300,000	46.0%
Qatar	2,200,000	78.7%
Saudi Arabia	13,100,000	38.8%
United Arab Emirates	8,600,000	87.9%

Source: Based on data retrieved from the Migration Data Portal, https://migrationdata
portal.org/?i=stock_abs_&t=2019&m=2&sm49=145.

poor housing conditions in overcrowded facilities provided by employers and often located in remote areas.[21] Together, these factors result in
a number of adverse health outcomes and particularly in high rates of
work-related accidents causing injury and death. However, precise estimates on work-related health consequences are lacking due to missing
reliable, systematic, and comprehensive statistics investigating labor practices across the region. Moreover, while engaged in hazardous work, such
as the construction of high-rises, laborers may face high rates of injury and
death with little assurance that their employers will cover their health-
care needs. Studies show that verbal abuse, isolation due to being cut off
from contact with family and friends, and cultural and language barriers
restricting engagement with society may compound health risks.[22,23,24,25,26]
A gender dimension emerges as specific risks exist for the many female
domestic workers employed in more secluded surroundings in private
homes. For these women, nonpayment of salaries, forced confinement,
isolation from wider society and from relatives abroad, food deprivation,
excessive workload, and instances of psychological, physical, and sexual
abuse are of particular concern.[27,28]

In terms of health status, migrant workers are overall in comparably
good health upon arrival to the GCC region, as they are recruited for
often physically demanding positions and frequently undergo very elaborate health screenings. Along with the work-related injuries and death
they may face, diseases that are prevalent in migrants' countries of origin
also affect their physical health following migration. Such diseases include
diabetes, cardiovascular diseases, and a wide range of infectious and non-
infectious diseases that may affect their health across the lifecourse.[29,30,31]
Studies have found higher rates of psychiatric morbidity, including depres-

sion and anxiety, and elevated suicide rates among migrants compared to nationals.[32,33,34,35] Despite the lack of detailed data, risk assessments show that the Covid-19 pandemic has disproportionally affected migrants in the region due to the combination of precarious jobs, financial insecurity, unsafe living and working conditions, and lack of access to testing and treatment.[36]

Access to and quality of health-care services for the diverse and growing migrant population are not well-described. However, overall, migrants are likely to face substantial barriers due to reduced coverage caused by limited health insurance for those in low-income jobs. Timely access to quality health care for migrants is further restricted by the context, as health-care systems in the GCC countries are pressured by increasing populations that are furthermore facing a quadruple disease burden that includes communicable and noncommunicable diseases, mental health issues, and accidental injuries.[37] These issues, combined with geographical, cultural, and language barriers, all point to substandard health-care provision for migrants.

Human rights violations are a particular concern that underpin much of the health vulnerabilities affecting low-income migrants in the GCC. The rapidly changing sociodemographic profiles of these societies are challenging policies and practices, and responses have been failing to secure adequate protection of the large numbers of migrants. The challenges brought about by a large influx of migrants have to a large extent been addressed by protecting the rights of nationals, for example, through sponsorship laws, mandatory migrant health screenings upon arrival, and restrictions on the settlement of migrants.[38] Human trafficking involving the financial exploitation of migrants through complex networks of middlemen operating across countries is a particular concern, as are issues related to restricted rights of movement and freedom of speech for migrant populations. Engagement and representation of perspectives of migrant workers in societal discussions and political developments are limited, partly also due to poverty, unemployment, and in some circumstances lack of safety in their home countries, making migrants less able to voice their needs. Critiques by key international human rights organizations have emerged and, based on my experiences living in the region, have oftentimes been dismissed by some GCC audiences as insensitive to the situation faced by the region, where reliance on migrant workers is seen as a temporary phenomenon. Concerns for the economic, social, and political rights of migrants persist, despite certain encouraging developments, such as movement toward the outlawing of employer confiscation of worker passports; changes to the rules related to sponsorships; and bans on recruitment fees and withholding of wages.[39,40,41] The creation of welfare codes to promote better quality of life and the construction of new housing units and health-care facilities that cater to migrants are additional steps being taken to improve their living conditions, health status, and access to health care. However, there is reason for concern about the lack of enforcement of these laws, which are often only partially and inconsistently implemented in governance structures that are pressured in rapidly changing societies.[42,43]

4.0 Where Do We Go from Here?

Despite the somewhat fragmented evidence base, overall low-income migrants living in the Persian Gulf region are exposed to a number of health risks, particularly due to inadequate occupational health and safety measures, and substandard living conditions, compounded by barriers to health-care services and examples of violations of basic human rights. To reduce these health inequalities for the benefit of migrants as well as societies in the region, a range of improvements that build on and accelerate current changes in policy and practice are needed. These changes must target immediate health risks, as well as the root causes of these inequalities.

Some key next steps include:

1. Monitoring migrant health: Standardized and comparable data on migrant population demographics, health, quality of life, and access to quality health-care services are needed across the region. For example, population-based health profiles should include migrant workers, who are at present typically excluded, and provide detailed information needed for adequate stratification of data on burden of disease, living circumstances, and access to health-care services according to ethnicity, sex, and occupation.[1-3] This will enhance both the scarce research base and accountability.

2. Ensuring migrant-sensitive health-care systems: All health-care services, ranging from health promotion, disease prevention, diagnosis, and treatment to rehabilitation and end-of-life care should be accessible to migrants. Insurance schemes must cover health-care needs, and services should be delivered to migrants in a culturally and linguistically appropriate way with adequate training

of health-care staff to ensure a comprehensive and coordinated response to migrant health-care needs.[2] Given current insights, particular emphasis needs to be given to addressing mental health problems, occupational safety, and the most prevalent communicable and noncommunicable diseases among different subgroups of migrants.[44,45]

3. Enforcing protection of human rights through policy and legal frameworks: National laws should be reviewed to ensure adequate reflection of the migrant population in terms of securing good living conditions and occupational health and safety standards and ensuring freedom of movement and speech, access to health-care services, and improved social security. Implementation of laws should be overseen, and mechanisms should be developed to protect against discrimination to overcome lack of citizenship for long-term migrants and/or their offspring and to enable family reunification. Representation of migrants in political and public debates is of key importance to ensure social justice. Global dimensions should be considered in terms of increasing bilateral collaboration between GCC countries and workers' countries of origin to protect against exploitation prior to emigration and to enforce internationally recognized standards and national policies outlining labor rights.

5.0 Conclusion

The Persian Gulf region has emerged as one of the world's most ethnically diverse areas, but it is also one of the most unequal. While countries across the region experience different developments, overall, the number of migrants is expected to grow in the coming decades. Growing evidence points to a range of health disparities, inadequate living conditions, and suboptimal access to quality health-care services for migrants in the region, concerns that are situated in a wider context of insufficient protection of basic human rights. Despite changes in recent years, facing up to this challenge remains critical not only for health-care policy and practice, but for the wider range of public and private sectors influencing the living circumstances of migrants. With the swift developments in the region, there is need for progress to be made to reduce health inequalities and fulfill the health rights of the many low-income migrant workers living in the region.

CHAPTER THIRTY-FOUR

South Africa

Jo Vearey

South Africa is the main migrant-receiving country within the Southern African Development Community (SADC), a region associated with a high communicable disease burden and historical and contemporary population movements. Long associated with various forms of migrant labor and livelihood-seeking mobility, large numbers of South Africans move within the country for short and longer periods, with most found in the Gauteng Province—home to the City of Johannesburg—where nearly half of the population was born in other South African provinces.[1] With approximately 7 percent of a population of fifty-nine million estimated to be a noncitizen—that is, someone born in another country, mostly from elsewhere in SADC—South Africa receives the largest number of migrants in the region.[2]

1.0 Background

While the relationship between migration and health is increasingly recognized globally,[3] South Africa and SADC have failed to effectively design and implement migration-aware public health-care systems—a whole-system response whereby population movement is embedded as a central concern in the design of interventions, policy, and research.[4]

As a result, health-system responses—including the prevention, treatment, and control of communicable (infectious) and noncommunicable diseases—do not adequately engage with migration and mobility. Failing to engage with migration and mobility affects public health interventions, as their design is based on the assumption that populations are static, that they can be continuously accessed at one geographical location, and that health-care users will access care and treatment at a single facility over time. Evidence indicates otherwise: health-care users in South Africa—both citizens and noncitizens alike—are mobile and are moving for reasons other than seeking health care.[5]

Recent years have, however, seen some attempts by international organizations—including the International Organization for Migration (IOM), Save the Children (STC), and Medécins Sans Frontières (MSF)—and local nongovernmental organizations, often in partnership with local government, to develop responses to health and migration in South Africa. These initiatives have mostly taken the form of pilot projects and have focused on communicable diseases—notably HIV, tuberculosis, and malaria—and involved engagement with migrants working in the mines and commercial farms, in inner-city Johannesburg, and at formal border crossings with a focus on people moving between Zimbabwe and South Africa, including long-distance truck drivers.[6]

Bilateral initiatives established at the local level across borders[7] and attempts to develop a coordinated national response to migration and health through the development of Migrant Health Forums (MHFs) have had varying levels of success.[8] Regional-level responses have thus far been lacking, with the Framework on Communicable Diseases and Population Mobility of 2009 still in draft form,[9] again suggesting the need for bilateral coordination across borders.

While the need to engage with diverse population movements to improve global health programming is increasingly recognized, including by international organizations such as the World Health Organization (WHO) and the IOM,[10] South Africa continues to lag in its response.[11] The current political climate in South Africa—associated with increasingly anti-foreigner and xenophobic sentiments from political leaders and civil society alike—is driving uninformed, non-evidence-based, and potentially dangerous international migration policy discussions and processes that may pose a threat to local, regional, and global health. This has more recently been demonstrated through the Covid-19 pandemic, whereby, as has been previously identified,[12] preparedness plans in South Africa and SADC have failed to engage with migration and migrant populations.[13] The longer-term impacts of this, particularly in relation to ongoing disease control measures and vaccine rollout, remain to be seen.

2.0 Key Migration and Health Concerns in South Africa

As outlined in table 34.1, there are four key interlinked and complex concerns that must be considered when exploring migration and health in South Africa. These contextual realities, which will be briefly discussed below, need to be better understood by all key stakeholders involved in the development, financing, and delivery of public health-care interventions. Improving knowledge of the historical and contemporary role of migration and mobility in South and Southern Africa is essential, as is gaining a clearer understanding of the ways in which persistent structural violence further impacts the effectiveness of health-system responses.

TABLE 34.1 **Migration and health in South Africa: Four key concerns**

1. South Africa is associated with mixed migration flows:

   Internal migration is far greater than the movement of people across borders yet is not considered in the framing of migration and health.
   The majority of people move in search of improved livelihoods; a far smaller number are forced migrants.
   South Africa has an urban refugee policy whereby asylum seekers and refugees are expected to self-settle and earn their own income; they receive no benefits from the state.
   Urban spaces are associated with marginalized and hidden migrant groups.

2. Current public health responses do not engage with migration and mobility:

   Serious implications for communicable disease control (especially TB, HIV, malaria); chronic treatment continuity; and pandemic preparedness planning.

3. Public health and social welfare systems are overburdened and struggling:

   Challenges are raised in a context of high inequality and inequity, where citizens reliant on the public health-care system are also struggling to access their basic rights.

4. Structural violence: Xenophobic attitudes and anti-immigrant policies and practice

   Xenophobic and anti-foreigner sentiments from political leaders and wider society increasingly drive policy making and practice.
   Noncitizens face challenges in accessing the health care to which they are entitled.
   Immigration and refugee policies are becoming more restrictive, making it increasingly difficult for noncitizens to obtain and maintain the documents required to be in the country legally.
   Border management approaches are increasingly securitized, including the building of fences, the deployment of army personnel, and the use of drones to monitor border areas.

2.1. Mixed Migration

2.1.1 POPULATION MOVEMENT WITHIN SOUTH AFRICA.   South Africa is a
country long associated with the movement of people, including the historical forced movements—from the 1860s until the mid-1980s—of people from former homelands to work on commercial farms and in gold and
diamond mines, as well as in urban centers.[14] This system resulted from the
need to bring cheap black labor into areas designated as "white" during
the colonial and apartheid era. The negative impacts of this unjust system
of migrant labor, which involved various forms of segregation to prevent
black workers from residing permanently in these areas and from mixing
with the white population, persist today.[15] While the system is no longer
officially in place, many within the country continue to move in order to
access work, including those who continue to work in the agriculture and
mining sectors that remain associated with low wages, poor housing and
working conditions, and resultant poor health. Some move for long periods of time, others for shorter periods. Many will regularly return home to
visit families and friends during holiday periods, particularly over Easter
and Christmas. These patterns of movement are found within many sectors across the country, including in the South African public health-care
system. Many South Africans who are employed in the public health-
care system have moved from their home to train in nursing colleges and
medical schools, moving again to undertake internships and professional
training, with further—and often continuous—movements to access jobs
in different parts of the country. These movements are similar to those of
other South Africans who migrate in search of work and education within
the country. Most South African migrants are found in the Gauteng Province, where nearly half of the population was born in other South African
provinces.[16]

2.1.2 MOVEMENT FROM OTHER COUNTRIES TO SOUTH AFRICA.   In addition
to these important movements within the country, South Africa is also
home to another migrant population: those who are born in other countries, mostly from elsewhere within SADC.[17] This population is much
smaller than the numbers of South African migrants who move within the
country. Approximately 7 percent of the population are estimated to be
noncitizens,[18] a figure far lower than often assumed. One reason for this
is that the media and government officials will often exaggerate figures
or misinterpret the data.[19] Just like South African migrants, the majority

of cross-border migrants find themselves in the Gauteng Province, the most densely populated province in South Africa. The Western Cape receives the second largest number. This means that in parts of Gauteng and the Western Cape, in central Johannesburg or Cape Town, for example, the numbers of cross-border migrants will be far greater than in other provinces, such as in the Eastern Cape or the Northern Cape. This can make it appear that there are more noncitizens in South Africa than there really are.

2.2 Current Public Health Responses Do Not Engage with Migration and Mobility

These population movements—both within the country and from other countries—can, if not engaged with properly, present some challenges to the public health-care system that need to be resolved.[20] Based on existing evidence, there are two priority concerns that the public health-care system needs to address in relation to migration.

First, it is very difficult to maintain continuous access to care and treatment for health-care users who are moving within South Africa or from another country. As a result, people who move can struggle to access care and treatment, which could have negative effects for the health of everyone living in South Africa. A central concern here relates to the management of TB and HIV: continued access to care is essential, but if somebody is moving between two different areas of the country for work, this can be difficult to maintain. In turn, this can contribute to treatment interruptions and resistance to first-line treatments, with subsequent impacts on the suppression of viral load. It is thought that this could be a key issue currently overlooked in HIV programming in South Africa and the region. This is also a challenge when thinking about other chronic conditions, like hypertension and diabetes. Evidence shows that South African migrant women who are pregnant can face many challenges when they choose to access prenatal care in the city but return home to deliver. It is very difficult for these women to check in for delivery and care in their home areas, and this has a range of negative consequences, including for the health and well-being of expectant mothers.

Second, noncitizens often face specific challenges when trying to access public health care, despite the law being very clear; as outlined in table 34.2, the denial of access to health care for *anyone*, including noncitizens, is unlawful.

TABLE 34.2 **The legal obligation to provide health care to all**

The law on migrant access to health-care services is quite clear. Denial of access to health-care services to anyone, including migrants, is unlawful. Section 27(1)(a) of the Constitution states that "everyone" has the right to have access to health care services. Subsection 3 further states that "no one" may be refused emergency medical treatment.

The National Health Act 61 of 2003 in section 4(3)(b) states that subject to any condition prescribed by the Minister, the State and clinics and community health centers funded by the State must provide all persons, except members of medical aid schemes and their dependents and persons receiving compensation for compensable occupational diseases, with free primary health-care services. In addition, all pregnant or lactating women and children under the age of six are entitled to free health-care services (at any level).

The Refugees Act 130 of 1998 provides for access to basic health-care services by refugees (and by implication asylum seekers).

The Uniform Patient Fee Schedule exempts certain categories of non–South Africans from being full paying patients. These exempted categories are immigrants who permanently reside in South Africa but have not attained citizenship, non–South African citizens with temporary residence or work permits, and persons from Southern African Development Community (SADC) states who do not have the documentation required to be in the country legally. The exemption of these categories of non–South Africans from paying full amounts for accessing health-care services clearly implies that all health facilities, including clinics, should be providing health-care services even to foreign nationals.

The South African law and policy on this issue is in line with the SADC Protocol on Health in terms of which SADC states agreed to treat citizens of other SADC states like citizens of their own country.

Notices posted in hospitals requiring "foreign nationals" to pay for health-care services are contrary to the policies explained above and are unlawful. The only time that a refugee, asylum seeker, or undocumented migrant from an SADC state should have to pay for health-care services is when he or she does not qualify for free health services in terms of a means test. In that case, like for South Africans, there are sums of money that the patient can be asked to pay, depending on the care required and the type of health facility.

Source: Johannesburg Migrant Health Forum, "Fact Sheet on Migration and Health in the South African Context," 2015, http://goo.gl/7N4yYM.

While the law is clear, as noted above, it is often not implemented. In recent years, an increase in challenges faced by noncitizens has been reported; these are outlined in table 34.3. These challenges may be linked to difficulties in communicating due to the different languages spoken but can also be the result of the way that they are treated by frontline health-care staff. Evidence suggests that there are increasingly xenophobic and anti-foreigner sentiments being displayed by health-care staff, resulting in noncitizens facing multiple hurdles when trying to access the care to which they are legally entitled.[21] A key concern relates to issues of documentation. It seems that the frontline staff requesting this information may fail to clearly communicate what they need and how it can be provided. Instead, they sometimes ask for a South African Identity Booklet or an asylum-seekers or refugee permit, and patients who are unable to

TABLE 34.3 **Key challenges in the implementation of law and policy**

1. A demand for the up-front payment of fees by non-nationals in need of maternal health care, including at time of delivery, with reports suggesting that the babies of non-national mothers are not released to the mother until full fees are paid.
2. A demand for up-front payment of fees before emergency treatment will be provided.
3. The misclassification of non-nationals when calculating co-payments, including documented refugees and asylum seekers being incorrectly categorized as full fee-paying patients.
4. Miscommunication when demanding proof of ID and proof of income.

Sources: Johannesburg Migrant Health Forum, "Fact Sheet on Migration and Health in the South African Context"; Vearey, J., Modisenyane, M., and Hunter-Adams, J., "Towards a Migration-Aware Health System in South Africa: A Strategic Opportunity to Address Health Inequity South African," *South African Health Review*, 2017.

provide that document are turned away. These patients are not told that they can provide other forms of ID (such as a foreign passport or affidavit, for example). Additionally, there are problems at the declaration of income stage, which is necessary for higher levels of care where copayments are required; some noncitizens are not given an opportunity to declare their income and instead get classified as full-fee-paying patients.[22]

2.3 Public Health and Social Welfare Systems Are Overburdened and Struggling

South Africa's historical injustices are today visible through struggling public health-care and social-welfare systems.[23] Citizens who are reliant on public health care—around 85 percent of the population—face multiple challenges in accessing care; thus, the ambitions of universal health coverage (UHC) are far from being realized,[24] and, while the ambitions of a national health insurance (NHI) are welcomed, there are many obstacles to its effective implementation.[25] Frontline health-care workers in the public sector are underpaid and forced to contend with the daily challenges presented by inadequate human resources and a poorly functioning system. These structural challenges are experienced by all public health-care users; while noncitizens may face additional challenges (as outlined above), there is a common, shared experience that is often overlooked.

2.4 Structural Violence: Xenophobic Attitudes and Anti-Immigrant Policies and Practice

As discussed, noncitizens face specific challenges associated with their nationality, documentation status, and/or language when trying to access the health care to which they are entitled. In addition to the pressures faced by public health-care workers, some attitudinal issues are a symptom of a more disturbing and prevalent social and political attitude to foreign nationals in South Africa. Xenophobic and anti-foreigner sentiments from political leaders and wider society increasingly drive policy making and practice,[26] with immigration and refugee policies becoming ever-more restrictive, making it more difficult for noncitizens to obtain and maintain the documents required to be in the country legally.[27] The proposed NHI will, according to the draft NHI Bill released in July 2018, decrease access to public health care for some noncitizens.[28] Not only could this have negative consequences for the health of all who live in South Africa if access to preventative methods (including vaccinations, for example, in the context of Covid-19), testing, treatment, and care for communicable diseases is restricted, but it will also prevent progress toward achieving the international health targets associated with UHC.[29] Additionally, border management approaches are increasingly securitized, including the building of fences, the deployment of army personnel, and the use of drones to monitor border areas; these approaches increase health risks by pushing international migrants into unsafe migratory routes that might entail irregular border crossings and a reliance on smugglers.[30]

3.0 The Way Forward

We need to find ways to respond to these challenges in order to ensure that we are upholding our responsibilities to provide health care to all; the urgency of this has been demonstrated by the limited engagement with migration and mobility in pandemic preparedness plans and in the response to the Covid-19 pandemic.[31] The health-care system needs to be responsive to the movement of people—both within the country and across borders. This requires migration-aware and mobility-competent health-system responses. By developing migration-aware health-system responses and using the strategic opportunities for a more inclusive approach offered by the ambitions of UHC, we will be improving access to health care for all—including citizens and migrants who come from other countries.[32]

CHAPTER THIRTY-FIVE

Migration and Health in China

Bingqin Li

1.0 Introduction

Migration may affect people's health status and pose new unmet health needs. People may face health issues associated with their migration experience[1] or with the negative consequences of the migration of close family members.[2] Since the economic reform in the 1970s, China has shifted away from the Central Planning System through a series of continuous social and economic reforms. As a result, people migrated voluntarily without formal arrangements or involuntarily as part of the resettlement plans. A large body of literature emerged on the health implications of migration in the post-reform era, and there are several systematic reviews and some meta-analyses describing the health implications of migration in China.[3,4,5,6,7] These publications principally consider rural-to-urban migration. This chapter argues that since 1978, China has experienced a series of structural changes, and each of them resulted in a large number or even new types of migrants. These migrants face very different health issues; some are related to their migration experience, some result from their current lifestyle, and some are institutional constraints that made it challenging to meet their health needs. The following sections of this chapter first map out the structural changes that lead to migration and then discuss the health issues associated with migration.

2.0 Structural Changes and Migration

Structural changes in this chapter mean shifts or changes in the ways a market or economy functions, resulting in a redistribution of resources among social groups or regions. In the context of China, structural changes are central parts of the development process, which is often discussed in contrast to the structural arrangements of the Central Planning era (1953–1978). Since 1978, the Central Planning System (the structure with which the state controlled resource allocation) has been continuously realigned to sustain economic growth in China.[8] Each readjustment of the structure impacted economic sectors and regions differently, resulting in labor market changes and leading to migration.

Table 35.1 shows the timeline, nature, and types of migration since 1949. During the Central Planning era, large numbers of migrants were relocated by the government for such purposes as national defense and reconstruction (army troop for farming), relieving urban employment pressure (educated youth to rural areas), resettlement of skilled labor force to newly developed industrial areas (construction of third-tier cities), and construction of water reservoirs. It is commonly recognized that migration during this period was state initiated and involuntary, and the government played an active role in the resettlement and servicing of the migrants (table 35.1).

Beginning in 1978, China started to liberalize the economy gradually. The government undid some of the migration policies in the past. Many educated youths who were enlisted to develop the countryside returned to cities in the 1980s. A large number of returnees shocked the urban labor market; many could not find jobs in cities.

At the same time, the country also went through several major economic transitions:

1) Privatization of state enterprises and the relaxed control of the labor market made it possible for people to move between cities. Large quantities of skilled labor resettled to southern cities, where the economy was booming.[9]
2) The development of the private sector and the later participation of the World Trade Organization (WTO) resulted in massive urbanization of the rural labor force. Farmers left rural areas and worked in cities.
3) Cities expanded through the acquisition of rural land occupied initially by farmers, leading to the resettlement of peri-urban farmers.[10]
4) Major projects, such as reservoirs and projects to respond to climate change or environmental degradation, resulted in eco-migration.[11]

While table 35.1 is not a comprehensive list of the total number of migrants in China over time, it illustrates a wide range of structural changing forces that resulted in migration in the pre–post-reform era (1978 on). It is essential to highlight that although migration took place in the process of economic transition, this does not mean that the state played a less critical role in creating the conditions for migration. The roles of the state include enacting policies to strengthen or relax the control of the economy, such as regulating the price of consumer goods; controlling over access to urban labor market and farmers' markets; establishing rural and urban development strategies that redefine rural and urban areas; and launching major projects that aim to transform the country's energy supply and the efforts to attract skilled labor.[12,13] The policy-driven migration means that a large proportion of the migration was not voluntary. Some people migrated because of household strategies. However, these are also frequently related to the broader changes in economic and social policies.[14,15] What makes post-reform migration different from pre-reform migration is that the government has not always assumed the responsibility to resettle the migrants as they did in the past. Labor migration relies on employers and the market to provide accommodation.[16] Other types of migration involve some government compensation or resettlement arrangements but not all.

In some cases, the compensation is not sufficient for resettlement.[17,18] The nature of migration in China is not always one direction and permanent. Some can be long-term, and some can be short-term or circular.[19]

3.0 Migration and Health

The health issues that migrants face can be a result of the process of migration, the activities they engage in, the destination, and their lifestyle.

3.1 Mental Health Issues

Migration in China has been shaped by government planning, directly or indirectly. After the Cultural Revolution, educated youth were initially eager to return to cities. However, these youth soon found that they were not competitive in the labor market,[20] and many of them had to live with their parents again. Although some were recruited by universities, they were often considered to be not as well trained as older or younger uni-

TABLE 35.1 **Types of migration in China**

Year	Name of the project	Type	Direction	No. of people	Driving force	Sectors
1954–1971	Production and Construction Troupes (shengchan jianshe bingtuan)	Soldiers and their families, farmers	Central locations to twelve provinces	4.8 million	Government	Farming
1950s–1991	Reservoir migrants	Rural + urban	Rural to urban, urban to urban	12 million	Government	Miscellaneous
1950s–END OF 1970s	Go to the mountainous areas and villages (Shangshan Xiaxiang)	Educated youth	Urban to rural	17–18 million	Government	Farming
1964–1980	Third-tier construction (Sanxian Jianshe)	Skilled labor	Urban to urban	4 million	Government	Industries
1980s	Returning Educated Youth (zhiqing fancheng)	Educated youth	Rural to urban	14 million	Government + market	Miscellaneous
1978–NOW	Rural–urban migrant workers (nongmin gong)	Unskilled labor	Rural to urban	290.8 million[1]	Government + market	Miscellaneous
1984–	Marketization reform (xiahai), talent attraction in recent years	Skilled labor, university graduates, ex-state enterprise employees	Urban to urban (often to southern provinces)		Government + market	Miscellaneous
1993	Urban expansion, Land acquisition (shidi nongmin)	Farmers	Rural to urban	40–100 million[2]	Government + market	Miscellaneous
1992–	Three Gorges Dam (sanxia)	Farmers and urban population	Rural to urban, urban to urban	1.31 million[3]	Government	Miscellaneous
1980s–	Poverty reduction (ecological migration)	Farmers	Rural to urban	9.47 million[4]	Government	Miscellaneous
2010–	Returning to rural areas (fanxiang)	Migrant workers	Urban to rural	30 million[5]	Government + market	Farming or rural industries

Sources and notes: Compiled by the author.

[1] NBS PRC, "The 2019 Statistical Bulletin of the People's Republic of China on National Economic and Social Development," 2019, http://www.stats.gov.cn/tjsj/zxfb/202002/t20200228_1728913.html.

[2] There are no official statistics of land loss farmers in China. The data on this is all estimation, ranging from forty million to one hundred million.

[3] Office of the Leading Group for Poverty Alleviation and Development of the State Council, "Say Goodbye to Absolute Poverty in the Three Gorges Reservoir Area," 2020, https://www.thepaper.cn/newsDetail_forward_8261662.

[4] National Development and Reform Commission, "Relocation for Poverty Alleviation and Relocation has Achieved 9.47 Million Residents," 2020, http://www.xinhuanet.com/politics/2020-04/23/c_1125897368.htm.

[5] *Xinhua News*, "Nearly 30 Million Migrant Workers Have Left Their Homes or Returned Home for the Second

versity graduates. Some recent surveys showed that on the whole, returned educated youth had less happy marriages, lower-quality social networks, and lower level of happiness.[21]

Zhong et al.'s (2016) meta-analysis of forty-eight cross-sectional surveys suggested that rural–urban migrant workers in China suffered from more severe psychological symptoms in almost all perspectives than the general population.[22] The distress is nonspecific, showing that it is a result of hard life rather than particular psychopathology. The causes of psychological distress include perceived social stigma, discriminatory experience, and low life quality.[23,24] Newer studies looked into the issues by the types of migration. Yang, Dijst, et al. (2018) used a cross-sectional survey (N=855) from Shenzhen and found that temporary migrants were at higher risks of experiencing mental problems than both migrants and nonmigrants.[25] Wang and Hu (2019) analyzed the 2010 China General Social Survey (N=1,660) and found that voluntary migrants had better mental health than rural residents with no migration intention.[26] Migrant women workers are at a higher risk for significant depressive symptoms. Interpersonal discrimination, acculturative stress, and institutional discrimination are some of the risk factors.[27] The discrimination experienced by migrant parents have also affected the family relations and lead to more depressive symptoms of the children.[28]

Displaced and resettled migrants have also been shown to suffer from serious mental health challenges. For some years, the land acquisition process was often traumatic. Local authorities did not give farmers sufficient time to leave and did not provide adequate compensation. Displacement often ended up in violence and forceful eviction.[29,30,31] Although there is little systematic research on the mental health impacts of displacement, some reports show that the resettled migrants were likely to complain about the resettled communities, as they felt they were victims of displacement.[32,33] After resettlement, migrants often found it hard to get jobs. The inability to lead an active life as laborers and the difficulties integrating into the urban society that they moved to have been associated with depression. This is the case for both farmers whose land was acquired by the government and people who were resettled for building reservoirs.[34,35] Landless farmers, marginalized by unfair and nonparticipatory land appropriation processes, suffer from livelihood adaptation difficulties characterized by long-term unemployment, even if they've received financial compensation.[36]

Migration has spillover impacts on children and the family members who are left behind in the poorer regions. Research by Tang et al. (2018)

found a higher risk of mental health problems among Chinese left-behind children. They have been shown to suffer from low self-esteem and depression, and symptoms have been more severe in those who have been separated from their parents longer. School bullying experienced by these children has been more prevalent, which results in trauma and consequent mental health challenges. Female left-behind children are at higher risk of panic symptoms than males.[37] Ge, Se, and Zhang (2015) examined the situation of the left-behind children in urban areas and found that a much larger proportion of them suffered from internet addiction, which also contributed to mental health issues.[38] Sun et al. (2017) found that more left-behind children reported psychotic-like experiences (PLEs) than other students.[39] They scored higher on the frequency of PLEs, the severity of childhood trauma, and the perceived psychological impact of trauma. Children looked after by their grandparents reported less severe impacts of trauma than the children looked after by other people. Migration with parents, rather than separation from parents, is better for the mental health of the children.[40]

3.2 Physical Health Issues

3.2.1 OCCUPATIONAL INJURIES AND DISEASES.   According to the National Health and Family Planning Commission (NHFPC), over 975,000 cases of occupational diseases had been reported until 2018 for the whole working population. Between 2010 and 2018, there were on average 28,000 cases per year. The actual incidence should be even higher than the reported number.[41] Eighty-seven percent (87.3%) were cases of pneumoconiosis (90% of which are migrant workers).[42] The majority of rural-to-urban migrants work in manual jobs that often involve hard labor or long working hours. It was estimated that around two hundred million employees in twelve million factories were exposed to risks of occupational diseases. Forty-three percent of migrant workers are exposed to risk factors such as dust, noise, high temperature, radiation, and vibration.[43] Often employers do not offer proper protection. As a result, occupational injuries are frequent. A systematic review conducted by Fitzgerald et al. (2013) showed that migrants suffer from disproportionately high rates of injury.[44] In hospitals in industrial areas and construction areas of cities, rural-to-urban migrants are the majority of patients of traumatic injuries. Occupational injury-related mortality occurs mainly among migrant workers who work in the poorly regulated private mining, construction, and manufacturing firms. They also suffer from chronic diseases resulting from work—for example, pneumoconiosis among construction workers.[45] There are also large numbers of cases in garment and shoemaking factories or factories using inferior-quality chemicals.[46]

3.2.2 INFECTIOUS DISEASES.   Tuberculosis is much more common among migrants than locals. Migrants are also less likely to seek treatment for active pulmonary tuberculosis.[47] They often seek quick treatment, which results in aggressive care and multidrug resistance.[48,49,50,51] Migrants suffered from a higher level of sexually transmitted diseases such as HIV/AIDS. A meta-analysis by Lei Zhang and colleagues (2013) shows that migrants living in urban areas were 6.7 times more likely to be infected with HIV than average; female migrants in this group were 12.2 times more likely.[52] Between 70 and 95 percent of female sex workers were rural–urban migrants. HIV-infected migrants were less likely to return to the villages than other people suffering from serious illnesses. A follow-up study by Xia Zou and colleagues (2014) showed that rural–urban migrants had a higher risk of STIs and hepatitis than average. However, there was no significant difference in STIs and hepatitis between female sex workers (FSWs), men who have sex with men (MSM), and drug users (DUs) and their migrant counterparts.[53] In recent years, there has been a growing number of migrants suffering from tuberculosis and HIV coinfection.[54]

3.2.3 CONTROL OF CHRONIC AND NONCOMMUNICABLE DISEASES.   There is no chronic disease control and management program for migrant workers. However, migrant workers are not less likely to suffer from chronic diseases, in particular hypertension, that are related to their lifestyle choices (for example, heavy drinking).[55] The inadequate management of chronic diseases put the migrant population in a more vulnerable situation, even if they had lower prevalence of the diseases than the urban population. Unaffordable health care made it more difficult to receive treatment when there was an emergency.[56]

3.2.4 REPRODUCTIVE HEALTH.   Women migrants from rural-to-urban areas suffered from much higher maternal mortality rates than residents in urban areas. This was because of lower health literacy,[57] lack of familiarity with the urban health-care services,[58] and lower financial affordability.[59]

3.2.5 HEALTH OF CHILDREN.   Left-behind children whose parents migrate to cities are vulnerable to safety accidents, injuries, and even death, with girls and younger children more vulnerable than average.[60] They are more likely than urban children to suffer from accidental injuries, such as traffic accidents, drowning, electric shock, fighting, dog bites, and food poisoning.[61,62] These are mostly a result of insufficient guardianship and the need to travel a long distance to school. Li, Liu, and Zang (2015) found that left-behind children in rural areas are more likely to get sick or develop chronic conditions than those living with their parents.[63] For the children following their parents to cities, there is low age-appropriate immunization coverage of migrant children in densely populated areas in cities.[64] Migrant children in cities also have poorer oral health compared with urban children, partly due to dietary changes (e.g., more processed food and sweets intake) and partly related to low health literacy.[65]

4.0 Conclusion

There are multiple types of migration in China, all of which are shaped by government policy, directly or indirectly. A large proportion of the migrants are in that position involuntarily and are particularly vulnerable to mental health issues associated with anxiety and the inability to adapt to life after migration. The voluntary migrants experienced more physical issues associated with their job and lifestyle. There are a range of health outcomes associated with the migration experience. Perceived discrimination and unfair treatment, long-term unemployment, and high work pressure have been associated with difficulties in adaptation to a new life after migration. This is the case for both adults and children or both rural–urban and urban–urban migrants. Lower affordability of health care, poorer health literacy, and lifestyle changes may result in physical health issues or health-care service usage that is not the best for health maintenance.

The health consequences of large-scale migration can be mitigated through efforts on multiple fronts. Integrated and equitable services at the community level to improve health literacy and mental health and to better manage chronic disease are essential. The lack of access to quality health-care services is a major hurdle to dealing with medical issues in a timely manner. In China, a key challenge is that quality health-care resources are highly concentrated in the best hospitals in the largest cities, and the marketization of health care has made it increasingly unaffordable to lower-income families.[66,67] These issues with the health-care system mean that migrants who are not high earners would avoid hospital services as much as possible and resort to non-prescribed medication.[68] When they do seek care, they prefer aggressive treatment to minimize the time spent in hospitals.[69] There is continuous health-care system reform in China that aims to grapple with the challenges of expensive and challenging health care and the improved insurance system. The social health insurance system may help some migrants to cover part of their health-care costs.[70] However, health-care reform is far from being complete, and there are still major gaps in public health and medical-care services to meet the health needs of migration in China.

CHAPTER THIRTY-SIX

Asian Immigrants in New Zealand

Eleanor Holroyd and Jed Montayre

1.0 Background

Contemporary New Zealand is composed of diverse populations; the European ethnic group (Pakeha) makes up the majority of the New Zealand population (70%), with Māori—the Tangata Whenua (16.5%), the Indigenous people—being the largest of the minority groups, followed by Asian (15.3%) and Pacific (9%).[1] To date, an emerging literature on health equity has highlighted health in Māori,[2] Pacific,[3] and more recently in Asian and African migrant communities.[4] The increasing number of overseas-born residents in New Zealand reflects the growing and steady flow of immigrants from different parts of the world.

Immigrants to New Zealand are required to be in a reasonable and good state of health as one of the main requirements in the application for immigration. While New Zealand guarantees its temporary and permanent migrants access to health care,[5] it was noted that some immigrants to New Zealand have a greater burden of poor health than do native-born residents.[6] Asian populations make up the largest non-Anglo-Saxon group of migrants to New Zealand. The authors will present here case studies about the largest Asian migrants groups (Chinese, Indian, and Filipino) living in New Zealand. The following case studies will focus on specific health issues and challenges that are linked to the consequences of migration.

2.0 Treaty of Waitangi and New Zealand Health-Care System

An understanding of health in New Zealand must rest on an appreciation of the foundations of health provision in the country. New Zealand is
unique among the world's countries in its government's efforts to honor
the principles of its founding document, the Treaty of Waitangi.

The Treaty of Waitangi—*te Tiriti o Waitangi*—embeds principles of protection, participation, and partnership with Māori, the indigenous population of New Zealand, and has, to date, underscored New Zealand's health
policies, priorities, and delivery of services.[7] Several New Zealand health
policies, such as the New Zealand Primary Health Care Strategy, have
been challenged in terms of their alignment with and whether they serve
the true essence of the te Triti o Waitangi, which is to affirm "Māori sovereignty and guaranteed the protection of *hauora* (health)."[8]

In New Zealand, the majority of health services are free or subsidized
and publicly funded, ensuring universal health care to all citizens and
permanent residents. This includes free hospital treatment, twenty-four-
hour accident and emergency services, heavily subsidized prescriptions,
maternity care, medical care for children under five years old, outpatient
care, and rest home and older adult care in acute hospital settings. Primary Health Organizations (PHOs) cater to the health needs of the local
communities and populations through a network of general practitioners
(GP) clinics and some nurse-led clinics.[9]

3.0 New Zealand Asian Immigrants

A quarter of the New Zealand population identifies as overseas born.[10]
This is reflected in the increasingly diverse and multiethnic makeup of the
New Zealand population, particularly in the major cities such as Auckland. The fastest growing ethnic group is the Asian–New Zealander population and is predicted to reach 1.38 million by 2038.[11] The growth of the
Asian population in New Zealand has been facilitated by the availability
of permanent residency following immigration and by family reunification
pathways. Asian groups from Chinese and Indian ethnicities are the two
largest Asian groups in New Zealand, and, in recent years, there has been
an increasing number of new Filipino and Korean immigrating to the
country. Asian immigrants in New Zealand represent a substantially diverse group in terms of culture, language, and cultural beliefs.

3.1 Asian Immigrants' Access to Health-Care Services

The establishment of growing Asian communities in New Zealand has led to several government initiatives and policies designed to meet the health needs of these populations.[12] Asians living in New Zealand in general have better health than other ethnic groups and commonly better health than other Asians globally.[13] These positive health trends, however, belie a complex pattern of heterogenous health service engagement and health-care outcomes among Asian immigrant populations residing in New Zealand.[14]

3.1.1 NEW ASIAN IMMIGRANTS' EMERGENCY DEPARTMENT VISITS. A body of scientific scholarship has documented Asian migrants' understanding and experience of New Zealand's health-care systems. Centrally, it has been shown that Asian immigrants are using emergency departments (EDs) disproportionately for respiratory illnesses, particularly asthma, that instead would be best provided for in primary-care clinics.[15] While asthma is a common respiratory condition and is prevalent in Asia—explaining its presence in many Asian migrant communities—ED attendance due to respiratory illnesses highlights new immigrants' health-seeking expectations and prior experiences as well as a health systems failure to support migrants to navigate the New Zealand health system.

Some recently arrived Asian immigrants—those who have lived in New Zealand for five years or less—explained that their rationale for accessing EDs was due to the lack of understanding and information about where to go for services, which was evidenced by the low enrollment rates at their primary health clinics.[16] Moreover, it was further noted that new Asian immigrants were not familiar with terminologies such as *GP* or *general practitioner* and were unaware that they needed to enroll at a GP clinic,[17] hence their rationale for visits to EDs for minor illnesses like coughs and colds. Aiming to address this challenge, staff in emergency services have started to direct new immigrants to enroll with their GP and access these services in their community. The local district health boards, particularly in populous cities, such as Auckland, have created dedicated centers for Asian and migrant health services. One of the many initiatives is "Your Local Doctor," which provides information in different languages to address the knowledge gap among migrant communities in accessing health-care services in New Zealand.[18]

3.1.2 HIV/STI HEALTH PROMOTION AND SCREENING. New Asian immigrants, particularly LGBTI immigrants, in New Zealand face considerable challenges in accessing sexual health services. Earlier research in health promotion regarding HIV/STI prevention in Chinese and South Asian populations in New Zealand revealed variable testing practices for HIV/ STIs.[19] Testing practices are influenced by personal beliefs and literacy in knowledge seeking about access to testing services. Of further note is Asian immigrants' reluctance to discuss sexual practices with their GPs, which is a barrier to sexual health promotion and testing for sexually transmitted diseases. Duration of residence in New Zealand has been shown to be an enabling factor in promoting the appropriate use of sexual health services; with an increase in testing documented among those who have lived in New Zealand for more than five years.[20] This pattern of health-seeking behaviors and years of residence in the host country holds true for newer waves of Asian immigrants to New Zealand, such as the Filipino populations, where low levels of engagement with HIV testing was observed due to limited access to health-promotion resources.[21] Understanding the health-care system and sexual-health services in New Zealand is key to promoting sexual health among Asian immigrants from LGBTQI groups. However, the cultural barriers to accessing STI/ HIV testing and sexual-health services continue to affect Asian LGBTQI members. Stigma against homosexuality and nonbinary orientation are still prevalent in many Asian families. In New Zealand, these factors continue to limit access to health promotion and prevention initiatives as well as to early treatment among Asian LGBTQI migrants.

3.2 Mental Health

Poor mental health has been on the rise among immigrant populations globally.[22] Culturally based factors such as causation beliefs and treatment remedies among Asians with mental health issues and their families have led to delayed diagnoses, preventing them from seeking timely professional help and services. Research has shown that mental health emergency services encounter higher levels of physical aggression linked to mood disorders and schizoaffective cases in Chinese groups compared to non-Chinese patient cohorts.[23] It has also been suggested that Chinese families prefer to contain mental health issues and behaviors within the family as long as possible, commonly resulting in late presentation to emergency services, when many of their symptoms of mental illness are advanced and more complex to manage.[24]

As another example, the authors have noted substantial changes in alcohol drinking patterns in Asian populations, leading to poor physical and mental ill health.[25] In a recent study about one-third of Asian adults and Asian young adults in New Zealand reported drinking in the month prior to the study.[26] Asian adults were more likely to report at least one harmful drinking related experience when compared to European/Other respondents (15% vs 21%). Asian students who had been in New Zealand five or fewer years were more likely to buy alcohol for themselves than New Zealand–born students.[27] This further adds to the burden of adverse behavioral health outcomes faced by Asian migrants in New Zealand.

Both these examples suggest that cultural influences play a critical role in shaping mental health and well-being among Asian immigrants in New Zealand and highlight the need for prioritizing health-care system literacy as a key determinant of good health outcomes in this group.

3.3 Aging and Asian Immigrants in New Zealand

Critical to this case study is the intersection of migration journeys, belief systems, health-seeking behaviors, and lifecourse and their impact on health-care behaviors and decisions. This perhaps plays out most vividly with older Asian populations, particularly those who arrived in New Zealand as later-life migrants.[28] A contemporary issue of some concern in migrant health and well-being in New Zealand is the growing challenge of adequate living arrangements and late-life care for aging migrants. Because of the increasingly diverse migrant ethnic groups, the number of aging migrants in New Zealand is expected to rise. Recent evidence has identified three main focus areas in terms of how living arrangements in advanced age could potentially affect health and well-being of older immigrants: reconfigured filial expectations in both parents and adult children; aging immigrants' acceptance of institutionalized living and care arrangements in old age; and health-facility structures that allow cultural diversity.[29]

Filipino migrants provide a good case study of changing care arrangements among older migrants to New Zealand. The adult children of Filipino migrants, despite being conflicted with cultural norms of filial reciprocity to aging parents, report the possibility of needing to resort to institutionalized long-term care (aged-care facilities) for their parents due to their personal and family commitments. Aging parents are also starting to accept the reconfigured filial duties of adult children.[30] These changing patterns of living arrangements and care in advanced age have been seen as consequences of the migration process and reconfigured care options in the host country.[31]

These shifts suggest that the relevant aged-care industries must be responsive to the cultural needs of aging immigrants, particularly those admitted into long-term care. Such attention would be consistent with the United Nations Special Report 2020, which highlighted living arrangements as an important factor affecting the well-being of aging populations.[32] New Zealand's aged-care sector is highly privatized. While there are small, privately owned, ethno-specific, long-term care facilities, the increasing number of aging immigrants might benefit from a national health strategy to address the diverse needs of aging immigrants. The future of aged care in New Zealand will be challenged to provide culturally appropriate services for aging populations from different immigrant and cultural backgrounds.

4.0 Conclusion

In New Zealand, a culturally diverse nation, empirical research on migrant communities, associated health risks, health needs, and access to and acceptability of service providers remains limited. There is scarce attention given to issues of heightened vulnerability, such as poverty, intersectionality, gender-related outcomes, and efficacy of services. For New Zealand's migrant Asian communities, more culturally appropriate information is needed to inform health-care professional curriculums and policy implementation and guide service providers on effective health-care delivery across the lifecourse. A comprehensive understanding of migrants' life choices and family needs can enhance health-care and health-policy decisions and improve migrant health in New Zealand in the coming decades. Sound prevention strategies are further needed that are informed by an understanding of evolving conditions for migrants along the continuum of the migration process during their time in New Zealand.

CHAPTER THIRTY-SEVEN

Mobility and Health in the Pacific Islands

Celia McMichael

1.0 Human Mobilities in the Pacific Islands

The Pacific region is home to twenty-two Pacific Island Countries and Territories (PICTs). They have a combined population of approximately 8.2 million people, distinct cultures, and substantial differences in population sizes; for example, around 5.2 million people live in Papua New Guinea, whereas Niue and Tokelau have fewer than 2,000 residents.[1] The region includes high volcanic islands and low-lying coral and atoll islands. These Pacific Islands are home to less than 1 percent of the world's population, but they are spread across an area equivalent to 15 percent of the earth's surface. Beyond their terrestrial boundaries, the Pacific Islands are further defined by Exclusive Economic Zones that delineate ocean boundaries and access to fishing and other resources that are vital to people and populations.[2] For example, Kiribati consists of thirty-three coral atolls spread over 3.5 million square kilometers of ocean—an area larger than India.

The Pacific Islands are divided into three subregions: Polynesia (including the Cook Islands, Niue, Samoa, Tonga and Tuvalu, and eight dependencies and territories); Micronesia (including the Federated States of Micronesia, Kiribati, the Marshall Islands, Nauru and Palau, and the US territories of Guam, Northern Marianas, and Wake Island); and Melanesia (including Fiji, Papua New Guinea, the Solomon Islands, Vanuatu, and the special territory of New Caledonia).

Since human settlement, mobility has been a feature of life in the Pacific "sea of islands."[3] During precolonial times, garden rotation, marriage, complex trading networks for foods and resources, and at times conflict meant that there was considerable intraisland and interisland mobility.[4] Colonial empires transformed the Pacific Islands by establishing new types of mobility that served the interests of colonial administrations, such as the relocation of workers, and by imposing boundaries between islander trade routes, leading to what Hau'ofa refers to as "the contraction of Oceania."[5] The era of so-called black birding (1840s to 1930s) and Pacific labor trade extracted more than one hundred thousand Pacific Islanders to work in the guano mines of Peru, Guatemala, and Mexico and in plantations in Queensland, Fiji, New Caledonia, Samoa, and Hawaii. Today, there are extensive migration flows across the Pacific Island region that link rural areas with urban areas, outer islands with main islands, different Pacific Island countries, and other countries in the Pacific Rim and beyond.

First, international migration has been significant in Pacific Island development, particularly for the smaller island states of Micronesia and Polynesia. Migration has shifted the population profiles of some smaller Pacific Island countries as people move to the Pacific Rim countries, particularly New Zealand and Australia. More Cook Islanders, Niueans, Tokelauans, and Samoans live permanently in the Pacific Rim than in their island homes.[6] In 2006, the Pacific Island–born population in Australia, New Zealand, and the United States was just under 350,000 people; by 2013, it had increased to 400,000 people.[7] By 2019, the number of international emigrants was 123,600 (1.1% of total population) in Melanesia, 68,400 (10.1%) in Polynesia, and 118,000 (21.7%) in Micronesia.[8] So, international migration among Pacific Islanders is rapidly increasing. It is expected that in the coming decades, major migration trends in the Pacific will include increasing opportunities for Melanesians to work in Australia and New Zealand and ongoing international migration from Polynesia and Micronesia.[9] Much international migration in the Pacific is driven by employment and education, with high youth unemployment underpinning a growing interest in exploring migration pathways.[10]

Second, there is accelerating rural–urban migration.[11] Yet movements of people within Pacific Island countries and territories are less well measured; limited data identify the scale and trends of internal migration. However, rural–urban migration is increasing from smaller islands to larger islands, from smaller villages to larger centers, and from remote interior

TABLE 37.1 **Urbanization and urban growth in the Pacific**

Region	% Population in urban areas			% Increase in urban population	
	1960	2000	2050	1960–2000	2000–2050
Melanesia	9.0	19.0	32.9	406.8	310.1
Micronesia	37.5	65.7	88.4	372.5	96.9
Polynesia	28.9	41.1	58.0	181.1	96.8
Pacific	12.7	23.5	36.3	380.6	245.4
Australia	87.5	87.2	85.9	99.5	61.3
New Zealand	76.0	85.9	85.6	83.8	46.7

Source: Adapted from ILO, *International Labour Migration Statistics: A Guide for Policymakers and Statistics Organizations in the Pacific*, 2015, http://www.ilo.org/wcmsp5/groups/public/---asia/---ro-bangkok/---ilo-suva/documents/publication/wcms_371837.pdf.

regions to coastal towns.[12] This is evident in the increasing proportion of urban populations across the Pacific Islands region (see table 37.1).

Third, small island countries, including the Pacific Islands, will be among the most affected by climate change, including slow onset events such as sea-level rise and ocean acidification, and increases in the severity of environmental disasters.[13] Migration, displacement, and relocation are expected to increase in climate-change-affected areas, although some populations may be unable or unwilling to move. Migrant remittances may help build the adaptive capacity of communities to cope with climate-change impacts.[14]

2.0 Pacific Islands, Health, and Human Mobility

Pacific Island populations face a triple disease burden: a rapidly rising epidemic of noncommunicable diseases, persistent and emerging infectious diseases, and the health impacts of climate change. These population health challenges threaten the sustainable development of Pacific Island communities.[15] They are further shaped by the variable and dynamic nature of migration and mobility, such as rising rates of noncommunicable diseases associated with dietary change among rural–urban migrants and infectious disease risks in the contexts of environmental disaster and displacement. Broadly, health is influenced by the structural nature and experiences of the migration process, access to health services, and the characteristics of mobile people and populations. Migration can be a positive experience that creates opportunities for health and development, including access to health services, healthier diets, cleaner environments, health-promoting economic benefits, and increased opportunities for social mobility in places of destination. And yet, as discussed below, health risks and vulnerabilities exist for migrants, including via their living and working conditions (e.g., inadequate water and sanitation for rural–urban migrant populations living in peri-urban poor areas or the psychosocial impacts of disrupted place attachments where people relocate away from low-lying sites of coastal risk).

The following subsections focus on the population health aspects of three key migration pathways within the Pacific Island countries and territories: international labor migration, internal migration to urban areas, and environmental and climatic change and human mobility.

2.1 Labor Migration and Health

Many Pacific Island countries have diaspora populations living in Australia, New Zealand, and the United States. Some countries have over half of their populations living overseas.[16] Citizens of some Pacific Island states have entry rights into Australia, New Zealand, and the United States. These rights include citizenship, right of entry, and quotas for permanent migration or participation in seasonal worker schemes.[17] Recently, a growing number of Pacific countries have begun to develop national labor migration policies and plans to increase labor migration opportunities.[18] Figure 37.1 illustrates key international mobility flows of Pacific Island countries and territories.

Since 2007, seasonal labor migration policies have helped to relieve underemployment in the Pacific Islands, including New Zealand's Recognised Seasonal Employer scheme and Australia's Seasonal Worker Programme. While providing employment opportunities for Pacific Islanders and promoting economic development in home countries, these programs also aim to meet labor needs, including in the horticulture and viticulture industries in Australia and New Zealand. During 2017 and 2018, over 9,600 people from the Pacific Islands were granted visas under New Zealand's Recognised Seasonal Employer scheme and more than 8,000 under Australia's Seasonal Worker Programme. In 2018, the Pacific Labour Scheme (PLS) was established for low- and semiskilled jobs in rural and regional Australia, including in the meat-processing and agricultural industries.[19]

The health and well-being of migrant workers is related to their working and living conditions and influenced by broader social conditions.[20]

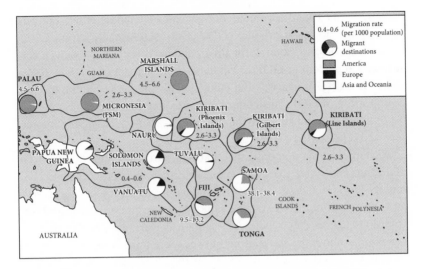

FIGURE 37.1. Pacific migration rates and major destinations for migrants, c. 2006

Source: Hugo, G., and R. Bedford, "Pacific Islands, Migration 18th Century to Present," in *The Encyclopedia of Global Human Migration*, edited by I. Ness, Hoboken, NJ: Wiley-Blackwell, 2013.

There is limited understanding of the health of Pacific workers engaged in labor migration schemes. While Pacific migrant workers typically arrive in good health, common health complaints include dental problems, skin infections, and poor diet due to a reliance on cheap and nutritionally inadequate foods. Despite being charged compulsory health insurance fees in Australia, some Pacific workers have found insurance difficult to use and have reportedly paid large out-of-pocket expenses.[21] Yet health outcomes among Pacific migrant workers have not been studied in any detail. So, while seasonal work provides the valued opportunity to earn high incomes in a relatively short period, there are challenges and health risks that need to be better understood and addressed.

The emigration of laborers also affects economies and development in Pacific Island countries. Some studies highlight a loss of skilled health workers and an increased burden on those who remain; conversely, others argue that international labor migration encourages development-enhancing remittances, knowledge transfers, and the return of migrants with greater skills and savings.[22] For example, remittances—financial or in-kind transfers made by migrants directly to families or communities in their countries of origin—are considered a key strategy for development in many Pacific Island economies and societies. Remittances, as a percentage of gross domestic product (GDP), vary substantially across Pacific Island countries; for example, in 2019, personal remittances received constituted 5.0 percent of GDP in Fiji versus 37.6 percent of GDP in Tonga. Indeed, in 2019, Tonga was the country with the largest remittances as a proportion of GDP. This compares, for example, to the Philippines—a well-known remittance-receiving economy—where personal remittances received represented 9.9 percent of GDP in 2019.[23]

Recent research demonstrates that migration and remittances in Fiji and Tonga contribute to development objectives at a household and community level, including via poverty reduction, funds for health services and education, improved housing, raised consumption standards, and contributions for disaster relief.[24] Yet caution is warranted before drawing conclusions about the associations between remittances and development in source communities. For example, in rural Vanuatu, homes improved through income from international labor migration are viewed as better and sturdy yet disruptive to social relationships, as they create social inequalities and undermine communal values.[25] So, while there is limited evidence of the impact of remittances on population health in Pacific Island countries, these studies suggest both positive and problematic effects.

2.2 Urbanization and Health

Significant internal migration to urban areas has occurred in the Pacific Islands in recent decades (see table 37.1). Many Pacific Island countries are experiencing urbanization rates more than three times the global average.[26] The term *urban* in Pacific Island context can refer to a relatively small town or city or a series of islets, and the global trend toward urbanization is clearly visible in Pacific Island countries.[27] New settlement forms, such as informal and squatter settlements, have become a feature of many Pacific towns and cities. In Papua New Guinea, for example, the informal settlement population has increased at an annual rate of 7.8 percent over the last decade, and in the Solomon Islands, the annual urban growth rate between 1999 and 2009 was approximately twice the national population growth rate, indicating rapid urbanization.[28] Due to changing gender relations—which include increasing opportunities for women in education and nonagricultural livelihoods—a growing number of girls and women are internally migrating to urban areas in the Pacific Islands.[29]

Nauru, Palau, and the Marshall Islands have urban populations that represent more than 70 percent of their total population. The largest urban settlements are in the Melanesian Pacific capitals: Honiara, Port Moresby, Port Vila, and Suva. In Port Moresby, 50 percent of the population live in urban village settlements. These peri-urban settlements are typically located in sites that have been deemed unsuitable for planned urban development, often on the edges of rivers, lagoons, estuaries, electricity easements, mangrove wetlands, and waste-disposal sites. Settlements range from groupings of disparate households to settlements similar to rural villages, with their own governance structures and microeconomic systems.[30]

Urban living can provide access to a wider range of health-care services, education, participation in cash economics, and livelihood opportunities. Yet settlements in Pacific towns and cities are also associated with overcrowding, unemployment, altered diets, crime, poverty, land disputes, social exclusion, environmental degradation, traffic congestion, inadequate housing and living conditions, exposure to flooding and cyclones, and pressures on health and other services such as water and sanitation and garbage disposal.[31] Such wide-ranging issues pose population health problems, including for rural–urban migrants living in these expanding informal settlements.

For example, informal settlements in the Pacific Islands experience challenges to water, sanitation, and hygiene (WaSH). There is often little formal provision of WaSH infrastructure and services, which are often self-built and self-managed. Research has reported unreliable standpipes and/or lack of access to piped water, unhygienic pit latrines, an absence of wastewater treatment, and open defecation in informal settlements in the Pacific Islands.[32] Health consequences of inadequate WaSH include diarrheal diseases, intestinal worms, respiratory infections, and vector-borne diseases (such as dengue). In 2013, there was a dengue outbreak in several Pacific Island countries. In Fiji, there was high dengue incidence in informal settlements with high population density and limited sanitation and public services.[33] The delivery of adequate WaSH is required in order to upgrade informal settlements and as a foundation for good health. Such efforts are underway, including in settlements in Fiji, Vanuatu, Papua New Guinea, and the Solomon Islands.[34]

The effects of climate change could worsen WaSH conditions, such as in low-lying atoll nations, where scarce groundwater resources are threatened by sanitation pollution and water extraction or where extreme weather disrupts WaSH services. There is the likelihood not only that climate change will increase mobility among Pacific Island populations (see section below), but also that people will move into sites of climatic risk. On Majuro atoll in the Marshall Islands, for example, rapid urban development and out-migration from traditional settlements have resulted in movement into climate-vulnerable locations on the island. Similarly, on Fongafale Island, the capital of Tuvalu, rapid development and urban population growth have led to the settlement of shoreline and swampland areas with heightened vulnerability to climate impacts, such as worsening WaSH conditions.[35]

Further, some urban informal settlements are prone to environmental hazards, including flooding, tropical cyclones, and sea-level rise, and associated health risks. In 2016, Tropical Cyclone Winston swept through informal settlements in Suva, Fiji, with substantial damage to housing; emergency shelter and sanitation were a priority. In 2014, flooding in informal settlements of Honiara, in the Solomon Islands, led to the pollution of drainage systems, inadequate sanitation, and the risk of landslide in populated areas.[36] Half the population in Kiribati and Tuvalu live in overcrowded urban areas with limited access to water and land and are experiencing impacts of sea-level rise, saltwater intrusion, and drought.

Despite these trends, urban planning and development is only now emerging as a priority for many PICs. Though all Pacific Island countries are different, they nonetheless face some similar challenges arising from rapid urbanization.[37] The Fifth Pacific Urban Forum, held in 2019, stressed the importance of local governments taking a leadership role in building sustainable, safe, resilient, and inclusive human settlements in the region. The Solomon Islands, Samoa, and Papua New Guinea have begun to develop urban policies.[38] There is a need for careful planning to support the sustainable development of informal settlements and effective urban policies so that the health and well-being of residents, including rural–urban migrants, are supported and promoted. This is of particular importance for the larger Melanesian capitals of Honiara, Port Moresby, Port Vila, and Suva, all of which have growing informal settlements.[39] But urban planning is also significant for the health and well-being of smaller urban populations in the Pacific Islands; for example, Nauru is among the world's most urbanized small island development states, with its entire (albeit small) population defined as urban.[40] Policy options for Pacific Island countries include the promotion of compact urban forms that can achieve resource efficiency, protect natural areas, and encourage walking, cycling, and transit-oriented development; settlement upgrading; the provision of affordable and adequate housing; and access to infrastructure and services.[41]

2.3 Environmental Disaster, Displacement, and Health

Climate change is expected to increase the severity and/or frequency of some environmental disasters in the Pacific Island regions, including both slow-onset and sudden-onset disaster. Five Pacific Island countries rank among the world's top fifteen countries at risk of environmental disaster, including Vanuatu, Tonga, the Solomon Islands, Papua New Guinea, and Fiji.[42] Environmental disasters do not inevitably lead to forced displacement (as displacement is determined by the underlying vulnerabilities of populations in conjunction with exposure to hazards), but the scale of disaster-related displacement relative to population size is high in the Pacific Islands. In 2018, 61,000 people in Papua New Guinea were displaced by an earthquake; volcanic activity displaced 13,000 people in Vanuatu in 2017/2018; in Fiji in 2016, Cyclone Winston affected 40 percent of the population, with approximately 7,000 evacuees; and in 2015, following Cyclone Pam, nearly 25 percent of the population in Vanuatu fled their homes and 55 percent of Tuvalu's population were displaced.[43]

While migration is often regarded as a source of resilience for Pacific communities because of the additional resources that can be accessed in host countries, forced displacement can have negative consequences. Health concerns due to disaster-related displacement include the risk of injury, infectious disease linked to unsanitary conditions, gender-based violence, disruption of health services, and mental health impacts. For example, in several Pacific Island countries, including Fiji and Samoa, flooding following cyclones and prolonged rainfall has contributed to outbreaks of vector-borne diseases (e.g., dengue) and waterborne bacterial diseases (e.g., leptospirosis, shigellosis, typhoid), including in crowded shelters and displaced populations.[44] In 2012, Fiji experienced widespread flooding resulting in substantial population displacement and significant increases in leptospirosis cases; conservative estimates place the number of cases at three hundred and the number of deaths at twenty-five.[45] Although Pacific Island states have established institutions and frameworks to support disaster response and risk reduction, particular pressures include their relative remoteness and large geographical spread, which can lead to higher transportation costs for essential post-disaster resources, the need for external aid particularly in those countries that have had difficulty achieving sustained economic growth and human development, and limitations in the provision of infrastructure and human resources.[46] However, limited research has focused on the health effects of post-disaster displacement, including in the Pacific Islands region.[47]

While migration and displacement can be a sign of vulnerability, human mobility can be a means to adapt to climate risk and promote security, especially when it is voluntary and planned. There is growing discussion—including among policy makers, national and regional organizations, academic researchers, media, and local communities—focused on the need for migration and the planned relocation of people and communities away from sites of environmental risk or from areas that are no longer inhabitable.[48] The Government of Fiji has been working with villages to support the retreat and relocation of households and communities identified as highly vulnerable to environmental risk. For example, Vunidogoloa is a small low-lying Indigenous village in Fiji that moved inland in 2014, within the boundaries of their customary land, in response to coastal flooding and erosion, saltwater intrusion, and the failure of seawalls. Potential health benefits of their relocation include better access to health services and improved sanitation; however, health risks include adverse psychosocial impacts of disrupted place attachment, reduced access to fish and seafood, and increased use of packaged and processed foods that come with greater proximity to a road.[49] So, Vunidogoloa's relocation has brought both health benefits and risks. However, there are as yet few cases of relocation that can unequivocally be linked to climate-change impacts; indeed climate-related mobility is always shaped by political, economic, sociocultural, demographic, and legislative factors that affect people's need, ability, and willingness to move. And few assessments of climate-related relocation address population health issues. Further research is needed to understand the health opportunities and risks of climate-related relocation and migration.

3.0 Addressing Human Mobility and Health in the Pacific Islands

Human mobility within and from the Pacific Islands is diverse, dynamic, and complex. Migration is widely viewed as an inevitable and largely beneficial phenomenon that is a consequence of and catalyst for the progressive transformation of Pacific Island societies and economies.[50] However, there are both health opportunities and threats associated with human mobility. Migration and mobility shape the determinants of health and well-being among Pacific Islanders—both those on the move and those who remain.

In the Pacific Islands region, attention to migrant health is key to advancing Universal Health Coverage and the Sustainable Development Goals (SDGs). There are various policy frameworks that address migrant health and/or broader determinants of health that are relevant to migrant populations in the wider Western Pacific Region, a region that includes the

Pacific Islands. For example, *Universal Health Coverage: Moving Towards Better Health—Action Framework for the Western Pacific* outlines an approach to improving health-system performance with a focus on people and communities, including migrants and displaced populations.[51] The *Regional Action Agenda on Achieving the SDGs in the Western Pacific* underlines the economic, environmental, political, and social factors that may create or perpetuate ill health, including among migrants.[52] And the urban health agenda is highlighted via the *Regional Framework for Urban Health in the Western Pacific 2016–2020: Healthy and Resilient Cities*, which aims to support efforts to anticipate, mitigate, and adapt to new urban health challenges.[53] There are growing opportunities in the convergence of efforts in Pacific Island countries and territories to address climate-change adaptation, sustainable development, human mobility, and labor migration, all of which are foundational to health and well-being.[54] For example, the International Organization for Migration's Regional Strategy for Asia and the Pacific (2017–2020) seeks to strengthen the governance of migration, address the drivers and consequences of forced migration in disaster contexts, protect migrants in vulnerable situations, promote migrant health and universal access to health care, protect migrant workers, support the development of migration policies, and address the migration/environment/climate-change nexus.[55]

Much concern has been expressed over the past decade about the impact that population mobility bears for population health.[56] As discussed above, mobile and migrant populations moving within and from the Pacific Islands face diverse health challenges and opportunities but may also enjoy significant benefits. As such, it is less useful to consider mobile people in general as a vulnerable risk group; instead, mobility should be looked at as a phenomenon involving many demographic groups, places, and socioeconomic processes. The health needs of people on the move in the Pacific Islands might be served through collaborative and multisectoral efforts to address—for example—disaster preparedness, urban health challenges, and labor schemes. This means shifting beyond a focus on the *migrant* and approaching and responding to mobility in the Pacific Islands as part of broader and dynamic systems.

CHAPTER THIRTY-EIGHT

Venezuela and Latin America

Oscar A. Bernal Acevedo, Jovana A. Ocampo Cañas, Jhon Sebastian Patiño Rueda, Laura Baldovino-Chiquillo, and Salma S. Baizer Cassab

1.0 Introduction

The region of the Americas has seen a large flow of migration recently.[1] In 2017, the United Nations estimated an approximate 258 million people migrated globally, representing 3 percent of the world population.[2] Out of these, the Economic Commission for Latin America and the Caribbean (ECLAC) estimates thirty million migrants were in Latin America.[3]

However, the phenomenon of migration is not new in Latin America, a region where there have been several waves of migration over time. In the 1930s, for example, this migration was largely triggered by the economic crisis and labor movement, with much migration from the countryside to the cities.[4] In the 1960s, on the other hand, the migration between neighboring countries was principally related to political, economic, social, and political conflicts, such as the civil wars in the countries of Colombia, Guatemala, Cuba, and the Dominican Republic.[5] In the 1980s, a new wave began that was related to globalization and included migration to the United States and Europe.[6]

Armed conflicts have also played a role in migration of communities in the Americans. For example, armed conflicts in Central America from the 1970s to the 1990s led to a mass migration of men, women, and children to Mexico and the United States. It is estimated that more than eight million people from the Latin American and Caribbean region migrated to the United States during these decades.[7] Additionally, Colombia's armed conflict from 1960 to the peace agreement with revolutionary armed forces of Colombia (FARC) in 2016 also led to the forced migration of its population inside and outside the country.[8] Consequently, Colombia has one of the largest populations of internally displaced persons—approximately 5.8 million, according to the Global Internal Displacement Observatory (GIDO).[9]

Most recently, since the 2010s, there has also been a mass migration of people from Venezuela, which has been considered the largest human mobilization in the recent history of Latin America.[10] According to the United Nations High Commissioner for Refugees (UNHCR), more than 4.6 million men, women, and children left Venezuela between 2016 and 2019, and this number continues to rise.[11] Furthermore, more than 80 percent of them have settled in Latin American countries.[12] The causes of this migration include a humanitarian and economic crisis in Venezuela, concern about public safety, and a sharp decline in living standards.[13]

2.0 Context of Venezuelan Migration in Colombia

While the challenges facing migrating communities in Central and South America are diverse and complex, for the purposes of this chapter, we will focus on the recent migration of Venezuelans into Colombia and discuss its broader implications on the region and beyond.

The history of migration in and from Colombia and Venezuela are different, despite the fact that the countries are neighbors.[14] Colombia's recent history has been characterized by the departure of Colombians to other parts of the world, mostly due to internal violence.[15] On the other hand, during most of the twentieth century, Venezuela was receiving people from other countries, especially Europeans and Latin Americans.[16] Since the 1980s, Venezuela was involved in a series of social, political, and economic crises that caused those who were immigrants from other countries (e.g., Colombians) in Venezuela to return to their homelands.[17]

After Hugo Chávez came to power in 1999, implementing constitutional change and revolutionary socialism, some sectors of Venezuelan society saw this as a risk and decided to leave the country. Ten years after the beginning of the Chavez presidency, in 2010, 521,620 Venezuelans immigrated to other countries.[18] This emigration was further accentuated by the arrival of Nicolás Maduro to power in 2013.[19] Venezuelan migrants left their country principally because of the socioeconomic challenges that included problems of food insecurity, low access to health services, and violations of human rights, among others.[20]

Colombia, as a neighbor, became the country that received most Vene-zuelans, especially through its border in Cúcuta, Norte de Santander.[21] Ac-cording to data from Migración Colombia, by June 2020, at least 1,748,716 Venezuelans were in Colombia,[22] mainly in Bogotá, Distrito Capital, with 19.62 percent of the migrant country's population, followed by Norte de Santander, with 11.32 percent.

Migrants to Colombia can be divided into two categories based on the legal status of their residence: regular and irregular migrants.[23] Regular mi-grants are those who are authorized to enter by state authorities (foreign students, temporary workers), and irregular, or undocumented, migrants are people who entered Colombia *without* legal authorization or whose residence permit has expired (772,857 regular migrants vs 985,859 irregu-lar migrants).[24] It is important to note that undocumented migrants consti-tute a heterogeneous group of individuals who have avoided deportation, had their visas revoked or terminated, or entered the country illegally or who are children whose parents have irregular immigration status.[25]

Venezuelan migrants who fell into this category of irregular migrants unfortunately suffered stigmatization, discrimination, and verbal, physi-cal, and sexual violence during their time in Colombia.[26] Over the past de-cade, Venezuelan migrants in Colombia have been blamed for different problems that afflict Colombian society, from unemployment to insecurity and crime.[27]

In addition to xenophobia, Venezuelan migrants have also experienced substantial human rights violations during their passage through and stay in several South American countries, with the right to health being one of their rights that is often violated.[28] The following sections will delve into the socioeconomic problems and violations of the right to health of Vene-zuelan migrants.

3.0 Economic and Social Challenges Facing Venezuelan Migrants

Migration in Latin America has long been motivated by conflicts and vio-lence, much like migration in other regions of the world.[29] For example, during the 1990s, 20 percent of the Colombian population that emigrated to other countries belonged to the poorest segments of society that were most affected by violence.[30] Similarly, the general violence in Mexico and El Salvador caused high rates of migration to the United States.[31] Vene-zuelan migration followed a similar pattern after the economic collapse and the humanitarian crisis that emerged in 2017, generating the largest exodus in the recent history of Latin America.[32]

According to UNHCR, since 2014, there has been an 8,000 percent increase in the application by Venezuelans for refugee status, mainly in the Americas.[33] Moreover, in a monitoring study carried out by UNHCR on 19,600 Venezuelan refugees and migrants in Latin American countries from January to June 2019, it was found that 50.2 percent of the families interviewed had at least one member who was or is at risk, due to their specific demographic profile or because they had to resort to serious negative coping mechanisms, such as sex for survival, begging, or sending children under fifteen years of age to work.[34]

Venezuelan migrants also experience higher rates of unemployment and engagement with an informal labor market.[35] According to the UNHCR, approximately 48 percent of Venezuelan migrants in Latin America have informal jobs. Moreover, according to the National Administrative Department of Statistics (DANE), the unemployment rate for Venezuelan migrants in Colombia between September 2018 and August 2019 was 19.2 percent, compared to 10.2 percent for the national total.[36] This percentage of unemployment increased by 1.5 percentage points between August and September 2019.[37] The above has been resulting in Venezuelan migrants having lower income and, when employed, low levels of job satisfaction.[38] This has also made meeting basic needs difficult for many Venezuelan migrants[39] and exposed many to the risks of sexual and labor exploitation[40] and participation in criminal activities as a means of subsistence.[41]

4.0 Venezuela Migrants and Health

The political, social, and economic problems that are ongoing in Venezuela have resulted in the collapse of its health-care system and the reemergence of previously controlled infectious diseases in the country.[42] Consequently, there has been an increase in cases of malaria,[43] tuberculosis, vaccine-preventable diseases, and sexually transmitted diseases such as HIV in Venezuela and subsequently in countries that receive most Venezuelan migrants (mainly countries of the Americas).[44] The influx of a poorly vaccinated population with high mobility places both the Venezuelan migrants and the host populations at risk of infectious diseases.[45]

Additionally, medical care, vaccination, and treatments add a burden on health-care systems of receiver countries that are relatively poor, unprepared, and unequipped to create health programs for the migrant population.[46] For example, in Colombia, a total of 1,157,732 doses of biologicals have been applied to Venezuelans from 2017 to 2019. This represents a cost greater than 18,366 million Colombian pesos in vaccines (approximately US$5 million), plus the resources and efforts made by territorial entities.[47]

Mental health issues, chronic conditions (e.g., diabetes, hypertension, and asthma),[48] limited access to programs such as organ transplantations, and immunological and oncological diseases have also been challenges facing Venezuelan migrants that have further strained the health-system capacities of host countries.[49] In addition, Venezuelan migrants face barriers to health-services access,[50] complicating their ability to receive adequate health care and increasing their health burden.

5.0 Migration and Venezuelan Women

The health of Venezuelan girls, adolescents, and women, particularly their sexual and reproductive rights (SRR), is precarious.[51]

Venezuelan women have limited access to contraceptives and lack the financial resources to purchase them.[52] Also, the crisis in the health sector[53] is accompanied by insufficient medical and paramedic personnel who can provide accurate information and adequate care to the migrants. This situation makes it impossible for the Venezuelan migrant population to access comprehensive sexual and reproductive health services, which has repercussions for access to and use of contraceptive methods.[54] This situation also affects decision-making on the number of children, the interruption of pregnancy, and the quality of delivery care.[55] This burden of poor reproductive health borne by Venezuelan women is worsened by a migration process that often exposes them to violence, abuse, sexual coercion, and unwanted pregnancies.[56]

According to research carried out by Profamilia and the International Planned Parenthood Federation (IPPF), the main needs to guarantee the SRR of the Venezuelan migrant population in Colombia by 2019 included access to family planning services, the prevention of sexually transmitted infections, safe abortion services, postabortion care, the prevention of adolescent pregnancy, youth-friendly services, access to maternal and child health services, and effective and comprehensive care for sexual violence.[57]

In response to the above-mentioned situation, Colombia has implemented comprehensive care strategies and public policy instruments that seek to respond to the health needs of Venezuelan migrants. One of the most recent of these is the Health Sector Response Plan to the Migration Phenomenon of 2019, carried out by the Ministry of Health and Social Protection.[58] This document sets out the guidelines, policies, and actions for the comprehensive health care of migrants from other countries or Colombians returning to the country that must be adapted and adopted by the different territories within the country.[59] However, very few actions are evident in this document to respond to the specific sexual and reproductive health needs of migrant women that guarantee their sexual and reproductive rights.[60]

6.0 Conclusion

The challenges faced by Venezuelan migrants in Colombia require comprehensive strategies that can guarantee them improved access to care and better overall health. In addition, such a response must include multiple sectors—health, education, justice, and so on—that are all committed to guaranteeing the well-being of the migrant population.

A comprehensive approach to ensuring the health of Venezuelan migrants in Colombia should be designed, implemented, and articulated within the framework of multilateralism; the Venezuelan migration situation will not stop if the socioeconomic conditions of Venezuela are not resolved. Recognizing this, ECLAC[61] has suggested that the crisis can only be resolved if the guarantee of human rights for all Venezuelans is respected throughout the region, including a guarantee of the right to health and social security for all Venezuelans.

Providing adequate health care to Venezuelan migrants is not possible without an intersectoral approach in which civil society organizations, academia, the government, and the private sector are involved in the creation of policies that are based on evidence, are inclusive, and are adapted to the context of each society to improve the health conditions of the Venezuelan migrant population in Latin America. This will help Venezuelan migrants not only in Colombia, but also in other countries hosting a significant Venezuelan population (e.g., Ecuador and Peru). Furthermore, Colombia has the opportunity to create a robust system that can help its own population, which is in need of a quality health system after four decades of civil war. Finally, we note that the Colombian model—rooted in empathy and multilateralism—can provide a blueprint for other countries in the region, both in the present and in the future.

CHAPTER THIRTY-NINE

The South Asian Context

Muhammad H. Zaman, Reshmaan Hussam, and Hulya Kosematoglu

1.0 Introduction

The South Asian subcontinent is comprised of the countries of Pakistan, India, Bangladesh, Nepal, Maldives, Bhutan, and Sri Lanka and spans an area of nearly two million square miles. Home to over 1.9 billion persons, it is among both the most populated and the most densely populated regions in the world, and migration into and within the subcontinent has featured prominently in its modern historical development.[1] The movement of bodies due to trade, economic opportunity, conflict, and foreign invasion has profoundly shaped the political, economic, and social institutions of the subcontinent and, in turn, the health and well-being of its people.[2]

While the release of India from British colonial rule in 1947 led to one of the world's largest mass migrations within the subcontinent, the last half century has been witness to enormous migration into the region, with the forcible displacement and in-migration of nearly twenty million persons.[3] From the west, the 1979 Soviet invasion of Afghanistan, subsequent political crises, and the US-led "War on Terror" of 2001–2014 has led to upward of two million Afghan citizens seeking new livelihoods in Pakistan.[4] While some have returned, over one million Afghan refugees remain in the country.[5] From the east, the decades-long oppression and the 2017 genocide of the Rohingya in Myanmar has drawn more than two million Rohingya into Bangladesh, making the Rohingya refugee camps in Cox's Bazar the largest in the world as of 2020.[6]

This chapter explores the health and health-care challenges faced by these two migrant populations on the opposing flanks of the subcontinent.

In this chapter, we deliberately do not focus on other prominent forms of internal and external migration—among them, the temporary migration of millions of laborers to the Gulf States, the seasonal migration of agricultural workers in rural regions into urban centers during lean seasons, and the internal displacement of climate migrants leaving salinized lands for new livelihoods.[7] We argue, however, that the vulnerabilities experienced by Afghan migrants in Pakistan and the Rohingya in Bangladesh span a wide spectrum, offering a valuable lens into the multitude of health challenges faced by migrants in South Asia.

2.0 False Dichotomies

We first encourage a reframing of the standard narrative of migration in the policy world—one that produces what we argue is a false dichotomy between the forcibly displaced refugee and the migrant who chooses to leave and a parallel false dichotomy between the migrant community and native populations.

2.1 The Forcibly Displaced and the Economic Migrant

While the Afghans and Rohingya are largely considered to be forcibly displaced due to violence and ethnic persecution, the line between the forcibly displaced refugee and the economic migrant (who is supposedly endowed with greater agency in the decision to migrate) is often a blurry one. In both the context of Afghanistan and Myanmar, oppressive economic conditions preceded and followed violent conflict, compelling millions to traverse porous borders into South Asia. The use of the term *refugee* to describe all Afghan migrants has itself been actively debated in the literature.[8] The migration of Afghans into Pakistan's northwest province (now known as Khyber Pakhtunkhwa) dates back hundreds of years, with strong cultural, religious, and ethnic ties that transcend the geographical borders separating the two countries.[9] Similarly, Rohingya have been migrating to Bangladesh for decades, both in response to episodes of ethnic violence and persecution from the Myanmar army and in search of greater economic opportunity. Prior to the violent expulsion out of Myanmar in 2017, approximately 1.5 million Rohingya had already made Bangladesh their home in search of alternative livelihoods.[10] We emphasize that *force* and its converse, *choice*, are arguably an illusion for the bulk of these migrants, whether they be refugees of persecution or refugees of poverty.

As such, while some health challenges, such as psychological trauma from violence and persecution, may be unique to the forcibly displaced, most of the vulnerabilities make no distinction between motives for migration.

2.2 *The Migrant and the Local Community*

Policy makers often consider the migrant or refugee in isolation: refugee populations are treated as if they reside in segregated communities distinct from those of local populations. Both within the Afghan and Rohingya populations, however, such boundaries are fluid. As much as 68 percent of the Afghan migrant population in Pakistan lives in urban settings among the local population;[11] in Bangladesh, Rohingya have resided among the Bangladeshi population for decades, and the recent construction of the camps in response to the 2017 influx has resulted in both a large inflow of old Rohingya into the camps and an outflow of new Rohingya into local communities. An improved understanding and redressal of the health vulnerabilities of migrants in South Asia therefore requires a systems-level analysis—one that does not see the migrant in a vacuum, but rather recognizes the interplay between the health state of the local community and that of the migrant.

3.0 Health Vulnerabilities of the Migrant

Transcending these two dichotomies expands our understanding of the health state of the migrant, a state that is often prone to a third reductionist focal point, particularly in South Asia, of communicable diseases alone. While communicable diseases remain important health concerns within concentrated migrant populations,[12] we argue that this focus is a consequence of policy makers' tendency to view migrant populations as a collective mass, rather than as individuals with meaningful histories and futures. A more holistic consideration of the health state of migrants requires a complementary understanding of migrants' psychological health, access to health care in their points of origin, safety within the family, and security within the local community.

3.1 *Communicable Disease*

When refugees move to a host country, they are more likely to be affected by disease relative to local community members, as they have not developed immunity to native strains of communicable diseases.[13] Between 2012 and 2018, almost 50 percent of Afghan refugees in Pakistan suffered from viral respiratory tract infections, often complemented by dysentery, skin disease, typhoid, measles, and reproductive tract infections.[14] Sexually transmitted infections (STIs) are highly prevalent among Rohingya refugees in Bangladesh, exacerbated by the widespread presence of STIs within the native population of Myanmar,[15] gender-based violence, the lack of basic living facilities, higher injection drug usage, and the substandard treatment of STIs in Bangladesh.[16] Containment of such communicable diseases requires an agile health system that is able to move quickly in times of rapid spread; a slow response not only has significant physical health consequences, but also costly mental health consequences, from prolonged segregation to a reinforcing of xenophobic fears around contamination among the local community.

3.2 Psychological Health

Mental and psychosocial health remain an underappreciated, poorly funded, but rapidly growing public health challenge among migrant populations in South Asia. The sources of poor mental health are numerous, ranging from post-traumatic stress disorder (PTSD) from violence experienced in the source country or the migration journey (with rates as high as 70% among the adult Rohingya population and 20% among children),[17] grief and lack of grounding from the loss of home, family, or ancestral lands,[18] feelings of inadequacy and loss of dignity from long-term unemployment,[19] and profound uncertainty regarding the future, spanning matters of daily living to existential survival.[20] Pervasive malnutrition among refugee children, in addition to its impacts on physical development, further contributes to greater likelihood of mental health challenges during adolescence and adulthood.[21] Beyond the direct effects of poor mental health on well-being, such challenges can lead to suboptimal investments in community, physical health, and education or employment, all of which may have intergenerational consequences and exacerbate the challenges of adjusting and integrating into local communities.[22] While some qualitative work in these spaces exist, rigorous data collection efforts around the psychological well-being of migrant populations is severely lacking. Meaningful developments in psychosocial well-being will require greater involvement of local research teams who are better equipped to design culturally appropriate surveys and engage in nuanced interpretation of such data.

3.3 Health State in Source Country

Often neglected by policy makers is a recognition of the state of health from which migrants come. In the case of the Rohingya, prior to the 2017 expulsion, the community faced what some term a "slow-burning genocide" in Rakhine State, Myanmar, where the deliberate deprivation of economic and medical resources was extreme. Northern Rakhine, where most Rohingya resided, had one physician per 158,000 individuals; child mortality was approximately 180 per 1,000 births and acute malnutrition at 25 percent (relative to 77 per 1,000 births and 14% in neighboring non-Rohingya regions).[23] The majority of children (62%) received no vaccinations, with only 2 percent receiving the WHO recommended dosage.[24] In parallel, health conditions in Afghanistan are ranked by WHO as among the poorest in the world. Maternal mortality in 2002 was 1,600 per 100,000 live births per year, with total fertility rates of 6.3 children per birth mother.[25] Decades of conflict have debilitated the health-care infrastructure, accompanied by a severe shortage of skilled health-care providers: a 1996 study in Kabul documented two doctors and 3.4 hospital beds available per 10,000 Afghans. The study also identified profound mental health challenges among women, with 42 percent of the women in the study reporting symptoms of PTSD and 97 percent reporting symptoms of major depression; this was precisely the population that would later seek refuge in Pakistan.[26] Having emerged from such a context, not only health itself but health literacy is likely to be low. Medical missions aimed at improving health must be complemented by appropriate literacy efforts in order to achieve sustainable improvements in the health of migrants and, inextricably, that of local populations.

3.4 Gender-Based Violence

Intimate partner violence (IPV) is a significant concern among refugees for whom poor access to mental health treatment, a patriarchal structure, congested living conditions, an absence of economic opportunities, and few social services make domestic challenges particularly acute. The problem is exacerbated by the absence of options for legal recourse available to the abused, particularly if those who suffer lack citizenship rights.[27] According to a report by the Reproductive Health for Refugees Consortium within Afghan refugee camps in Pakistan, 79 percent of the women reported having been beaten by their husbands.[28] Qualitative work in the

Rohingya camps highlights a similar ubiquity of IPV, although accurate statistics are challenging to gather, given the sensitivity of the topic.[29]

3.5 Xenophobia

Refugees and migrants face safety concerns not only within the household, but also in relation to host communities. Hostility from host communities is a common fear articulated by both the Rohingya and Afghan migrants.[30] Fears of communicable disease by locals paired with the lack of economic security and health literacy of migrants fuel xenophobic narratives. Such xenophobia has both immediate and long-term implications: it jeopardizes the immediate health and well-being of already-vulnerable migrant populations and contributes to a deeper cycle of isolation and dehumanization, which can be used to reinforce the deprivation of basic rights and resources to these otherized communities.

4.0 Demand for Health Care

The vulnerable health state of Rohingya refugees and Afghan migrants underscores both the necessity for adequate health-care provision to migrant communities and the opportunity to alleviate easily preventable sources of morbidity and mortality.[31] However, social and institutional barriers along both the supply and demand sides of health care make this a challenging exercise.

While the migrant may recognize his or her need for health care, a lack of trust in local authorities and a fear of xenophobic backlash contribute to underinvestment in health. Afghan refugees, like other vulnerable communities, are wary of local health-care institutions due to fear of persecution and lack of formal identification.[32] As such, these communities often seek health care through informal channels that increase their risk of relying on poor quality, substandard, and counterfeit medicines. Reliance on informal channels can have severe consequences: the rapid rise of malaria in the northwestern region of Pakistan in the early 2000s among Afghan refugees was connected to the wide prevalence of poor-quality medicines.[33] As hospitals and public health facilities are often overburdened and underfunded, competition for resources and ensuing xenophobia further dissuade refugees from seeking out public facilities. They are faced with a choice of paying out-of-pocket for substandard health care from unqualified informal providers or risking physical, emotional, and mental harm by venturing to public facilities.[34]

5.0 Supply of Health Care

The quality of health-care provision in the local communities of Northwest Pakistan and Southern Bangladesh, where Afghan and Rohingya refugees respectively reside, is at baseline poor.[35] Vulnerable refugee communities are exposed to further disruptions to an already weak health-care infrastructure. With increasing anti-migrant public sentiment, governments have made little investment in providing adequate quality care for migrants, with investment in mental health services being particularly weak.[36] In the absence of robust local investment, most services for refugees are donor funded and suffer from the ebb and flow of international agencies' funding capacity and fluctuating priorities, depriving already unstable migrant livelihoods of a reliable and stable source of health care.[37]

6.0 Policy Recommendations

Given the landscape described, we offer three policy recommendations to address the state of health and health-care provision among migrants in the South Asian subcontinent. First, we encourage the design of more integrated health-care systems. Historically, governments in the region have created parallel health systems for locals and migrants,[38] resulting in health infrastructure for the latter being underfunded and understaffed. Integrated models such as the Shaukat Khanum Hospital for cancer care, which provides services for both citizens and noncitizens, are necessary for building robust communities.[39] While the average refugee expects to return home within a year of displacement, he or she typically remains displaced for seventeen years,[40] a duration in which some form of engagement and integration with the host community—whether desired or not—is inevitable. As such, receiving countries would do well to be attentive to the economic and health needs of these populations as if they are their own.

Second, we underscore the necessity of concerted efforts to combat xenophobic rhetoric that undermines the safety of refugees. In recent years, government institutions have either remained complacent or been complicit as nationalist rhetoric grows louder.[41] Dehumanizing rhetoric manifests in dehumanizing treatment. Without a home, refugees not only lack the physical protection that local communities enjoy, but also the psychosocial security of an established identity. Having dehumanized them, it is easier to label such communities as undeserving of basic health care, education, or protection. These labels and deprivations can persist across generations, eroding trust between migrants (or children of migrants) and host communities, leading to poor physical and mental health conditions, an increase in informal channels of health-care provision, and an undermining of the public health system.

Finally, we note that neither Bangladesh, Pakistan, nor India are signatories to the 1951 Refugee Convention, whose clause on *non-refoulement* protects refugees from forced repatriation. Signatories to this convention have a responsibility to provide refugees with, among other rights, identity documents and equal access to public resources such as education and health care. These nations of the subcontinent are purportedly wary of participation in the convention, lest it encourage greater migrant flows or threaten security.[42] As we have done throughout this chapter, we stress that the vast majority of migration flows into and within South Asia are acts of necessity rather than choice. While certainly true for those fleeing violence and persecution, necessity also drives those seeking employment in response to crippling poverty or refuge from destroyed livelihoods due to climate change. Notably, the 1951 Refugee Convention is limited to refugees of conflict or political persecution, excluding these economic or climate migrants who will grow substantially in share and in vulnerability in the years ahead.[43]

We therefore encourage policy makers across the subcontinent to not only become party to the existing Refugee Convention, but also to extend the rights of non-refoulement, identity documents, and access to public resources to economic and climate migrants across the South Asian subcontinent, as well.

PART VI

The Future of Migration and Health

CHAPTER FORTY

Preparing the Next Generation of Scholars in Migrant Health

Zelde Espinel and James M. Shultz

1.0 Introduction

As the study of migration and population health comes into full flower as a field of inquiry, the future of the field lies squarely with the next generation of scholars who will study migration and population health. This chapter discusses the state of the science in teaching about migration and population health to illustrate how we may best contribute to the creation of the next generation of scholars in the field.

We are both educators, and one of us (ZE) is a clinician and immigrant. Opportunities to train graduate students in public health (JS) and medical students and resident physicians (ZE, JS) have provided us with an appreciation of the importance of participatory engagement of learners. The study of migration and population health is rich with possibilities for stimulating student involvement. In that spirit, we shall discuss the process of creating migrant health coursework, bringing the reader along as an unseen colleague and cocreator. We will start by asking and answering several framing questions as we proceed to outline the structure of a potential course.

We are fortunate that our remit for this chapter is supported by three remarkable and contemporary resources. Balancing at the intersection of population health and migration, we are buoyed by recent edited texts in both spheres: *Teaching Public Health*,[1] *Migration and Health*,[2] and a pedagogical framework, *The Re-Imagining Migration Guide to Creating Curriculum: A Planning Tool to Support Quality Teaching for a World on the Move*,[3] that has continuously evolved and flourished from its inception in 2017.

2.0 The Quick Approach for Creating a Well-Evaluated Migration and Health Course

The field of migration and population health is sufficiently compelling in breadth and complexity that a talented instructor, laboring within time constraints, can assemble a course quickly, deliver the course, and likely receive high ratings. There is no magic here: select key topics from resources that canvass the field, deliver dazzling didactics, invite fascinating guest speakers, carefully curate a selection of videos and podcasts, provide a list of relevant web-based resources, and propel a high-energy classroom environment throughout the semester. Instructor charisma helps. This formula has frequently worked well in university settings to present content that is inherently captivating. The theme of migration and health certainly qualifies.

Unfortunately, this too-common approach to course creation and presentation reflects content delivery devoid of pedagogy. The most important contributor to coursework on migration and health—the learner—is reduced to a receptacle for a sampler of engrossing content. Migration and health cannot be taught well with learners in spectator mode; they must be personally involved. Our learners' experiences are important for "norming" the migrant experience. Learners themselves are emissaries from a world on the move.

3.0 Five Framing Questions for a Learner-Invested Curriculum

Educators at *Re-Imagining Migration* employ evidence-based methods to solidify the teaching of migration while creating opportunities for advancement of both teaching faculty and learners of all ages.[4] Their focus on migration does not purposefully incorporate the population-health perspective, so that is something that we will add. When planning a migration curriculum, the team at *Re-Imagining Migration* asks a sequence of five interrelated questions that provide the scaffolding, or, as they describe it, the "framework" for educators. Here we both modify and adapt these questions to fit our focus on migration and population health:[5]

1) Who are the learners we are teaching about migration and health?

2) What are the most important perspectives for teaching about the nexus of migration and health in the context of our ongoing engagement with a world on the move?

3) How can we teach about migration and health by asking the types of questions that invite active learner participation in the telling of moving stories?

4) How do we create engaging, experiential learning environments for students, realizing that we cohabit a world on the move?

5) How do we empower educators to teach migration and health for a world undergoing continual transformation?

We will expand on each of these questions in sequence.

4.0 Framing Question 1: Who Are the Learners We Wish to Teach about Migration and Health?

Perhaps the most self-evident question that arises whenever an educational experience is being forged is *who are we teaching*? On the population-health front, *Teaching Public Health* has an entire section devoted to best practices for learners throughout their educational lifecourse, starting with adolescents and young adults and progressing through undergraduate, masters, and doctoral levels, as well as chapters on interprofessional education — a natural fit for migration and health — and lifelong learning. On the migration front, *Re-Imagining Migration* supports training for younger learners during their formative years when they encounter and react to sharing classrooms and educational experiences with immigrant and non-immigrant children.[6] Yet *Re-Imagining Migration*'s well-designed structure is adaptable for application at all levels beyond secondary education.

Regardless of academic level, when teaching on migration, we must remember that students are the most valuable resources in our courses and classrooms. Their ongoing lived experiences provide critical material for class discussions and team assignments.

4.1 Learners' Fields of Study

When designing lessons, courses, or entire curricula on migration and health, consider where students are in their educational trajectories. In which programs of studies are they enrolled? *Re-Imagining Migration* considers that, in secondary education, this topic might be integrated into a lesson plan, a unit, or a course, or interspersed throughout an entire curriculum.[7]

For learners at the undergraduate or graduate levels, would migrant health be core or elective coursework within a particular school or major field of study? This is important. One of us (ZE) completed masters-level degree programs both in public health and in population and development—at different institutions on different continents. While both programs could easily accommodate a course on migrant health, the teaching would be very different. Public health, international studies, race and ethnicity studies, civil rights and immigration law, labor and workforce studies, and population and development are examples among many of disciplines that could readily embrace migrant health coursework.

4.2 Learner Experiences with Migration

We consider the composition of our class as one of the most important assets. While the composition of the class may be unknown prior to the first day of class, most instructors can surmise quite a bit about the likely makeup of the class based on learners enrolled in the school, the department, or the overarching program of study. When developing the syllabus, it is useful to consider the following: Will there be international students in class? Immigrant students? Students whose family members have been employed as migrant and seasonal farm workers (MSFWs)? Will diverse cultures be represented? How long will learners have resided in the area? How will our students have been affected by migration? What are our students' motivations to learn about migration and health?

Some questions can be addressed early through surveys distributed prior to the first day of class. Starting on day one, anonymous in-class polling can jump-start discussion prior to students gaining confidence and a sense of safety and comfort and expressing themselves in the class setting. Polling will be useful all semester when potentially sensitive questions are asked.

Studying migration draws upon vivid, ongoing, lived experience. Each student in migration and health studies is a potential story capsule. *Re-Imagining Migration* uses a clever device—"moving stories"—to describe autobiographical accounts shared by the learners themselves. Each of us has a personal story of migration.[8] Hearing others' migration stories enlightens us to their experiences and reflects back on our own. One of our current public-health students picked berries in the fields from the ages of seven to seventeen; she aspires to become a physician serving MSFWs. Sharing moving stories also creates opportunities for learners to expand their own repertoire of interpersonal and communication skills in the areas of understanding, empathy, and compassion. The moving stories approach brings migration down to a deeply personal level, with each learner living out their own case example.

The classroom can become a "collaboratory" for expanding upward from individual experience to enhance population-health thinking skills that are so avidly trained in public-health education. Apprehending and appreciating the stories of diverse fellow learners help to reduce prejudice and stigma toward marginalized persons, including those of immigrant origin. This is where instructors can incorporate two mainstays of public-health teaching: the multilevel (eco-epidemiological) perspective and the lifecourse dimension.[9]

4.3 Learner Migration Experiences from the Eco-epidemiological Perspective

Teaching migration and population health provides the opportunity to expand beyond personal experience to the nested levels in which each learner is embedded—family, social networks, neighborhoods, communities, nations. This eco-epidemiological perspective is a foundational element when teaching public-health and population-health science. Early class sessions train and practice skills in population-health thinking. Throughout the semester, connections can be made repeatedly that link personal stories to larger communities and, conversely, connect case examples of population mobility down to individual experience. Within several class sessions, instructor and students should be able to glide smoothly among these multiple levels.

Population-health education is frequently enriched by using case studies, yet too often case studies are presented as fascinating tales that are external to the personal experience of learners. Students react to scenarios to which they may have no direct connection. Fortunately, migration and health studies represent the exception to this, because "we are all in this together."

Migration and Health serves as a rich resource, replete with case studies from many population subgroups from every continent.[10] When teaching migration and health, it is useful to look at the broad panorama of migration on a global and regional scale, to examine what is happening within more circumscribed communities, and also, at the moving stories level, to connect teaching to our individual learners and their student teams.

As this volume reveals, migration patterns are much broader and more nuanced than forced migration alone. Nor is migration simply a point A to point B proposition. High proportions of migrants worldwide engage in cyclical labor migration, flowing from one harvest to the next or one seasonal job to another. Elsewhere, migration patterns are pendular, as is happening for Venezuelan migrants who enter Colombia and return back to Venezuela multiple times each year. Migration patterns globally provide a richness of examples, and many are captured in this volume.

4.4 Learner Migration Experiences from the Lifecourse Perspective

Migration and Health dedicates several chapters to describing migration in the context of the lifecourse.[11] While migration—populations on the move—necessarily features the *place* perspective, the lifecourse perspective brings the *time* dimension to the forefront for understanding how health is produced.

When teaching public health, the eco-epidemiological and lifecourse perspectives serve as orthogonal dimensions that together create a matrix. This matrix is a useful teaching tool for visually summarizing how migration affects health at relevant levels ranging from individuals (potentially including our students!) to their families, communities, and nations—across the lifecourse from the youngest young to the oldest old.

5.0 Framing Question 2: What Are the Most Important Perspectives for Teaching about the Nexus of Migration and Health in the Context of Our Ongoing Engagement with a World on the Move?

As elucidated in one section of *Migration and Health*, there are multiple academic perspectives for understanding the migration-health crossroads. Both content and pedagogy are interdisciplinary and interprofessional. Multiple lenses are brought to bear on the subject matter and the learner experiences.[12]

What *Re-Imagining Migration* injects into this conversation is a "shift in mindset" regarding educational outcomes.[13] Teaching migration and health draws upon riveting current events and case examples, a wealth of fascinating subject matter sufficient to produce a valued, well-regarded course. However, there is an entirely different level on which this material can be taught, one that transitions teaching to a higher plane. Considering compelling content as just the foundation, *Re-Imagining Migration* educators envision teaching that transforms learner "dispositions." Here are "five dispositions for living in a world on the move," each preceded by the phrase: "*Capacity, sensitivity, and inclination to —*."[14]

- *Understand own and others' perspectives with empathy.* This disposition focuses on self-awareness and on empathizing and respecting the dignity of others in the context of migration and health studies.
- *Inquire about human migration with care and nuance.* This disposition stimulates curiosity and exploration about our shared human story, including the causes and consequences of migration at multiple levels (individual, community, nation).
- *Communicate and build relationships across differences.* This disposition focuses on developing a repertoire of communication skills: active and empathic listening coupled with respectful expression and culture-straddling dialogue when discussing migration and health.
- *Recognize power and inequities in human experience and migration.* This disposition acknowledges and clarifies power disparities that dovetail with racial/ethnic, class, and gender inequities and intersect in complex ways with migration and health.
- *Take action to foster inclusive and sustainable societies.* This disposition challenges instructors to devise assignments and activities that give agency to learners to become a voice and an advocate for the health and safety of migrants.

These five dispositions are essentially competencies that can be developed through teaching in a manner that achieves enculturation.

6.0 Framing Question 3: How Can We Teach about Migration and Health by Asking the Types of Questions that Invite Active Learner Participation in the Telling of Moving Stories?

Collaborative, experiential learning is strongly promoted in the field of public health. Active learning places students in participatory roles and involves them in analysis, synthesis, and creation activities. Particularly during graduate education, students can assume leadership roles in the presentation of course materials in a manner that stimulates energized involvement from classmates. Team presentations are well suited for this, particularly when the presenting team has prepared polls and asks questions tailored to encourage audience interaction. Strategies like *think-pair-share*, where learners initially tackle a question solo, then in a dyad with one other class member, and then with a larger team or the entire class, are applicable to a question-driven migration/health curriculum. Affinity mapping, problem-based learning, and team-based learning are also amenable to migration and health subject matter.

However, the application of a range of pedagogic techniques to facilitate student engagement on content delivery is just one piece. The *Re-Imagining Migration* team has developed a conceptualization that they call The Learning Arc that focuses on learners developing a deeper, personalized understanding of migration.[15] This is highly relevant in a world where more than one billion people are on the move and one in four of these—250 million persons—are currently living outside of their countries of origin. The magnitude of global mobility and the mixture of push-and-pull factors that impel or attract people to mobilize mean that interactions with persons on the move is now normative. However, we need to know more. As examples, was migration forced or voluntary? Reactive or proactive? Short-term or long-term? What drivers were moving people to move? Employment? Climate change? Poverty? Persecution? Armed conflict?

Teaching migration and health goes far beyond documenting population movements and attendant implications for health. It now becomes important to personalize the arc of migration itself. Questions are helpful to decipher the nature of the migratory experience. Much like the approach used throughout this chapter, guided by five practical and potentially transformative queries, the strategy for modifying our learners' dispositions is also based on asking questions related to the phases of migration (pre-, peri-, post-migration). *Re-Imagining Migration*'s preferred alternative phrasing uses the terms *life before migration, the journey*, and *adjustment*.[16] To set the moving story in motion, begin with the prompt: *We all have a migration story*. During this semester we hope to explore two complementary questions: *What is my story?* and *What is your story?* Although deceptively simple, these are perhaps the most important questions of the semester. Follow-up questions examine each phase in the trajectory of migration.

7.0 Framing Question 4: How Do We Create Engaging, Experiential Learning Environments for Students, Realizing That We Cohabit a World on the Move?

The field of migration and health undergoes constant, dynamic flux. This interdisciplinary field should be a delight to teach because it is so current and complex. What is outlined here, with gratitude for the vision and foresight of the *Re-Imagining Migration* professionals who have provided a pedagogic wagon for teaching about migration on which to hitch the population-health dimension, is a much deeper educational experience that brings out personal moving stories and attempts to transform student dispositions.[17]

This requires the creation of an educational environment that is, above all else, safe for learners. Migration and health must be taught with conscious focus on infusing all class activities and experiences with respectful and empathic regard for culture, diversity, equity, inclusion, and self-examination of our layers of biases and misunderstandings. Classes must emphasize what is scientifically known, what is evidence-based, and what is truthful. Classes should provide secure spaces for learning and sharing the stories that shape each of us.

8.0 Framing Question 5: How Do We Empower Educators to Teach Migration and Health for a World Undergoing Continual Transformation?

Teaching migration and health requires investment of time, talent, creativity, and considerable courage to take a more sensitized approach to course preparation and a more intensive approach to course delivery in order to showcase learners' moving stories. Asking educators and learners to share their own stories and examine their views and actions toward migrants takes some hard self-reflection that includes grappling with our own preconceptions, biases, and prejudices. School systems and universities, including specific departments sponsoring these educational offerings, can do much to support the professional development of educators who seek the opportunity—and privilege—to teach about migration and health.

Future symposia and conference themes focusing on the migration and health nexus can spark conversations about how to mutually support educators venturing into this domain. The good news is that the process of self-selection—with educators interested in this theme rising to teach fascinating content to enlightened learners who bring their own experiences to class—will identify a community of professionals who will further refine the field, energize the pedagogy, and encourage one another.

9.0 Distilling Guidance into Course Structure

To end on a practical note, we have created an outline for a fifteen-week-semester course on Migration and Population Health, with master's of public health (MPH) students or advanced bachelor's in public health (BSPH) students in mind (table 40.1). Consider this to be an illustrative

TABLE 40.1 **Example of a fifteen-week course on migration and population health for undergraduate and graduate public-health students**

Session	Session themes	Team presentations: Migration current events Team presentations: Migration health consequences	Active learner activities/ migration case studies
1	Course overview Key concepts in migration Migration current events Key concepts in population health	Meet in teams / class introductions Moving stories 1	A world on the move: International students
2	Migration history Hunter-gatherer mobility Transcontinental migration Agricultural civilizations Industrial age / The Anthropocene	Team: Migration current events Moving stories 2	2021 climate change and indigenous peoples: Yaqui Tribe water wars
3	Global drivers of migration Adaptation / employment / natural disaster / armed conflict / climate migration / ecological degradation / regime change with economic collapse	Team: Migration current events Moving stories 3	Famine and conflict in Drylands: South Sudan Migrant workers and the spread of Covid-19 in India
4	Phases of migration Premigration/migration/ post-migration Life before migration/the journey/adjustment	Team: Migration current events Team: Migration and food insecurity	Internal displacement in Colombia due to fifty-two-year armed conflict

TABLE 40.1 *(continued)*

Session	Session themes	Team presentations: Migration current events / Team presentations: Migration health consequences	Active learner activities/ migration case studies
5	Migration epidemiology Numbers, trends, geography The role of economic/ labor migration	Team: Migration current events Team: Migration and reproductive health	International migration trends
6	Eco-epidemiological perspectives Lifecourse perspectives on migration Multilevel/lifecourse matrix	Team: Migration current events Team: Migration and child development	2017 separating migrant children at US southern border
7	Dimensions for defining migration Level of preparedness: reactive/proactive Level of coercion: forced/ voluntary Duration: short-term/ long-term	Team: Migration current events Team: Migration and employment for children/ adults	2019 ethnic cleansing: Rohingya refugees seeking refuge in Bangladesh
8	International migration organizations	Team: Migration current events Team: Migration and older adults	2004 international response to the Southeast Asia tsunami
9	"Natural" disasters: short-term migration	Team: Migration current events Team: Migration and infectious disease exposure	2020 Cyclone Amphan in Bangladesh and India during Covid-19
10	Migration and technological/ecological disasters	Team: Migration current events Team: Migration and chronic disease rates	2011 Fukushima Daiichi nuclear power plant meltdown during Great East Japan disaster
11	Climate migration	Team: Migration current events Team: Migration and mental health/ substance use	Small island states: 2019 Hurricane Dorian— inability to migrate, environmental injustice
12	Conflict-induced displacement and migration	Team: Migration current events Team: Migration and exposure to violence	Armed conflict: Syrian/ European migrant crisis
13	Regime change/economic implosion as a driver of migration	Team: Migration current events Team: Migration during Covid-19	Regime change/economic collapse: Venezuelan diaspora
14	Immobility: When adaptive migration is not an option	Team: Migration current events Team: Migration and exposure to environmental hazards	Migrant and seasonal farm workers: exposure to extreme heat
15	Complex extreme events/ compound disasters and implications for migration	Team: Migration current events Team: Migration and future health threats	2020 California climate-driven wildfires during Covid-19 pandemic

structure for packaging course content that will be reworked for the specific purposes and preferences of each instructor.

The sequence of topics draws from multiple sources including, prominently, *Migration and Health*.[18] The selection of case studies is based on salient examples, including events about which we have published or have participated in the response. Instructors will substitute their own preferred choices.

Much in-class activity has potential to be student-led. For larger classes, student teams might be ideal. Migration is always a current event, so we suggest that teams present salient news of the week. We also have teams presenting a broad spectrum of health consequences throughout most of the fifteen sessions. Responsibilities for presenting selected case studies can be delegated to individual students, teams, or the instructor. Not included here are sessions that feature guest speakers, but certainly invited expertise would be a valuable addition.

In summary, we challenge instructors to consider the wise guidance from educators who have specialized in migration, fusing this with equally critical material from population health. Instructors have the opportunity to present coursework that is rich in content within the context of a class environment that is safe and conducive to having learners share their moving stories, as we stimulate meaningful, engaged participation from each of our students to optimize their educational experiences.

CHAPTER FORTY-ONE

Migration and Health

Taking Stock and Looking to the Future

Muhammad H. Zaman, Catherine K. Ettman, and Sandro Galea

A s we write these words, the burden of the Covid-19 pandemic continues to have a disproportionate impact on those who are socio-
economically disadvantaged, vulnerable, historically marginalized, and
without health safety nets.[1] From New York to New Delhi, we see these
patterns reinforced. In many ways, Covid-19 has brought to the fore the inequality and cracks in the health system that have always been there.[2] Not
only are the mortality and morbidity significantly higher among vulnerable groups, but access to care — and in particular access to vaccinations —
remains divided globally and locally among the haves and have-nots. Migrants, by and large, are among the have-nots. As of May 2021, nearly forty-
six million migrants had been excluded from national Covid-19 vaccination
programs around the world.[3]

Covid-19 is just one of the many lenses that allows us to look at the
challenges facing individuals and populations on the move. This volume
aims to present this and other lenses that range from geographic to demographic and economic in articulating and understanding the myriad issues
that migrant communities have to tackle as they are moving. The preced-
ing chapters describe health challenges and barriers to accessing health
care faced by migrants during the journey and in their new places of residence, whether that residence is temporary or permanent. As has been
described in several chapters, the drivers for migration differ significantly
across the globe and even within a single country. Conflict, climate change,
and economic factors remain some of the major drivers, but these factors

can often coincide, and the separation between them may be arbitrary at times. For example, climate change can work in tandem with conflict, as in Yemen and South Sudan, or economic reasons and climate change may converge for farmers who are no longer able to cultivate the lands they have historically resided in. Social exclusion on the basis of race, religion, and sexual orientation and government policies remain a major driver for economic migration, but policies in the new and host countries are just as responsible for access (or lack thereof) to health care. However, just as migration does not always means crossing international borders (for example, in the case of internally displaced), it is also not limited to extreme circumstances driven by conflict in low- and middle-income countries. The chapter on migration in old age (sunset migration) describes an important but underappreciated aspect of the need for health care among the elderly who migrate in high-income countries and have needs that are distinct from other groups.

In addition to discussing the drivers of migration and the harrowing realities of the journey, several chapters have carefully described the challenges faced by migrants in accessing health care. Xenophobia, exclusion, and racism continue to affect migrants' access to health care. Violence against migrants remains a permanent threat, and women and children often suffer heavily, both during the journey and in their new environments. In some instances, access to health care has been used as a political tool by governments, which is both disturbing in and of itself and completely antithetical to the goals of dignified, equitable, and quality health care. Upon reaching a new environment, language and cultural barriers can further exacerbate these challenges. In the recent past, nativist, nationalist, and anti-immigrant sentiments in the United States, Europe, Australia, and elsewhere have created further complications and limited the access to migrant communities who are in new environments. These communities often have limited financial resources and are lacking in social networks that facilitate access to health care. Some scholars have also argued that the impact of migration is not limited to migrants themselves, but also to the family and community that are unable to, or choose not to, migrate. Studies on migrant labor from South Asia and the Philippines to the Gulf countries have shown that while migration helps with remittances to the local communities, mental health issues continue to rise among the family members who are left behind. The movement of migrant labor back to the communities also correlates with high rates of domestic violence. The complex and underappreciated challenges of mental health have been noted by several contributors, as have the associated risks of substance abuse and domestic violence. Stigma, a lack of awareness, and the poor allocation of resources make mental health a continued and growing challenge faced by migrant communities of all age groups, as well as their extended families who may not migrate. The trauma of migration, anxiety from being in a new and potentially unwelcoming environment, and limited social and financial capital have been highlighted as issues that need urgent and sustained attention. Among the health challenges, it is also important to note that at times the separation between chronic and infectious diseases is a false separation, and these challenges not only manifest themselves together (e.g., Covid-19 and mental health), but may also reinforce each other.

Just as several chapters highlighted both the drivers and the intersecting health challenges, contributors to this volume also discussed various policy recommendations along with their limitations. Health-care access and its provision to migrants is simultaneously a human right, economic issue, and legal issue. Domestic and international legal structures are critical for dignified and equitable care that meets an international standard of quality. Landmark international treaties may serve as a starting point to address some of the glaring gaps in health-care access to those who migrate. Yet, agreement across nation states on what constitutes a basic standard varies, and implementing treaties is often just as complicated as creating them. Nation states, whose policies may be the reason for driving people out in the first place, may not be eager to sign or enact treaties that may highlight their own negligence and the victimization of specific communities. Scholars contributing to this volume have also noted that while international treaties are important to create a global safety net that provides health care to migrants, local legal structures are just as important. Inequity, xenophobia, racism, and exclusion affect health care not just during the journey, but also within the borders of the new home. This is particularly true for communities that may not have the formal or permanent legal status.

In this case, the role of civil society and nongovernmental organizations is also important to provide guidance, support, and services to the migrants and to raise awareness and argue for stronger legal protection for the vulnerable. Health—as discussed by some scholars—cannot be separated from other social services, such as meaningful employment and education. Therefore, the need for legislation at the local level that takes a more holistic view of health and well-being is important for sustainable access to health care. Contributors to this volume note that universal health coverage (UHC) remains a potent tool in improving access, yet we also note that it is part of the bigger picture and may have a larger impact in some areas (such as equitable and affordable perinatal care) than others. Nonetheless, despite political and economic challenges, we believe that UHC should remain an important piece of the solution landscape. Technology also has an important role to play. Cell phones, rapid diagnostics, artificial intelligence, data-sharing, and telehealth services are becoming an integral part of any health system. Migrants are increasingly relying on WhatsApp, social media, and other applications to access information and health care throughout their journey and after reaching their destination. These technological tools are also important in creating and maintaining a sense of community. Technology therefore can make a real contribution in improving access to health care among migrants. Yet, these technological solutions are also at risk of manipulation and exploitation in the absence of a strong ethical and regulatory framework. Migrants, who may not enjoy a robust legal protection, may find their health and personal data and privacy compromised, thereby increasing their vulnerability and eroding trust between health-care providers and those who seek care. Ethics in legal structures, technology access, and policy development, therefore, must lay the foundations of any robust solution to the health-care challenges faced by migrants. An ethical approach, as our contributors have pointed out, relies on rigorously developed and analyzed case studies, is multidisciplinary, and reflects on the human condition. This, as noted by our contributors, needs to be implemented not just in practice, but also in training programs and curricula for health professionals and practitioners.

Despite the challenges, many of which have been thoughtfully described by contributors to this volume, we remain hopeful for the future. This volume highlights not only what we ought not to do, but also what has worked well in terms of policies, legal frameworks, social engagement by civil society, and technology development. Most importantly, we are hopeful because a dialogue across scholars and practitioners of various disciplines, across communities and geographies, is the basis of a marketplace of ideas for a better and more equitable world where the health and well-being of migrants is protected and nourished. This volume is a step in that direction.

Acknowledgments

We would like to acknowledge all our colleagues who have participated in conversations and meetings about this topic over the years; they have much sharpened our thinking about the field. Thank you to all the chapter authors who engaged with this project—we have learned from all of you. As always, we thank our families for their support as we took on this book amid many other ongoing projects. We would like to thank the migrants who have shared their stories, informing the scholarship presented in this book. And last, thank you to all who have welcomed migrants, moving the world forward.

Contributors

NADIA N. ABUELEZAM, Boston College, Chestnut Hill, USA

SERGIO AGUILAR-GAXIOLA, University of California, Davis, Sacramento, CA, USA

RICHARD ALDERSLADE, Health and Migration Programme, World Health Organization, Geneva, Switzerland

GEORGE J. ANNAS, Boston University, Boston, MA, USA

SALMA SOFÍA BAIZER CASSAB, Universidad de los Andes, Bogotá, Colombia

OSCAR A. BERNAL ACEVEDO, Universidad de los Andes, Bogotá, Colombia

JOSHUA BRESLAU, RAND Corporation, Pittsburgh, PA, USA

FRANCESCO CASTELLI, University of Brescia and ASST Spedali Civili, Brescia, Italy

CARLY CHING, Boston University, Boston, MA, USA

LAURA BALDOVINO-CHIQUILLO, Universidad de los Andes, Bogotá, Colombia

SONDRA S. CROSBY, Boston University, Boston, MA, USA

SÓNIA DIAS, National School of Public Health, New University Lisbon, Lisboa, Portugal

ZELDE ESPINEL, University of Miami, Miami, FL, USA

CATHERINE K. ETTMAN, Boston University, Boston, MA, and Brown University, Providence, RI, USA

AHSAN M. FUZAIL, Boston University, Boston, MA, USA

SANDRO GALEA, Boston University, Boston, MA, USA

ANA GAMA, National School of Public Health, New University Lisbon, Lisboa, Portugal

DIRGHA GHIMIRE, University of Michigan, Ann Arbor, MI, USA

STEVEN J. GOLD, Michigan State University, East Lansing, MI, USA

SABRINA HERMOSILLA, University of Michigan, Ann Arbor, MI, USA

ANDERS HJERN, Karolinska Institutet and Centre for Health Equity Studies (CHESS), Karolinska Institutet/Stockholm University, Stockholm, Sweden

ERIN HOARE, Deakin University, Victoria, Australia

ELEANOR HOLROYD, Auckland University of Technology (AUT) and AUT Centre for Migrant and Refugee Research, New Zealand Auckland, New Zealand

RESHMAAN HUSSAM, Harvard University, Cambridge, MA, USA

PALMIRA IMMORDINO, Health and Migration Programme, World Health Organization, Geneva, Switzerland

FELICE JACKA, Deakin University, Victoria, Australia

AYESHA KADIR, Save the Children UK, London, UK

HULYA KOSEMATOGLU, Harvard University, Cambridge, MA, USA

ALLAN KRASNIK, University of Copenhagen, Copenhagen, Denmark

MARIA KRISTIANSEN, University of Copenhagen, Copenhagen, Denmark

TILMAN LANZ, University of Groningen, Groningen, Netherlands

BINGQIN LI, University of New South Wales, Sydney, Australia

JUTTA LINDERT, University of Applied Sciences Emden / Leer, Emden, Germany

GUSTAVO LOERA, University of California, Davis, Sacramento, CA, USA

SANA LOUE, Case Western Reserve University, Cleveland, OH, USA

PATRÍCIA MARQUES, National School of Public Health, New University Lisbon, Lisboa, Portugal

CELIA MCMICHAEL, University of Melbourne, Victoria, Australia

MARÍA ELENA MEDINA-MORA, National Autonomous University of Mexico, Ciudad Universitaria and National Institute of Psychiatry RFM, Mexico City, Mexico

JANNA METZLER, Women's Refugee Commission, New York, NY, USA

JED MONTAYRE, AUT Centre for Migrant and Refugee Research, Auckland, New Zealand, and Western Sydney University, Sydney, Australia

YUDIT NAMER, Bielefeld University, Bielefeld, Germany

MARIE NORREDAM, University of Copenhagen, Copenhagen, Denmark

SONJA NOVAK-ZEZULA, Center for Health and Migration, Vienna, Austria

LIKA NUSBAUM, Ben-Gurion University of the Negev, Beer-Sheva, Israel

JOVANA A. OCAMPO CAÑAS, Universidad de los Andes, Bogotá, Colombia

ADRIENNE O'NEIL, Deakin University, Victoria, Australia

EBIOWEI SAMUEL F. ORUBU, Boston University, Boston, MA, USA

WENDY E. PARMET, Northeastern University, Boston, MA, USA

JHON SEBASTIAN PATIÑO RUEDA, Universidad de los Andes, Bogotá, Colombia

LILIAN G. PEREZ, RAND Corporation, Santa Monica, CA, USA

CARRIE J. PRESTON, Boston University, Boston, MA, USA

KARL PHILIPP PUCHNER, Aristotle University of Thessaloniki, Thessaloniki, Greece

OLIVER RAZUM, Bielefeld University, Bielefeld, Germany

ANDREAS RECHKEMMER, Hamad Bin Khalifa University, Doha, Qatar

SANTINO SEVERONI, Health and Migration Programme, World Health Organization, Geneva, Switzerland

JAMES M. SHULTZ, University of Miami, Miami, FL, USA

MELISSA SIEGEL, Maastricht University/UNU-MERIT, Maastricht, Netherlands

DENISE L. SPITZER, University of Alberta, Edmonton, Alberta, Canada

FELICITY THOMAS, Wellcome Centre for Cultures and Environments of Health, University of Exeter, Exeter, UK

EMILY TRELEAVEN, University of Michigan, Ann Arbor, MI, USA

URSULA TRUMMER, Center for Health and Migration, Vienna, Austria

AGIS D. TSOUROS, Imperial College London, London, UK, and Boston University, Boston, MA, USA

MICHAEL R. ULRICH, Boston University, Boston, MA, USA

JO VEAREY, Wits University, Johannesburg, South Africa

NICOLAS VIGNIER, Centre hospitalier de Cayenne, French Guiana, Université Sorbonne Paris Nord, Bobigny, Institut Convergences et Migration, Aubervilliers, and Institut Pierre Louis d'Épidémiologie et de Santé Publique (IPLESP), Sorbonne Université, Paris, France

TONY WARNES, University of Sheffield, Sheffield, UK

YANG XIAO, Tongji University, Shanghai, China

MUHAMMAD H. ZAMAN, Boston University, Boston, MA, USA

Notes

Chapter 1

1. John F. Cherry and Thomas P. Leppard, "Experimental Archaeology and the Earliest Seagoing: The Limitations of Inference," *World Archaeology* 47, no. 5 (October 20, 2015): 740–55, https://doi.org/10.1080/00438243.2015.1078739.

2. Marie McAuliffe and Binod Khadria, eds., *World Migration Report 2020* (Geneva: International Organization for Migration, 2019), https://publications.iom.int/system/files/pdf/wmr_2020.pdf.

3. Joop de Beer, James Raymer, Rob van der Erf, and Leo van Wissen. "Overcoming the Problems of Inconsistent International Migration Data: A New Method Applied to Flows in Europe," *European Journal of Population* 26, no. 4 (November 2010): 459–81, https://doi.org/10.1007/s10680-010-9220-z.

4. Paul Douglas, Martin Cetron, and Paul Spiegel, "Definitions Matter: Migrants, Immigrants, Asylum Seekers and Refugees," *Journal of Travel Medicine* 26, no. 2 (February 1, 2019), https://doi.org/10.1093/jtm/taz005.

5. Douglas et al., "Definitions Matter."

6. "International Migrant Stock 2019," United Nations Population Division, Department of Economic and Social Affairs, accessed January 19, 2021, https://www.un.org/en/development/desa/population/migration/data/estimates2/estimates19.asp.

Chapter 2

1. Centers for Disease Control and Prevention, "The Social-Ecological Model: A Framework for Prevention," January 29, 2021, https://www.cdc.gov/violenceprevention/about/social-ecologicalmodel.html; Nancy Krieger, "Epidemiology and the Web of Causation: Has Anyone Seen the Spider?," *Social Science and Medicine* 39, no. 7 (October 1994): 887–903, https://doi.org/10.1016/0277-9536(94)90202-x.

2. George A. Kaplan, "What's Wrong with Social Epidemiology, and How Can We Make It Better?," *Epidemiologic Reviews* 26, no. 1 (July 1, 2004): 124–35, https://doi.org/10.1093/epirev/mxh010.

3. Dolores Acevedo-Garcia et al., "Integrating Social Epidemiology into Immigrant Health Research: A Cross-National Framework," *Social Science and Medicine*, special issue, *Place, Migration and Health*, 75, no. 12 (December 1, 2012): 2060–68, https://doi.org/10.1016/j.socscimed.2012.04.040.

4. Jo Vearey, Charles Hui, and Kolitha Wickramage, "Migration and Health: Current Issues, Governance and Knowledge Gaps," *World Migration Report* (2020), 38.

5. Jessica Allen et al., *Social Determinants of Mental Health* (Geneva: World Health Organization, 2014), http://apps.who.int/iris/bitstream/10665/112828/1/9789241506809_eng.pdf?ua=1.

6. Andrea L. Roberts et al., "Posttraumatic Stress Disorder and Incidence of Type 2 Diabetes Mellitus in a Sample of Women: A 22-Year Longitudinal Study," *JAMA Psychiatry* 72, no. 3 (March 1, 2015): 203, https://doi.org/10.1001/jamapsychiatry.2014.2632.

7. Kaplan, "What's Wrong with Social Epidemiology?"

8. Kaplan, "What's Wrong with Social Epidemiology?"

9. Mina Fazel et al., "Mental Health of Displaced and Refugee Children Resettled in High-Income Countries: Risk and Protective Factors," *Lancet* 379, no. 9812 (January 21, 2012): 266–82, https://doi.org/10.1016/S0140-6736(11)60051-2.

10. Sol P. Juárez et al., "Revisiting the Healthy Migrant Paradox in Perinatal Health Outcomes through a Scoping Review in a Recent Host Country," *Journal of Immigrant and Minority Health* 19, no. 1 (February 2017): 205–14, http://dx.doi.org.ezproxy.bu.edu/10.1007/s10903-015-0317-7.

11. Steven Kennedy et al., "The Healthy Immigrant Effect: Patterns and Evidence from Four Countries," *Journal of International Migration and Integration* 16, no. 2 (May 2015): 317–32, http://dx.doi.org.ezproxy.bu.edu/10.1007/s12134-014-0340-x.

12. Kyriakos S. Markides and Sunshine Rote, "The Healthy Immigrant Effect and Aging in the United States and Other Western Countries," *The Gerontologist* 59, no. 2 (March 14, 2019): 205–14, https://doi.org/10.1093/geront/gny136.

13. Eran Shor, David Roelfs, and Zoua M. Vang, "The 'Hispanic Mortality Paradox' Revisited: Meta-Analysis and Meta-Regression of Life-Course Differentials in Latin American and Caribbean Immigrants' Mortality," *Social Science and Medicine* 186 (August 1, 2017): 20–33, https://doi.org/10.1016/j.socscimed.2017.05.049.

14. Zoua M. Vang et al., "Are Immigrants Healthier Than Native-Born Canadians? A Systematic Review of the Healthy Immigrant Effect in Canada," *Ethnicity and Health* 22, no. 3 (2017): 209–41, https://doi.org/10.1080/13557858.2016.1246518.

15. Yasser Moullan and Florence Jusot, "Why Is the 'Healthy Immigrant Effect' Different between European Countries?," *European Journal of Public Health* 24, no. 1 (August 2014): 80–86, https://doi.org/10.1093/eurpub/cku112.

16. Vang et al., "Are Immigrants Healthier?"

17. Anna Gkiouleka et al., "Depressive Symptoms among Migrants and Non-Migrants in Europe: Documenting and Explaining Inequalities in Times of Socio-Economic Instability," *European Journal of Public Health* 28, no. 5 (December 1, 2018): 54–60, https://doi.org/10.1093/eurpub/cky202.

18. Sarah Missinne and Piet Bracke, "Depressive Symptoms among Immigrants and Ethnic Minorities: A Population Based Study in 23 European Countries," *Social Psychiatry and Psychiatric Epidemiology* 47, no. 1 (January 2012): 97–109, https://doi.org/10.1007/s00127-010-0321-0.

19. Maria Roura, "Unravelling Migrants' Health Paradoxes: A Transdisciplinary Research Agenda," *J Epidemiol Community Health* 71, no. 9 (September 1, 2017): 870–73, https://doi.org/10.1136/jech-2016-208439.

20. Jeong-Ah Ahn et al., "Health of International Marriage Immigrant Women in South Korea: A Systematic Review," *Journal of Immigrant and Minority Health* 20, no. 3 (June 2018): 717–28, http://dx.doi.org.ezproxy.bu.edu/10.1007/s10903-017-0604-6.

21. Yeeun Lee and Subin Park, "The Mental Health of Married Immigrant Women in South Korea and Its Risk and Protective Factors: A Literature Review," *International Journal of Social Psychiatry* 64, no. 1 (February 1, 2018): 80–91, https://doi.org/10.1177/0020764017744581.

22. P. Priscilla Lui, "Intergenerational Cultural Conflict, Mental Health, and Educational Outcomes among Asian and Latino/a Americans: Qualitative and Meta-Analytic Review," *Psychological Bulletin* 141, no. 2 (March 2015): 404–46, https://doi.org/10.1037/a0038449.

23. Matthias Pierce et al., "Effects of Parental Mental Illness on Children's Physical Health: Systematic Review and Meta-Analysis," *British Journal of Psychiatry: Journal of Mental Science* 217, no. 1 (July 2020): 354–63, https://doi.org/10.1192/bjp.2019.216.

24. Gracia Fellmeth et al., "Health Impacts of Parental Migration on Left-behind Children and Adolescents: A Systematic Review and Meta-Analysis," *Lancet* 392, no. 10164 (December 5, 2018): 2567–82, https://doi.org/10.1016/S0140-6736(18)32558-3.

25. Lisa Merry, Sandra Pelaez, and Nancy C. Edwards, "Refugees, Asylum-Seekers and Undocumented Migrants and the Experience of Parenthood: A Synthesis of the Qualitative Literature," *Globalization and Health* 13, no. 1 (September 19, 2017): 75, https://doi.org/10.1186/s12992-017-0299-4.

26. Tsui-Sui Annie Kao, Chikwekwe Musonda Lupiya, and Susan Clemen-Stone, "Family Efficacy as a Protective Factor Against Immigrant Adolescent Risky Behavior: A Literature Review," *Journal of Holistic Nursing: Official Journal of the American Holistic Nurses' Association* 32, no. 3 (September 2014): 202–16, https://doi.org/10.1177/0898010113518840.

27. Rana Dahlan et al., "Impact of Social Support on Oral Health among Immigrants and Ethnic Minorities: A Systematic Review," *PloS One* 14, no. 6 (June 20, 2019): e0218678, https://doi.org/10.1371/journal.pone.0218678.

28. Russell Miller et al., "Mental Well-Being of International Migrants to Japan: A Systematic Review," *BMJ Open* 9, no. 11 (November 3, 2019): e029988, https://doi.org/10.1136/bmjopen-2019-029988.

29. Kerri E. McPherson et al., "The Association between Social Capital and Mental Health and Behavioural Problems in Children and Adolescents: An Integrative Systematic Review," *BMC Psychology* 2, no. 1 (2014): 7, https://doi.org/10.1186/2050-7283-2-7.

30. Roshanak Mehdipanah, Alexa Eisenberg, and Amy Schulz, "Housing," in *Urban Health*, ed. Sandro Galea, Catherine K. Ettman, and David Vlahov (New York: Oxford University Press, 2019).

31. Frank L. Farmer and Doris P. Slesinger, "Health Status and Needs of Migrant Farm Workers in the United States: A Literature Review," *Journal of Rural Health* 8, no. 3 (1992): 227–34, https://doi.org/10.1111/j.1748-0361.1992.tb00356.x.

32. Sara A. Quandt et al., "Farmworker Housing in the United States and Its Impact on Health," *New Solutions: A Journal of Environmental and Occupational Health Policy* 25, no. 3 (November 1, 2015): 263–86, https://doi.org/10.1177/1048291115601053.

33. Ben Marsh et al., "Understanding the Role of Social Factors in Farmworker Housing and Health," *New Solutions: A Journal of Environmental and Occupational Health Policy* 25, no. 3 (November 1, 2015): 313–33, https://doi.org/10.1177/1048291115601020.

34. Bukola Salami, Salima Meherali, and Azeez Salami, "The Health of Temporary Foreign Workers in Canada: A Scoping Review," *Canadian Journal of Public Health* 106, no. 8 (March 16, 2016): e546–554, https://doi.org/10.17269/cjph.106.5182.

35. Cindy D. Chang, "Social Determinants of Health and Health Disparities Among Immigrants and Their Children," *Current Problems in Pediatric and Adolescent Health Care* 49, no. 1 (January 1, 2019): 23–30, https://doi.org/10.1016/j.cppeds.2018.11.009.

36. Quandt et al., "Farmworker Housing in the United States."

37. Marsh et al., "Understanding the Role of Social Factors."

38. Salami et al., "The Health of Temporary Foreign Workers in Canada."

39. David R. Williams, "The Health of U.S. Racial and Ethnic Populations," *Journals of Gerontology: Series B* 60, no. 2 (October 1, 2005): S53–62, https://doi.org/10.1093/geronb/60.Special_Issue_2.S53.

40. Chang, "Social Determinants of Health."

41. Mark Edberg, Sean Cleary, and Amita Vyas, "A Trajectory Model for Understanding and Assessing Health Disparities in Immigrant/Refugee Communities," *Journal of Immigrant and Minority Health* 13, no. 3 (June 2011): 576–84, http://dx.doi.org.ezproxy.bu.edu/10.1007/s10903-010-9337-5.

42. Fazel et al., "Mental Health of Displaced and Refugee Children."

43. Sandraluz Lara-Cinisomo, Yange Xue, and Jeanne Brooks-Gunn, "Latino Youth's Internalising Behaviours: Links to Immigrant Status and Neighbourhood

Characteristics," *Ethnicity and Health* 18, no. 3 (2013): 315–35, https://doi.org/10.1080/13557858.2012.734278.

44. Rita Hamad et al., "Association of Neighborhood Disadvantage with Cardiovascular Risk Factors and Events Among Refugees in Denmark," *JAMA Network Open* 3, no. 8 (August 3, 2020): e2014196–e2014196, https://doi.org/10.1001/jamanetworkopen.2020.14196.

45. Benjamin Schilgen et al., "Health Situation of Migrant and Minority Nurses: A Systematic Review," *PloS One* 12, no. 6 (2017): e0179183, https://doi.org/10.1371/journal.pone.0179183.

46. Farmer and Slesinger, "Health Status and Needs of Migrant Farm Workers"; Marsh et al., "Understanding the Role of Social Factors."

47. Cecilia Arici et al., "Occupational Health and Safety of Immigrant Workers in Italy and Spain: A Scoping Review," *International Journal of Environmental Research and Public Health* 16, no. 22 (November 2019), https://doi.org/10.3390/ijerph16224416.

48. Antonio Sarría-Santamera et al., "A Systematic Review of the Use of Health Services by Immigrants and Native Populations," *Public Health Reviews* 37 (2016): 28, https://doi.org/10.1186/s40985-016-0042-3.

49. Judit Simon et al., *Public Health Aspects of Migrant Health: A Review of the Evidence on Health Status for Labour Migrants in the European Region*, WHO Health Evidence Network Synthesis Reports (Copenhagen: WHO Regional Office for Europe, 2015), http://www.ncbi.nlm.nih.gov/books/NBK379432/.

50. Niina Markkula et al., "Use of Health Services among International Migrant Children—A Systematic Review," *Globalization and Health* 14 (May 16, 2018), https://doi.org/10.1186/s12992-018-0370-9.

51. Amelia Seraphia Derr, "Mental Health Service Use Among Immigrants in the United States: A Systematic Review," *Psychiatric Services (Washington, DC)* 67, no. 3 (March 2016): 265–74, https://doi.org/10.1176/appi.ps.201500004.

52. Maria A. Monserud and Kyriakos S. Markides, "Changes in Depressive Symptoms during Widowhood among Older Mexican Americans: The Role of Financial Strain, Social Support, and Church Attendance," *Aging and Mental Health* 21, no. 6 (June 2017): 586–94, https://doi.org/10.1080/13607863.2015.1132676.

53. Sol Pía Juárez et al., "Effects of Non-Health-Targeted Policies on Migrant Health: A Systematic Review and Meta-Analysis," *Lancet Global Health* 7, no. 4 (2019): e420–35, https://doi.org/10.1016/S2214-109X(18)30560-6.

54. Alastair Ager and Alison Strang, "Understanding Integration: A Conceptual Framework," *Journal of Refugee Studies* 21, no. 2 (June 1, 2008): 166–91, https://doi.org/10.1093/jrs/fen016.

55. Chang, "Social Determinants of Health."

56. *Lancet*, "US Public Charge Rule: Pushing the Door Closed," *Lancet* 393, no. 10187 (June 1, 2019): 2176, https://doi.org/10.1016/S0140-6736(19)31233-4.

57. Angela Kalich, Lyn Heinemann, and Setareh Ghahari, "A Scoping Review of Immigrant Experience of Health Care Access Barriers in Canada," *Journal of*

Immigrant and Minority Health 18, no. 3 (June 2016): 697–709, http://dx.doi.org .ezproxy.bu.edu/10.1007/s10903-015-0237-6.

58. Goleen Samari, Héctor E. Alcalá, and Mienah Zulfacar Sharif, "Islamophobia, Health, and Public Health: A Systematic Literature Review," *American Journal of Public Health* 108, no. 6 (2018): e1–9, https://doi.org/10.2105/AJPH.2018.304 402.

59. Shazeen Suleman, Kent D. Garber, and Lainie Rutkow, "Xenophobia as a Determinant of Health: An Integrative Review," *Journal of Public Health Policy; Basingstoke* 39, no. 4 (November 2018): 407–23, http://dx.doi.org.ezproxy.bu.edu/10 .1057/s41271-018-0140-1.

60. Nadia Andrade, Athena D. Ford, and Carmen Alvarez, "Discrimination and Latino Health: A Systematic Review of Risk and Resilience," *Hispanic Health Care International: The Official Journal of the National Association of Hispanic Nurses* 19, no. 1 (May 8, 2020), 5–16, https://doi.org/10.1177/1540415320921489.

61. Abdulrahman M. El-Sayed and Sandro Galea, "The Health of Arab-Americans Living in the United States: A Systematic Review of the Literature," *BMC Public Health* 9 (July 30, 2009): 272, https://doi.org/10.1186/1471-2458-9-272.

62. Gilbert C. Gee et al., "Racial Discrimination and Health among Asian Americans: Evidence, Assessment, and Directions for Future Research," *Epidemiologic Reviews* 31 (2009): 130–51, https://doi.org/10.1093/epirev/mxp009.

63. Anne Sofie Borsch et al., "Health, Education and Employment Outcomes in Young Refugees in the Nordic Countries: A Systematic Review," *Scandinavian Journal of Public Health* 47, no. 7 (August 1, 2018): 735–47, https://doi.org/10.1177 /1403494818787099.

64. Kristin Toso, Paul de Cock, and Gerard Leavey, "Maternal Exposure to Violence and Offspring Neurodevelopment: A Systematic Review," *Paediatric and Perinatal Epidemiology* 34, no. 2 (2020): 190–203, https://doi.org/10.1111/ppe.12651.

65. Kathryn M. Yount, Ann M. DiGirolamo, and Usha Ramakrishnan, "Impacts of Domestic Violence on Child Growth and Nutrition: A Conceptual Review of the Pathways of Influence," *Social Science and Medicine* 72, no. 9 (May 1, 2011): 1534–54, https://doi.org/10.1016/j.socscimed.2011.02.042.

66. George C. Patton et al., "Our Future: A Lancet Commission on Adolescent Health and Wellbeing," *Lancet* 387, no. 10036 (June 11, 2016): 2423–78, https://doi .org/10.1016/S0140-6736(16)00579-1.

67. Debora Lee Oh et al., "Systematic Review of Pediatric Health Outcomes Associated with Childhood Adversity," *BMC Pediatrics* 18, no. 1 (February 23, 2018): 83, https://doi.org/10.1186/s12887-018-1037-7.

68. P. Curtis, J. Thompson, and H. Fairbrother, "Migrant Children within Europe: A Systematic Review of Children's Perspectives on Their Health Experiences," *Public Health*, special issue, *Migration: A Global Public Health Issue* 158 (May 1, 2018): 71–85, https://doi.org/10.1016/j.puhe.2018.01.038.

69. N. Leigh-Hunt et al., "An Overview of Systematic Reviews on the Public

Health Consequences of Social Isolation and Loneliness," *Public Health* 152 (November 2017): 157–71, https://doi.org/10.1016/j.puhe.2017.07.035.

70. Helena Honkaniemi et al., "Psychological Distress by Age at Migration and Duration of Residence in Sweden," *Social Science and Medicine* 250 (February 20, 2020): 112869, https://doi.org/10.1016/j.socscimed.2020.112869.

71. Teresa Saraiva Leão et al., "The Influence of Age at Migration and Length of Residence on Self-Rated Health among Swedish Immigrants: A Cross-Sectional Study," *Ethnicity and Health* 14, no. 1 (February 2009): 93–105, https://doi.org/10.1080/13557850802345973.

72. Markides and Rote, "The Healthy Immigrant Effect."

73. Markides and Rote, "The Healthy Immigrant Effect."

74. Shor, Roelfs, and Vang, "The 'Hispanic Mortality Paradox' Revisited."

75. Sepali Guruge and Hissan Butt, "A Scoping Review of Mental Health Issues and Concerns among Immigrant and Refugee Youth in Canada: Looking Back, Moving Forward," *Canadian Journal of Public Health* 106, no. 2 (February 3, 2015): e72–78, https://doi.org/10.17269/cjph.106.4588.

76. Jan Michael Bauer, Tilman Brand, and Hajo Zeeb, "Pre-Migration Socioeconomic Status and Post-Migration Health Satisfaction among Syrian Refugees in Germany: A Cross-Sectional Analysis," *PLoS Medicine* 17, no. 3 (2020): e1003093, https://doi.org/10.1371/journal.pmed.1003093.

77. Margaret Butler et al., "Migration and Common Mental Disorder: An Improvement in Mental Health over Time?," *International Review of Psychiatry* 27, no. 1 (February 2015): 51–63, https://doi.org/10.3109/09540261.2014.996858.

78. A. Jud, E. Pfeiffer, and M. Jarczok, "Epidemiology of Violence against Children in Migration: A Systematic Literature Review," *Child Abuse and Neglect* 108 (July 31, 2020): 104634, https://doi.org/10.1016/j.chiabu.2020.104634.

79. Ibrahim Abubakar et al., "The UCL-Lancet Commission on Migration and Health: The Health of a World on the Move," *Lancet* 392, no. 10164 (December 5, 2018): 2606–54, https://doi.org/10.1016/S0140-6736(18)32114-7.

80. Juárez et al., "Effects of Non-Health-Targeted Policies on Migrant Health."

81. Guruge and Butt, "A Scoping Review of Mental Health Issues."

82. J. Das-Munshi et al., "Migration, Social Mobility and Common Mental Disorders: Critical Review of the Literature and Meta-Analysis," *Ethnicity and Health* 17, no. 1–2 (2012): 17–53, https://doi.org/10.1080/13557858.2011.632816.

83. Christina Greenaway and Francesco Castelli, "Infectious Diseases at Different Stages of Migration: An Expert Review," *Journal of Travel Medicine* 26, no. 2 (February 1, 2019), https://doi.org/10.1093/jtm/taz007.

84. D. Bhugra, "Migration and Mental Health," *Acta Psychiatrica Scandinavica* 109, no. 4 (April 2004): 243–58, https://doi.org/10.1046/j.0001-690x.2003.00246.x; D. Bhugra, "Migration and Depression," *Acta Psychiatrica Scandinavica* 108 (October 2, 2003): 67–72, https://doi.org/10.1034/j.1600-0447.108.s418.14.x.

85. Heide Castañeda et al., "Immigration as a Social Determinant of Health,"

Annual Review of Public Health 36, no. 1 (March 18, 2015): 375–92, https://doi.org /10.1146/annurev-publhealth-032013-182419.

86. Marie Nørredam, "Migration and Health: Exploring the Role of Migrant Status through Register-Based Studies," *Danish Medical Journal* 62, no. 4 (April 2015): B5068.

Chapter 3

1. International Organization for Migration (IOM). "World Migration Report 2020." Accessed October 10, 2020. https://publications.iom.int/system/files/pdf/wmr _2020.pdf.

2. IOM, "World Migration Report 2020."

3. Mishal S. Khan, Anna Osei-Kofi, Abbas Omar, Hilary Kirkbride, Anthony Kessel, Aula Abbara, David Heymann, Alimuddin Zumla, and Osman Dar. "Pathogens, Prejudice, and Politics: The Role of the Global Health Community in the European Refugee Crisis." *Lancet Infectious Diseases* 16 (2016): e173–77. http://dx .doi.org/10.1016/S1473-3099(16)30134-7; Ibrahim Abubakar, Robert W. Aldridge, Delan Devakumar, Miriam Orcutt, Rachel Burns, Mauricio L. Barreto, Poonam Dhavan, Fouad M. Fouad, Nora Groce, Yan Guo, Sally Hargreaves, Michale Knipper, Jaime J. Miranda, Nyovani Madise, Bernadette Kumar, Davide Mosca, Terry McGovern, Leonard Rubenstein, Peter Sammonds, Susan M. Sawyer, Kabir Sheikh, Stephen Tollman, Paul Spiegel, and Cathy Zimmerman, on behalf of the UCL– Lancet Commission on Migration and Health. "The UCL–Lancet Commission on Migration and Health: The Health of a World on the Move." *Lancet* 392 (2018): 2606–54.

4. Francesco Castelli and Giorgia Sulis. "Migration and Infectious Diseases." *Clinical Microbiology and Infection* 23, no. 5 (2017): P283–89. https://doi.org/10.10 16/j.cmi.2017.03.012; Christina Greenaway and Francesco Castelli. "Infectious Diseases at Different Stages of Migration: An Expert Review." *Journal of Travel Medicine* 26, no. 2 (2019): taz007. https://doi.org/10.1093/jtm/taz007.

5. P. Douglas, Marty Cetron, and Paul Spiegel. "Definitions Matter: Migrants, Immigrants, Asylum Seekers and Refugees." *Journal of Travel Medicine* 26, no. 2 (2019). https://doi.org/10.1093/jtm/taz005.

6. Marianne Vervliet, Bruno Vanobbergen, Eric Broekaert, and Ilse Derluyn. "The Aspirations of Afghan Unaccompanied Refugee Minors Before Departure and On Arrival in the Host Country." *Childhood: A Global Journal of Child Research* 22, 3 (2015): 330–45. https://doi.org/10.1177/0907568214533976.

7. European Asylum Support Office (EASO). "Significant Pull/Push Factors for Determining of Asylum-Related Migration" (November 2016). Accessed October 4, 2020. https://op.europa.eu/en/publication-detail/-/publication/e68aa57d-c102 -11e6-a6db-01aa75ed71a1.

8. Everett S. Lee. "A Theory of Migration." *Demography* 3, no. 1 (1966): 47–57.

9. Stephen Castles, Hein de Haas, and Mark J. Miller. "The Age of Migration." New York: Palgrave MacMillan, 2014.

10. Nicholas Van Hear, Oliver Bakewell, and Katy Long. "Push-Pull Plus: Reconsidering the Drivers of Migration." *Journal of Ethnic and Migration Studies* 44, no. 6 (2018): 927–44. https://doi.org/10.1080/1369183X.2017.1384135.

11. Francesco Castelli. "Drivers of Migration. Why Do People Move?" *Journal of Travel Medicine* 25, no. 1 (2018). https://doi.org/10.1093/jtm/tay040.

12. United Nations Department of Economic and Social Affairs (UNDESA). "World Population Prospects 2019." Accessed October 11, 2020. https://population .un.org/wpp/Download/.

13. United Nations Development Programme (UNDP). "Human Development Index." Accessed October 4, 2020. http://hdr.undp.org/en/content/human-develop ment-index-hdi.

14. UN General Assembly Seventieth Session. "Transforming Our World: The 2030 Agenda for Sustainable Development." October 21, 2015. Accessed November 14, 2020. https://www.un.org/ga/search/view_doc.asp?symbol=A/RES/70/1&Lang=E.

15. Michael Clemens. "Does Development Reduce Migration?" Center for Global Development Working Paper 359. Washington, DC: Center for Global Development, 2014.

16. United Nations. "Declaration of Alma Ata." Accessed October 18, 2020. https:// www.who.int/publications/almaata_declaration_en.pdf.

17. Margaret Whitehead, Dahlgren Goran, and Evans Timothy. "Equity and Health Sector Reforms: Can Low-Income Countries Escape the Medical Poverty Trap?" *Lancet* 358 no. 9284 (September 8, 2001): 833–36. doi:10.1016/S0140-6736 (01)05975-X.

18. United Nations. "The Millennium Development Goals Report 2015." Accessed October 18, 2020. https://www.un.org/millenniumgoals/2015_MDG_Report /pdf/MDG%202015%20rev%20(July%201).pdf.

19. United Nations. "Sustainable Development Goals Report 2020." Accessed October 18, 2020. https://unstats.un.org/sdgs/report/2020/The-Sustainable-Develop ment-Goals-Report-2020.pdf.

20. The Intergovernmental Panel on Climate Change (IPCC). "Climate Change 2014: Synthesis Report. Contribution of Working Groups I, II and III to the Fifth Assessment Report of the Intergovernmental Panel on Climate Change." Edited by R. K. Pachauri and L. A. Meyer. IPCC, Geneva, Switzerland, 2014.

21. United Nation Development Programme (UNDP). "Human Development Report: Fighting Climate Change—Human Solidarity in a Divided World." New York: UN Development Programme, 2007.

22. Sharon Friel, Michael Marmot, Anthony J. McMichael, Tord Kjellstrom, and Denny Vågerö. "Global Health Equity and Climate Stabilisation: A Common Agenda." *Lancet* 372 (November 8, 2008): 1677–83.

23. Celia McMichael. "Climate Change-Related Migration and Infectious Disease." *Virulence* 6, no. 6 (2015: 548–53. https://doi.org/10.1080/21505594.2015.1021 539.

24. Kanta K. Rigaud, Alex de Sherbinin, Bryan Jones, Jonas Bergmann, Viviane Clement, Kayly Ober, Jacob Schewe, Susana Adamo, Brent McCusker, Silke Heuser, and Amelia Midgley. "Groundswell: Preparing for Internal Climate Migration." Washington, DC: World Bank, 2018. Accessed October 11, 2020. https://openknowl edge.worldbank.org/handle/10986/29461.

25. Stefanie Schütte, François Gemenne, Muhammad Zaman, Antoine Flahault, and Anneliese Depoux. "Connecting Planetary Health, Climate Change, and Migration." *Lancet Planet Health* 2, no. 2 (February 2018): e58–e59. https://doi.org/10 .1016/S2542-5196(18)30004-4.

26. International Organization for Migration (IOM), "Migration and Climate Change." IOM Migration Research Series 31 (2008). ISSN 1607-338X. International Organization for Migration, Geneva.

27. Celia McMichael. "Human Mobility, Climate Change, and Health: Unpacking the Connections." *Lancet Planet Health* 4, no. 6 (June 2020): e217–18. https://doi .org/10.1016/S2542-5196(20)30125-X.

28. Jochen Durr. "Sugar-Cane and Oil Palm Expansion in Guatemala and Its Consequences for the Regional Economy." *Journal of Agrarian Change* 17 (2017): 557–70.

29. Robert McLeman. "Migration and Land Degradation: Recent Experience and Future Trends." UNCCD Global Land Outlook Working Paper (2017). Accessed October 18, 2020. https://knowledge.unccd.int/sites/default/files/2018-06/8.%20Mi gration%2Band%2BLand%2BDegradation__R_McLeman.pdf.

30. Uppsala Conflict Data Program (UCDP). Department of Peace and Conflict Research, University of Uppsala. Accessed October 11, 2020. https://ucdp.uu .se/#/encyclopedia.

31. IOM, "World Migration Report 2020."

32. Daniela Del Boca and Alessandra Venturini. "Italian Migration." IZA Discussion Paper No. 938. Forschungsinstitut zur Zukunft der Arbeit Institute for the Study of Labor (November 2003). Accessed October 11, 2020. http://ftp.iza.org/dp 938.pdf.

33. Hein de Haas, Mathias Czaika, Marie-Laurence Flahaux, Edo Mahendra, Katharina Natter, Simona Vezzoli, and Maria Villares-Varela. "International Migration: Trends, Determinants and Policy Effects." *Population and Development Review* 45, no. 4 (2019): 885–922.

34. Stephen Castles and Simona Vezzoli. "The Global Economic Crisis and Migration: Temporary Interruption or Structural Change?" International Migration Institute. University of Oxford. *Paradigms* 2 (June 2009). Accessed October 18, 2020. https://www.migrationinstitute.org/files/news/castles-and-vezzoli_the-global-eco nomic-crisis-and-migration.pdf.

35. de Haas et al., "International Migration."

36. Line N. Handlos, Maria Kristiansen, and Marie Norredam. "Wellbeing or Welfare Benefits—What Are the Drivers for Migration?" *Scandinavian Journal of Public Health* 44 (2016): 117–19.

37. Hein de Haas. "The Determinants of International Migration. Conceptualising Policy, Origin and Destination Effects." University of Oxford International Migration Institute. Working Paper (2011).

38. Organization for Economic Co-operation and Development (OECD). "ODA 2019 Detailed Summary" (2020). Accessed October 10th, 2020. https://www.oecd.org/dac/financing-sustainable-development/development-finance-data/ODA-2019-detailed-summary.pdf.

39. Ben Edwards, Diana Smart, John De Maio, Michelle Silbert, and Rebecca Jenkinson. "Cohort Profile: Building a New Life in Australia (BNLA): The Longitudinal Study of Humanitarian Migrants." *International Journal of Epidemiology* 47, no. 1 (2018): 20–20h. https://doi.org/10.1093/ije/dyx218.

40. Philippe Fargues. "International Migration and Education—A Web of Mutual Causation." Paper commissioned for the Global Education Monitoring Report 2019 Consultation on Migration. Paris: UNESCO, 2018. Accessed October 18, 2020. https://cadmus.eui.eu/bitstream/handle/1814/47106/Fargues_International%20Migration%20and%20Education.pdf?sequence=2.

41. Clare Cummings, Julia Pacitto, Deletta Lauro, and Marta Foresti. "Why People Move: Understanding the Drivers and Trends of Migration to Europe." Working Paper n. 430. London: Oversea Development Institute, 2015. Accessed October 18, 2020. https://www.odi.org/sites/odi.org.uk/files/resource-documents/10485.pdf.

42. de Haas et al. "International Migration"; Kerilyn Schewel and Sonja Fransen. "Formal Education and Migration Aspirations in Ethiopia." *Population and Development Review* 44, no. 3 (2018): 555–87.

43. United Nations. "Global Compact for Safe, Orderly and Regular Migration." Co-facilitators' summary of the second informal session, May 22–23, May 2017. United Nations Headquarters, New York. Accessed October 4, 2020. https://refugeesmigrants.un.org/sites/default/files/ts2_cofacilitators_summary.pdf.

44. David Hollenbach. "Religion and Forced Migration." In *The Oxford Handbook of Refugee and Forced Migration Studies*, edited by Elena Fiddian-Qasmiyeh, Gil Loescher, Katy Long, and Nando Sigona (June 2014). https://doi.org/10.1093/oxfordhb/9780199652433.013.0008.

45. Refugee Studies Centre. "Sexual Orientation and Gender Identity and the Protection of Forced Migrants." *Forced Migration Review* 42 (April 2013). Accessed October 18, 2020. https://www.fmreview.org/sites/fmr/files/FMRdownloads/en/fmr42full.pdf.

46. Jorgen Carling and Francis Collins. "Aspiration, Desire and Drivers of Migration." *Journal of Ethnic and Migration Studies* (October 18, 2017). https://doi.org/10.1080/1369183X.2017.1384134.

47. Khalid Koser. *International Migration: A Very Short Introduction*. 2nd ed. New York: Oxford University Press, 2016.

Chapter 4

1. Benjamin S. Bradshaw and Edwin Fonner, "The Mortality of Spanish Surnamed Persons in Texas: 1969–71," in *Demography of Racial and Ethnic Groups*, ed. Frank D. Bean and W. Parker Frisbie (New York: Academic Press, 1978), 261–82.

2. Jacob S. Siegel and Jeffrey S. Passel, "Coverage of the Hispanic Population of the United States in the 1970 Census: A Methodological Analysis (No. 82)" (Washington, DC: US Census Bureau, 1979).

3. Kyriakos S. Markides and Jeannine Coreil, "The Health of Hispanics in the Southwestern United States: An Epidemiologic Paradox," *Public Health Reports* 101, no. 3 (1986): 253–65.

4. Anthony J. Swerdlow, "Mortality and Cancer Incidence in Vietnamese Refugees in England and Wales: A Follow-Up Study," *International Journal of Epidemiology* 20, no. 1 (1991): 13–19, https://doi.org/10.1093/ije/20.1.13.

5. John M. Ruiz, Patrick Steffen, and Timothy B. Smith, "Hispanic Mortality Paradox: A Systematic Review and Meta-Analysis of the Longitudinal Literature," *American Journal of Public Health* 103, no. 3 (March 2013): e52–60, https://doi.org/10.2105/AJPH.2012.301103.

6. Myriam Khlat and Nicole Darmon, "Is There a Mediterranean Migrants Mortality Paradox in Europe?," *International Journal of Epidemiology* 32, no. 6 (December 2003): 1115–18, https://doi.org/10.1093/ije/dyg308.

7. Myriam Khlat and Youssef Courbage, "Mortality and Causes of Death of Moroccans in France, 1979–91," *Population. An English Selection* 8 (1996): 59–94.

8. Oliver Razum, Hajo Zeeb, H. Seval Akgün, and Selma Yılmaz, "Low Overall Mortality of Turkish Residents in Germany Persists and Extends into a Second Generation: Merely a Healthy Migrant Effect?," *Tropical Medicine and International Health* 3, no. 4 (April 1998): 297–303, https://doi.org/10.1046/j.1365-3156.1998.00233.x.

9. Manuel Holz, "Health Inequalities in Germany: Is the Healthy Immigrant Effect Operative?," in *International German Socioeconomic Panel User Conference* (Berlin, 2018).

10. Martha F. Trulson, Robert E. Clancy, W. J. E. Jessop, R. W. Childers, and Frederick J. Stare, "Comparisons of Siblings in Boston and Ireland. Physical, Biochemical, and Dietary Findings," *Journal of the American Dietetic Association* 45 (September 1964): 225–29.

11. Michael G. Marmot, S. Leonard Syme, A. Kagan, H. Kato, J. B. Cohen, and J. Belsky, "Epidemiologic Studies of Coronary Heart Disease and Stroke in Japanese Men Living in Japan, Hawaii and California: Prevalence of Coronary and Hypertensive Heart Disease and Associated Risk Factors," *American Journal of*

Epidemiology 102, no. 6 (December 1975): 514–25, https://doi.org/10.1093/oxford journals.aje.a112189.

12. Michael G. Marmot and S. Leonard Syme, "Acculturation and Coronary Heart Disease in Japanese-Americans," *American Journal of Epidemiology* 104, no. 3 (September 1976): 225–47, https://doi.org/10.1093/oxfordjournals.aje.a112296.

13. Katerina Maximova, Jennifer O'Loughlin, and Katherine Gray-Donald, "Healthy Weight Advantage Lost in One Generation Among Immigrant Elementary Schoolchildren in Multi-Ethnic, Disadvantaged, Inner-City Neighborhoods in Montreal, Canada," *Annals of Epidemiology* 21, no. 4 (April 2011): 238–44, https:// doi.org/10.1016/j.annepidem.2011.01.002.

14. Anna Reeske, Jacob Spallek, and Oliver Razum, "Changes in Smoking Prevalence among First- and Second-Generation Turkish Migrants in Germany—An Analysis of the 2005 Microcensus," *International Journal for Equity in Health* 8, no. 1 (2009): 26, https://doi.org/10.1186/1475-9276-8-26.

15. Alexander Domnich, Donatella Panatto, Roberto Gasparini, and Daniela Amicizia, "The 'Healthy Immigrant' Effect: Does It Exist in Europe Today?," *Italian Journal of Public Health* 9, no. 3 (September 13, 2012), https://doi.org/10.2427/7532.

16. Barry R. Chiswick, Yew Liang Lee, and Paul W. Miller, "Immigrant Selection Systems and Immigrant Health," *Contemporary Economic Policy* 26, no. 4 (October 2008): 555–78, https://doi.org/10.1111/j.1465-7287.2008.00099.x.

17. Anthony J. McMichael, "Standardized Mortality Ratios and the 'Healthy Worker Effect': Scratching Beneath the Surface," *Journal of Occupational and Environmental Medicine* 18, no. 3 (March 1976): 165–68, https://doi.org/10.1097/000 43764-197603000-00009.

18. Karl Eschbach, Glenn V. Ostir, Kushang V. Patel, Kyriakos S. Markides, and James S. Goodwin, "Neighborhood Context and Mortality Among Older Mexican Americans: Is There a Barrio Advantage?," *American Journal of Public Health* 94, no. 10 (October 2004): 1807–12, https://doi.org/10.2105/AJPH.94.10.1807.

19. Oliver Razum and Dorothee Twardella, "Time Travel with Oliver Twist— Towards an Explanation for a Paradoxically Low Mortality among Recent Immigrants," *Tropical Medicine and International Health* 7, no. 1 (January 2002): 4–10, https://doi.org/10.1046/j.1365-3156.2002.00833.x.

20. Ariel Pablos-Méndez, "Mortality Among Hispanics," *JAMA* 271, no. 16 (April 27, 1994): 1237, https://doi.org/10.1001/jama.1994.03510400023017.

21. Razum et al., "Low Overall Mortality of Turkish Residents."

22. Matthew Wallace and Hill Kulu, "Low Immigrant Mortality in England and Wales: A Data Artefact?," *Social Science and Medicine* 120 (November 2014): 100–109, https://doi.org/10.1016/j.socscimed.2014.08.032.

23. Maria Roura, "Unravelling Migrants' Health Paradoxes: A Transdisciplinary Research Agenda," *Journal of Epidemiology and Community Health* 71, no. 9 (September 2017): 870–73, https://doi.org/10.1136/jech-2016-208439.

24. Edna A. Viruell-Fuentes, "Beyond Acculturation: Immigration, Discrimination,

and Health Research among Mexicans in the United States," *Social Science and Medicine* 65, no. 7 (October 2007): 1524–35, https://doi.org/10.1016/j.socscimed.2007.05.010.

25. Yudit Namer and Oliver Razum, "Convergence Theory and the Salmon Effect in Migrant Health," in *Oxford Research Encyclopedia of Global Public Health* (Oxford University Press, 2018), https://doi.org/10.1093/acrefore/9780190632366.013.17.

26. Amelie F. Constant, "The Healthy Immigrant Paradox and Health Convergence," GLO Discussion Paper (Maastricht, 2017).

27. Cristian Bartolucci, Claudia Villosio, and Mathis Wagner, "Who Migrates and Why? Evidence from Italian Administrative Data," *Journal of Labor Economics* 36, no. 2 (April 2018): 551–88, https://doi.org/10.1086/694616.

28. Rosa Weber and Jan Saarela, "Who Migrates in a Setting of Free Mobility? Assessing the Reason for Migration and Integration Patterns Using Cross-National Register Data from Finland and Sweden," Stockholm Research Reports in Demography (Stockholm, 2020), https://doi.org/https://doi.org/10.17045/sthlmuni.121360 83.v1.

29. Philip Anglewicz, Mark VanLandingham, Lucinda Manda-Taylor, and Hans-Peter Kohler, "Cohort Profile: Internal Migration in Sub-Saharan Africa—The Migration and Health in Malawi (MHM) Study," *BMJ Open* 7, no. 5 (May 17, 2017): e014799, https://doi.org/10.1136/bmjopen-2016-014799.

30. Philip Anglewicz, Mark VanLandingham, Lucinda Manda-Taylor, and Hans-Peter Kohler, "Health Selection, Migration, and HIV Infection in Malawi," *Demography* 55, no. 3 (June 27, 2018): 979–1007, https://doi.org/10.1007/s13524-018-0668-5.

31. Philip Anglewicz, Rachel Kidman, and Sangeetha Madhavan, "Internal Migration and Child Health in Malawi," *Social Science and Medicine* 235 (August 2019): 112389, https://doi.org/10.1016/j.socscimed.2019.112389.

32. Yao Lu, "Test of the 'Healthy Migrant Hypothesis': A Longitudinal Analysis of Health Selectivity of Internal Migration in Indonesia," *Social Science and Medicine* 67, no. 8 (October 2008): 1331–39, https://doi.org/10.1016/j.socscimed.2008.06.017.

33. Yao Lu and Lijian Qin, "Healthy Migrant and Salmon Bias Hypotheses: A Study of Health and Internal Migration in China," *Social Science and Medicine* 102 (February 2014): 41–48, https://doi.org/10.1016/j.socscimed.2013.11.040.

34. Elizabeth Nauman, Mark VanLandingham, Philip Anglewicz, Umaporn Patthavanit, and Sureeporn Punpuing, "Rural-to-Urban Migration and Changes in Health Among Young Adults in Thailand," *Demography* 52, no. 1 (February 21, 2015): 233–57, https://doi.org/10.1007/s13524-014-0365-y.

35. Guillermina Jasso, Douglas S. Massey, Mark Rosenzweig and James Smith, "Immigration, Health, and New York City: Early Results Based on the U.S. New Immigrant Cohort of 2003," *Economic Policy Review* 11, no. 2 (December 2005): 127–51, https://econpapers.repec.org/RePEc:fip:fednep:y:2005:i:dec:p:127-151:n:v.11 no.2.

36. Ilana Redstone Akresh and Reanne Frank, "Health Selection Among New Immigrants," *American Journal of Public Health* 98, no. 11 (November 2008): 2058–64, https://doi.org/10.2105/AJPH.2006.100974.

37. Jasso et al., "Immigration, Health, and New York City."

38. Holly E. Reed and Guillermo Yrizar Barbosa, "Investigating the Refugee Health Disadvantage Among the U.S. Immigrant Population," *Journal of Immigrant and Refugee Studies* 15, no. 1 (January 2, 2017): 53–70, https://doi.org/10.1080/15562948.2016.1165329.

39. Gilbert C. Gee, A. B. de Castro, Catherine M. Crespi, May C. Wang, Karen Llave, Eleanor Brindle, Nanette R. Lee, Maria Midea M. Kabamalan, and Anna K. Hing, "Health of Philippine Emigrants Study (HoPES): Study Design and Rationale," *BMC Public Health* 18, no. 1 (December 20, 2018): 771, https://doi.org/10.1186/s12889-018-5670-8.

40. A. B. de Castro, Anna K. Hing, Nanette R. Lee, Maria Midea M. Kabamalan, Karen Llave, Catherine M. Crespi, May Wang, and Gilbert Gee, "Cohort Profile: The Health of Philippine Emigrants Study (HoPES) to Examine the Health Impacts of International Migration from the Philippines to the USA," *BMJ Open* 9, no. 11 (November 14, 2019): e032966, https://doi.org/10.1136/bmjopen-2019-032966.

41. Brittany N. Morey, Adrian Matias Bacong, Anna K. Hing, A. B. de Castro, and Gilbert C. Gee, "Heterogeneity in Migrant Health Selection: The Role of Immigrant Visas," *Journal of Health and Social Behavior* 61, no. 3 (September 29, 2020): 359–76, https://doi.org/10.1177/0022146520942896.

42. Gilbert C. Gee, A.B.de Castro, Catherine Crespi, May Wang, Anna Hing, Adrian Bacong, and Karen Llave, "Pre-Acculturation as a Risk Factor for Obesity: Findings from the Health of Philippine Emigrants Study (HoPES)," *SSM—Population Health* 9 (December 2019): 100482, https://doi.org/10.1016/j.ssmph.2019.100482.

43. Karri Silventoinen, Niklas Hammar, Ebba Hedlund, Markku Koskenvuo, Tapani Rönnemaa, and Jaakko Kaprio, "Selective International Migration by Social Position, Health Behaviour and Personality," *European Journal of Public Health* 18, no. 2 (December 7, 2007): 150–55, https://doi.org/10.1093/eurpub/ckm052.

44. Amanda R. Cheong and Douglas S. Massey, "Undocumented and Unwell: Legal Status and Health among Mexican Migrants," *International Migration Review* 53, no. 2 (June 22, 2019): 571–601, https://doi.org/10.1177/0197918318775924.

45. Lori M. Hunter and Daniel H. Simon, "Might Climate Change the 'Healthy Migrant' Effect?," *Global Environmental Change* 47 (November 2017): 133–42, https://doi.org/10.1016/j.gloenvcha.2017.10.003.

46. Anglewicz et al., "Health Selection, Migration, and HIV Infection in Malawi."

47. Nauman et al., "Rural-to-Urban Migration."

48. Jasso et al., "Immigration, Health, and New York City."

49. Michelle A. Montgomery, Charlotte T. Jackson, and Elizabeth A. Kelvin, "Premigration Harm and Depression: Findings from the New Immigrant Survey,

2003," *Journal of Immigrant and Minority Health* 16, no. 5 (October 17, 2014): 773–80, https://doi.org/10.1007/s10903-013-9810-z.

50. de Castro et al., "Cohort Profile."

51. Damarys Canache, Matthew Hayes, Jeffery J. Mondak, and Sergio C. Wals, "Openness, Extraversion and the Intention to Emigrate," *Journal of Research in Personality* 47, no. 4 (August 2013): 351–55, https://doi.org/10.1016/j.jrp.2013.02.008.

52. Silventoinen et al., "Selective International Migration."

53. Swerdlow, "Mortality and Cancer Incidence."

54. Jacob Spallek, Hajo Zeeb, and Oliver Razum, "What Do We Have to Know from Migrants' Past Exposures to Understand Their Health Status? A Life Course Approach," *Emerging Themes in Epidemiology* 8, no. 1 (December 15, 2011): 6, https://doi.org/10.1186/1742-7622-8-6.

55. Roura, "Unravelling Migrants' Health Paradoxes."

56. Oliver Razum, "Commentary: Of Salmon and Time Travellers—Musing on the Mystery of Migrant Mortality," *International Journal of Epidemiology* 35, no. 4 (August 1, 2006): 919–21, https://doi.org/10.1093/ije/dyl143.

Chapter 5

1. International Organization for Migration, "World Migration Report 2020," Geneva, 2019, https://publications.iom.int/system/files/pdf/wmr_2020.pdf.

2. World Health Organization (WHO), "Migration and Health," Regional Office for Europe Copenhagen, https://www.euro.who.int/en/health-topics/health-determinants/migration-and-health.

3. National Immigration Forum, "Immigrants as Economic Contributors: Immigrant Entrepreneurs—National Immigration Forum." Accessed November 23, 2020, https://immigrationforum.org/article/immigrants-as-economic-contributors-immigrant-entrepreneurs/.

4. National Immigration Forum, "Immigrants as Economic Contributors."

5. World Bank, "KNOMAD, World Bank Group Migration and Remittances. Recent Developments and Outlook. Special Topic: Global Compact on Migration. Migration and Development Brief," April 27, 2017. Accessed November 23, 2020, http://pubdocs.worldbank.org/en/992371492706371662/MigrationandDevelopmentBrief27.pdf.

6. EU Science Hub—European Commission, "The Crucial Contribution of Migrant Workers to Europe's Coronavirus Response—EU Science Hub—European Commission." Accessed November 23, 2020, https://ec.europa.eu/jrc/en/news/crucial-contribution-migrant-workers-europes-coronavirus-response.

7. A. Swain, "Increasing Migration Pressure and Rising Nationalism: Implications for Multilateralism and SDG Implementation," Uppsala University, Sweden, Paper Prepared for the Development Policy Analysis Division of the United Nations, Department of Economics and Social Affairs, June 2019, https://www

.un.org/development/desa/dpad/wp-content/uploads/sites/45/publication/SDO _BP_Swain.pdf.

8. N. Pocock and C. Chan, "Refugees, Racism and Xenophobia: What Works to Reduce Discrimination?," United Nations University, 2019, https://ourworld.unu .edu/en/refugees-racism-and-xenophobia-what-works-to-reduce-discrimination.

9. UNHCR, "The 1951 Refugee Convention." Accessed November 23, 2020, https://www.unhcr.org/uk/1951-refugee-convention.html.

10. International Organization for Migration, "Who Is a Migrant?" Accessed November 23, 2020, https://www.iom.int/who-is-a-migrant.

11. The term includes a number of well-defined legal categories of people, such as migrant workers; persons whose particular types of movements are legally defined, such as smuggled migrants; and those whose status or means of movement are not specifically defined under international law, such as international students.

12. The present definition was developed by IOM for its own purposes and is not meant to imply or create any new legal category.

13. International Organization for Migration, "World Migration Report 2020," Geneva, 2019, https://publications.iom.int/system/files/pdf/wmr_2020.pdf.

14. UN Department of Economic Affairs, "The Number of International Migrants Reaches 272 Million, Continuing an Upward Trend in All World Regions, Says UN," September 17, 2019, https://www.un.org/development/desa/en/news/pop ulation/international-migrant-stock-2019.html#:~:text=The%20number%20of%20 international%20migrants%20globally%20reached%20an%20estimated%20272 ,by%20the%20United%20Nations%20today.

15. UNHCR, "Figures at a Glance," accessed May 13, 2022, https://www.unhcr .org/uk/figures-at-a-glance.html.

16. FAO, "Strengthening Sector Policies for Better Food Security and Nutrition Results Policy Guidance Note 10 Rural Migration," Rome, 2017. Accessed November 23, 2020, https://www.fao.org/3/i8166e/i8166e.pdf.

17. C. Zimmerman, L. Kiss, and M. Hossain, "Migration and Health: A Framework for 21st Century Policy-Making," *PLoS Med* 8, no 5 (2011): e1001034, https:// doi.org/10.1371/journal.pmed.1001034.

18. WHO, "Report on the Health of Refugees and Migrants in the WHO European Region," Copenhagen, 2018. Accessed November 23, 2020, https://web.ar chive.orghttps://web.archive.org/web/20201123133529/https://www.euro.who.int /en/publications/html/report-on-the-health-of-refugees-and-migrants-in-the-who -european-region-no-public-health-without-refugee-and-migrant-health-2018/en /index.html.

19. WHO Regional Office for Europe, "Improving the Health Care of Pregnant Refugee and Migrant Women and Newborn Children," 2018. Accessed November 23, 2020, https://www.euro.who.int/__data/assets/pdf_file/0003/388362/tc-mother -eng.pdf?ua=1.

20. Stateless Journeys, "Birth Registration and Children's Rights European

Network on Statelessness," https://statelessjourneys.org/main-issues/birth-registra
tion-and-the-childs-right-to-nationality/.

21. WHO, "Improving the Health Care of Pregnant Refugee and Migrant
Women."

22. WHO Regional Office for Europe, "Strategy and Action Plan for Refugee
and Migrant Health in the WHO European Region," Copenhagen, 2018, https://
www.euro.who.int/__data/assets/pdf_file/0004/314725/66wd08e_MigrantHealth
StrategyActionPlan_160424.pdf.

23. Euro Peristat, "The European Perinatal Health Report 2010." Accessed November 23, 2020, http://www.europeristat.com/reports/european-perinatal-health
-report-2010.html.

24. L. P. da Costa, S. F. Dias, and M. d. R. O. Martins, "Association between
Length of Residence and Overweight among Adult Immigrants in Portugal: A Nationwide Cross-Sectional Study," *BMC Public Health* 17, no. 316 (2017), https://doi
.org/10.1186/s12889-017-4252-5.

25. S. Toselli, E. Gualdi-Russo, D. N. K. Boulos, W. A. Anwar, C. Lakhoua, I. Ja-
ouadi, M. Khyatti, and K. Hemminki, "Prevalence of Overweight and Obesity in
Adults from North Africa," *European Journal of Public Health* 24, no. 1 (2014):
31–39, https://doi.org/10.1093/eurpub/cku103.

26. WHO Regional Office for Europe, "10 Facts on Refugee and Migrants Health:
Noncommunicable Diseases." Accessed November 23, 2020, https://www.euro.who
.int/en/health-topics/health-determinants/migration-and-health/migration-and
-health-in-the-european-region/10-facts-on-refugee-and-migrant-health/noncom
municable-diseases.

27. U. Fedeli, E. Ferroni, M. Pigato, F. Avossa, and M. Saugo, "Causes of Mortality across Different Immigrant Groups in Northeastern Italy," *PeerJ* 3 (2015): e975,
https://doi.org/10.7717/peerj.975.

28. S. Priebe, D. Giacco, and R. El-Nagib, "Public Health Aspects of Mental
Health among Migrants and Refugees: A Review of the Evidence on Mental Health
Care for Refugees, Asylum Seekers and Irregular Migrants in the WHO European
Region," *Health Evidence Network Synthesis Report* 47 (2016), WHO European
Regional Office. Accessed November 23, 2020, http://www.euro.who.int/__data
/assets/pdf_file/0003/317622/HEN-synthesis-report-47.pdf?ua=1,accessed30Octo
ber2018).

29. WHO Regional Office for Europe, "Mental Health Promotion and Mental Health Care in Refugees and Migrants," 2018, https://www.euro.who.int/__data
/assets/pdf_file/0004/386563/mental-health-eng.pdf?ua=1.

30. Laurence J. Kirmayer, L. Narasiah, M. Munoz, M. Rashid, A. G. Ryder,
J. Guzder, G. Hassan, C. Rousseau, and K. Pottie, "Common Mental Health Problems in Immigrants and Refugees: General Approach in Primary Care," *CMAJ*
183, no. 12 (September 6, 2011): E959–E967, https://doi.org/10.1503/cmaj.090292
https://www.ncbi.nlm.nih.gov/pmc/articles/PMC3168672/.

31. C. Moyce and M. Schenker, "Migrant Workers and Their Occupational Health and Safety," *Annual Review of Public Health* 39, no. 1 (2018): 351–65, https://www.annualreviews.org/doi/pdf/10.1146/annurev-publhealth-040617-013714.

32. ILO, "When the Safety of Nepali Migrant Workers Fails: A Review of Data on the Numbers and Causes of the Death of Nepali Migrant Workers," http://www.ilo.org/kathmandu/whatwedo/publications/WCMS_493777/lang--en/index.htm.

33. Royal College of Psychiatrists, "Detention of People with Mental Disorders in Immigration Removal Centres (IRCs)," London, April 2021, https://www.rcpsych.ac.uk/docs/default-source/improving-care/better-mh-policy/position-statements/position-statement-ps02-21---detention-of-people-with-mental-disorders-in-immigration-removal-centres---2021.pdf?sfvrsn=58f7a29e_6.

34. Office of the United Nations High Commissioner for Human Rights, "The Right to Health," Fact Sheet 31, Geneva, 2008, https://www.ohchr.org/documents/publications/factsheet31.pdf.

35. S. Malin, A. Depoux, S. Schutte, A. Flahault, and L. Saso., "Migrants' and Refugees' Health: Towards an Agenda of Solutions," *Public Health Review* 39 (2018): 27, https://doi.org/10.1186/s40985-018-0104-9 https://www.ncbi.nlm.nih.gov/pmc/articles/PMC6182765/.

36. WHO, "Universal Health Coverage," Geneva.

37. IOM, "Social Determinants of Migrant Health International Organization for Migration," Geneva, 2021, https://www.iom.int/migration-health.

38. A. Chiarenza, M. Dauvrin, V. Chiesa, S. Baatout, and H. Verrept, "Supporting Access to Healthcare for Refugees and Migrants in European Countries under Particular Migratory Pressure," *BMC Health Services Research* 19, no. 513 (2019), https://doi.org/10.1186/s12913-019-4353-1.

39. H. Bradby, R. Humphris, D. Newall, and J. Phillimore, "Public Health Aspects of Migrant Health: A Review of the Evidence on Health Status for Refugees and Asylum Seekers in the European Region," *Health Evidence Network Synthesis Report* 44 (2015), WHO Regional Office for Europe, https://www.euro.who.int/__data/assets/pdf_file/0004/289246/WHO-HEN-Report-A5-2-Refugees_FINAL.pdf.

40. WHO, "Health Services for Syrian Refugees in Turkey." Accessed November 24, 2020, https://www.euro.who.int/en/health-topics/health-emergencies/syrian-crisis/health-services-for-syrian-refugees-in-turkey.

41. WHO, *Health in Emergencies* 18 (December 2003), https://www.who.int/hac/about/12010.pdf.

42. Centre For European Reform, "Why Europe Needs Legal Migration And How To Sell It." Accessed November 23, 2020, https://www.cer.eu/publications/archive/policy-brief/2018/why-europe-needs-legal-migration-and-how-sell-it.

43. Global Migration Group, *Handbook for Improving the Production and Use of Migration Data for Development*, https://www.un.org/development/desa/pd/sites/www.un.org.development.desa.pd/files/unpd_cm15_201702_final_handbook_30.06.16_as4_0_0.pdf.

44. Bradby et al., "Public Health Aspects of Migrant Health."

45. UNHCR, "Global Compact on Refugees," 2018, https://www.unhcr.org/uk/the-global-compact-on-refugees.html.

46. UN, "Global Compact for Safe Orderly and Regular Migration," 2018, https://refugeesmigrants.un.org/migration-compact.

47. United Nations Network on Migration website. Accessed November 23, 2020, https://migrationnetwork.un.org/.

48. As declared in the preamble to the Constitution of the WHO. Also, the International Covenant on Economic, Social and Cultural Rights, Article 2.2 and Article 12, recognizes the right of everyone to the enjoyment of the highest attainable standard of physical and mental health without discrimination of any kind as to race, color, sex, language, religion, political or other opinion, national or social origin, property, birth, or other status.

49. Seventieth World Health Association, "Promoting the Health of Refugees and Migrants," https://www.iom.int/sites/default/files/our_work/DMM/Migration-Health/WHA_RES_70.15-Promoting-the-health-of-refugees-and-migrants.pdf.

50. WHO, "Promoting the Health of Refugees and Migrants: Framework of Priorities and Guiding Principles to Promote the Health of Refugees and Migrants." Accessed November 23, 2020, http://www.who.int/migrants/about/framework_refugees-migrants.pdf.

51. WHO, "Promoting the Health of Refugees and Migrants: Draft Global Action Plan, 2019–2023," Geneva, 2019, https://www.who.int/publications/i/item/promoting-the-health-of-refugees-and-migrants-draft-global-action-plan-2019-2023.

52. WHO, *International Health Regulations (2005)*, 3rd ed. Accessed November 23, 2020, https://www.who.int/publications/i/item/9789241580496.

53. WHO, "Promoting the Health of Refugees and Migrants: Draft Global Action Plan."

Chapter 6

1. D. Gil-González, M. Carrasco-Portiño, C. Vives-Cases, A. A. Agudelo-Suárez, R. Castejón Bolea, and E. Ronda-Pérez, "Is Health a Right for All? An Umbrella Review of the Barriers to Health Care Access Faced by Migrants," *Ethnicity and Health* 520, no. 5 (2015): 523–541, https://doi.org/10.1080/13557858.2014.946473.

2. World Health Organization (WHO), *Constitution of the WHO* (United Nations, 1946).

3. United Nations, *International Declaration of Human Rights* (United Nations, 1948).

4. United Nations, *International Covenant on Economic, Social and Cultural Rights* (United Nations, 1966); United Nations, *CESCR General Comment No. 14: The Right to the Highest Attainable Standard of Health (Art. 12)* (United Nations, 2000).

5. P. Braveman, S. Kumanyika, J. Fielding, T. Laveist, L. N. Borrell, R. Manderscheid,

and A. Troutman, "Health Disparities and Health Equity: The Issue Is Justice," *American Journal of Public Health* 101, no. 1 (December 2011): S149–55, https:// doi.org/10.2105/AJPH.2010.300062.

6. L. Stubbe Østergaard, M. Norredam, C. Mock-Munoz de Luna, M. Blair, S. Goldfeld, and A. Hjern, "Restricted Health Care Entitlements for Child Migrants in Europe and Australia," *European Journal of Public Health* 27, no. 5 (October 1, 2019): 869–73, https://doi.org/10.1093/eurpub/ckx083.

7. M. Winters, B. Rechel, L. de Jong, and M. Pavlova, "A Systematic Review on the Use of Healthcare Services by Undocumented Migrants in Europe," *BMC Health Services Research* 18, no. 1 (January 18, 2018): 30, https://doi.org/10.1186/s12 913-018-2838-y.

8. D. Biswas, M. Kristiansen, A. Krasnik, and M. Norredam, "Access to Healthcare and Alternative Health-Seeking Strategies among Undocumented Migrants in Denmark," *BMC Public Health* 11, no. 560 (July 13, 2011), https://doi.org/10.1186 /1471-2458-11-560.

9. C. Michaëlis, A. Krasnik, and M. Norredam, "Introduction of User Fee for Language Interpretation: Effects on Use of Interpreters in Danish Health Care," *European Journal of Public Health* 31, no. 4 (January 26, 2021): 705–07, https://doi.org /10.1093/eurpub/ckaa254.

10. A. Bischoff and K. Denhaerynck. "What Do Language Barriers Cost? An Exploratory Study among Asylum Seekers in Switzerland," *BMC Health Services Research* 10, no. 248 (2010): 1–7.

11. Z. D. Bailey, N. Krieger, M. Agénor, J. Graves, N. Linos, and M. T. Bassett. "Structural Racism and Health Inequities in the USA: Evidence and Interventions," *Lancet* 389, no. 10077 (April 8, 2017): 1453–63, https://doi.org/10.1016/S0140-6736 (17)30569-X.

12. WHO, "What Are the Roles of Intercultural Mediators in Health Care and What Is the Evidence on Their Contributions and Effectiveness in Improving Accessibility and Quality of Care for Refugees and Migrants in the WHO European Region?," *Health Evidence Network Synthesis Report* 64.

13. Bischoff and Denhaerynck, "What Do Language Barriers Cost?"

14. E. Satinsky, D. C. Fuhr, A. Woodward, E. Sondorp, and B. Roberts, "Mental Health Care Utilisation and Access among Refugees and Asylum Seekers in Europe: A Systematic Review," *Health Policy* 9, no. 123 (2019): 851–63, https://doi .org/10.1016/j.healthpol.2019.02.007.

15. G. Abdoli, M. Bottai, K. Sandelin, and T. Moradi, "Breast Cancer Diagnosis and Mortality by Tumor Stage and Migration Background in a Nationwide Cohort Study in Sweden," *Breast* 31 (February 2017): 57–65, https://doi.org/10.1016/j .breast.2016.10.004.

16. S. Hargreaves, L. B. Nellums, M. Ramsay, V. Saliba, A. Majeed, S. Mounier-Jack, and J. S. Friedland, "Who Is Responsible for the Vaccination of Migrants in Europe?," *Lancet* 391, no. 10132 (May 5, 2018):1752–54, https://doi.org/10.1016 /S0140-6736(18)30846-8; M. Vahabi, A. Lofters, E. Kim, J. P. Wong, L. Ellison,

E. Graves, and R. H. Glazier, "Breast Cancer Screening Utilization Among Women From Muslim Majority Countries in Ontario, Canada," *Preventive Medicine* 105 (December 2017): 176–83, https://doi.org/10.1016/j.ypmed.2017.09.008.

17. E. Ghreiz, "The Syrian Refugee Crisis in Jordan: Challenges and Future Opportunities for NGOs," in *Syrian Crisis, Syrian Refugees. Mobility and Politics*, edited by J. Beaujouan and A. Rasheed (Cham: Palgrave Pivot, 2020), http://link.library .eui.eu/portal/Syrian-Crisis-Syrian-Refugees--Voices-from/e7VMQEC1b2Q/.

18. L. S. Ostergaard and A. Krasnik, "Migrant Health Clinics: Hospital-Based Care Coordination in Denmark for Patients with Ethnic Backgrounds other than Danish," in *World Health Organization: Compendium of Health System Responses to Large-Scale Migration in the WHO European Region* (Copenhagen: WHO, Regional Office of Europe, 2018).

19. M. McKee, "What Can Health Services Contribute to the Reduction of Inequalities in Health?," *Scandinavian Journal of Public Health Suppl* 59 (2002): 54–58.

20. C. Seeleman, J. Suurmond, and K. Stronks, "Cultural Comptence: A Conceptual Framework for Teaching and Learning," *Medial Education* 43, no. 3 (March 2009): 229–37, DOI: 10.1111/j.1365-2923.2008.03269.x.

21. J. Sorensen, M. Norredam, J. Suurmond, O. Carter-Pokras, M. Garcia-Ramirez, and A. Krasnik, "Need for Ensuring Cultural Competence in Medical Programmes of European Universities," *BMC Medical Education* 19, no. 1 (January 15, 2019): 21, https://doi.org/10.1186/s12909-018-1449-y.

22. C. Agyemang, E. Beune, K. Meeks, E. Owusu-Dabo, P. Agyei-Baffour, A. de-Graft Aikins, and F. Dodoo et al., "Rationale and Cross-Sectional Study Design of the Research on Obesity and Type 2 Diabetes among African Migrants: The RODAM Study," *BMJ Open* 4, no. 3 (March 21, 2014): e004877, https://doi.org/10 .1136/bmjopen-2014-004877.

23. S. S. Jervelund, T. Malthesen, C. L. Wimmelmann, J. H. Petersen, and A. Krasnik, "Know Where to Go: Evidence from a Controlled Trial of a Healthcare System Information Intervention among Immigrants," *BMC Public Health* 18, no. 1 (July 11, 2018): 863, https://doi.org/10.1186/s12889-018-5741-x.

24. K. Bozorgmehr and O. Razum, "Effect of Restricting Access to Health Care on Health Expenditures among Asylum-Seekers and Refugees: A Quasi-Experimental Study in Germany, 1994–2013," *PLoS ONE* 10, no. 7 (2015); U. Trummer, S. Novak-Zezula, A. Renner, and I. Wilczewska, "Cost Savings through Timely Treatment for Irregular Migrants and EU Citizens without Insurance," *European Journal of Public Health* 28, no. 1 (May 2018).

Chapter 8

1. United Nations, "UN Summit for Refugees and Migrants 2016," accessed January 30, 2021, https://refugeesmigrants.un.org/summit.

2. International Organization for Migration (IOM), "World Migration Report 2020," https://www.iom.int/wmr/.

3. R. Thakur and T. G. Weiss, "Framing Global Governance, Five Gaps," in *The Global Studies Reader*, edited by M. Steger (New York: Oxford University Press, 2015) 27–40.

4. United Nations Development Programme, "Advancing Development Approaches to Migration: UNDP Position Paper on the Global Compact for Migration," 2019.

5. IOM, "Glossary on Migration (2019)," November 2, 2016, https://www.iom.int/glossary-migration-2019.

6. IOM, "World Migration Report 2020."

7. S. Martin and S. Weerasinghe, "Global Migration Governance: Existing Architecture and Recent Developments," in *World Migration Report 2018*, edited by M. McAuliffe and M. Ruhs (Geneva: IOM, 2017), 125–47.

8. United Nations Human Rights Office of the High Commissioner, "Protocol to Prevent, Suppress and Punish Trafficking in Persons," November 15, 2000, https://www.ohchr.org/EN/ProfessionalInterest/Pages/ProtocolTraffickingInPersons.aspx.

9. United Nations Human Rights Office of the High Commissioner, "International Convention on the Protection of the Rights of All Migrant Workers," December 18, 1990, https://www.ohchr.org/en/professionalinterest/pages/cmw.aspx.

10. United Nations Human Rights, "Status of Ratifications of Treaties," https://indicators.ohchr.org/.

11. IOM, "World Migration Report 2020."

12. United Nations, "UN Summit."

13. United Nations Sustainable Development, "United Nations Sustainable Development Goals: 17 Goals to Transform Our World," accessed January 30, 2021, https://www.un.org/sustainabledevelopment/.

14. United Nations, "Addis Ababa Action Agenda of the Third International Conference on Financing for Development," July 13, 2015, https://sustainabledevelopment.un.org/index.php?page=view&type=400&nr=2051&menu=35.

15. United Nations High Commissioner for Refugees, "The Global Compact on Refugees," December 17, 2018, https://www.unhcr.org/the-global-compact-on-refugees.html.

16. United Nations High Commissioner for Refugees, "Comprehensive Refugee Response Framework," accessed January 30, 2021, https://www.unhcr.org/comprehensive-refugee-response-framework-crrf.html.

17. United Nations High Commissioner for Refugees, "The Global Compact on Refugees."

18. Michaela Told, "Global Governance of the Migration System and Its Interface with Health," in *Health Diplomacy: Spotlight on Refugees and Migrants*, WHO Regional Office for Europe (2019): 38–51.

19. United Nations, "UN Summit."

20. "United Nations Network on Migration—Terms of Reference," accessed January 30, 2021, https://migrationnetwork.un.org/.

21. The Joint United Nations Programme on HIV/AIDS (UNAIDS), United Nations Economic, Social and Cultural Organization (UNESCO), the World Bank (WB), and the World Health Organization (WHO).

22. United Nations Network on Migration, "Migration Multi-Partner Trust Fund," December 2018, https://migrationnetwork.un.org/trustfund.

23. Told, "Global Governance."

24. D. Skiadas, *EU Migration Governance: Budgeting and Spending in Times of Crisis as Seen by the European Court Auditors* (Thessaloniki: University of Macedonia Press, 2020).

25. European Commission, "Communication from the Commission on a New Pact on Migration and Asylum," Brussels, September 23, 2020 (COM(2020) 609 final).

26. M. Giampaolo and A. Ianni, "Migration Governance in the European Union: The New Pact on Migration and Asylum," *Centro Studi Politica Internazionale* (2021).

27. P. De Bruycker, "The New Pact on Migration and Asylum: What It Is Not and What It Could Have Been," December 15, 2020, https://eumigrationlawblog.eu/the-new-pact-on-migration-and-asylum-what-it-is-not-and-what-it-could-have-been.

28. Merconsur Residence Agreement (Good Practice—MERCOSUR Residence Agreement (ilo.org)).

29. A. Montenegro Braz, "Migration Governance in South America: The Bottom Up Diffusion of the Residence Agreement of Merconsur," *Brazilian Journal of Public Administration* 52, no. 2 (March/April 2018): 303–20.

30. IOM, "Constitution and Basic Texts of the Governing Bodies," September 30, 2014, https://www.iom.int/constitution-and-basic-texts-governing-bodies.

31. Martin and Weerasinghe, "Global Migration Governance."

32. IOM, "Migration Governance Framework," https://www.iom.int/sites/default/files/about-iom/migof_brochure_a4_en.pdf.

33. United Nations High Commissioner for Refugees, "About Us," accessed January 30, 2021, https://www.unhcr.org/about-us.html.

34. International Labour Organization, "About the ILO," accessed January 30, 2021, https://www.ilo.org/global/about-the-ilo/lang--en/index.htm.

35. *ILO Multilateral Framework on Labour Migration: Non-Binding Principles and Guidelines for a Rights-Based Approach to Labour Migration* (Geneva: International Labour Office, 2006), https://www.ilo.org/global/topics/labour-migration/publications/WCMS_178672/lang--en/index.htm.

36. *ILO Multilateral Framework on Labour Migration: Non-Binding Principles and Guidelines for a Rights-Based Approach to Labour Migration* (Geneva: International Labour Office, 2006), https://www.ilo.org/global/topics/labour-migration/publications/WCMS_178672/lang--en/index.htm.

37. IOM, "World Migration Report 2018," https://publications.iom.int/books/world-migration-report-2018.

38. "NGO Committee on Migration," accessed January 30, 2021, https://ngo-migration.org/.

39. Global Forum on Migration & Development, "The GFMD and the GCM: Global Forum on Migration and Development," accessed January 30, 2021, https://www.gfmd.org/process/gfmd-and-gcm.

40. United Nations. "Transforming Our World: The 2030 Agenda for Sustainable Development,." United Nations, 2015, https://sustainabledevelopment.un.org/post2015/transformingourworld/publication.

41. Swiss Agency for Development and Cooperation SDC, "Migration and the 2030 Agenda for Sustainable Development," September 2018, https://www.odi.org/sites/odi.org.uk/files/resource-documents/12422.pdf.

42. WHO, "Promoting the Health of Refugees and Migrants," January 2017, https://www.who.int/migrants/about/framework_refugees-migrants.pdf.

43. United Nations, "Report of the United Nations High Commissioner for Refugees: Part II: Global Compact on Refugees," September 13, 2018, https://www.unhcr.org/gcr/GCR_English.pdf.

44. WHO, "Health of Migrants: Report by the Secretariat," April 7, 2008, https://apps.who.int/iris/bitstream/handle/10665/23467/A61_12-en.pdf;sequence=1.

45. WHO, "Promoting the Health of Refugees and Migrants."

46. IOM, "2nd Global Consultation on Migrant Health: Resetting the Agenda," December 19, 2016, https://www.iom.int/migration-health/second-global-consultation.

47. WHO, "Refugee and Migrant Health," accessed January 30, 2021, http://www.who.int/migrants/en/.

48. UHC2030, "Global Compact for Progress towards Universal Health Coverage," 2018, https://www.uhc2030.org/fileadmin/uploads/uhc2030/Documents/About_UHC2030/mgt_arrangemts___docs/UHC2030_Official_documents/UHC2030_Global_Compact_WEB.pdf.

49. Global Health Security Agenda, "Global Health Security Agenda," accessed January 30, 2021, https://ghsagenda.org/.

50. United Nations Children's Fund, "UNICEF's Agenda for Action for Refugee and Migrant Children," accessed January 30, 2021, https://www.unicef.org/eca/emergencies/unicefs-agenda-action-refugee-and-migrant-children.

51. *ILO Multilateral Framework on Labour Migration: Non-Binding Principles and Guidelines for a Rights-Based Approach to Labour Migration* (Geneva: International Labour Office, 2006), https://www.ilo.org/global/topics/labour-migration/publications/WCMS_178672/lang--en/index.htm.

52. IOM, "The Colombo Statement. Health of Migrants: Resetting the Agenda," Second Global Consultation on Migrant Health, Colombo, February 23, 2017, https://www.iom.int/sites/default/files/our_work/DMM/Migration-Health/colombo_statement.pdf.

53. WHO Regional Office for Europe, "WHO European Healthy Cities Network,"

accessed January 30, 2021, https://www.euro.who.int/en/health-topics/environment
-and-health/urban-health/who-european-healthy-cities-network.

54. Skiadas, *EU Migration Governance*.

55. M. McAuliffe and C. Bauloz, "Here's Why Coronavirus Could Be Devastating for Migrants," World Economic Forum, April 6, 2020.

56. WHO Regional Office for Europe, "How to Mitigate the Impacts of the COVID-19 Pandemic on Migrant Workers' Health," December 11, 2020, https://www.euro.who.int/en/health-topics/health-determinants/migration-and-health/news/news/2020/11/how-to-mitigate-the-impacts-of-the-covid-19-pandemic-on-migrant-workers-health.

57. H. H. P. Kluge, Z. Jakab, J. Bartovic, V. D'Anna, and S. Severoni, "Refugee and Migrant Health in the COVID-19 Response," *Lancet* 395, no. 10232 (2020): 1237–39, https://doi.org/10.1016/S0140-6736(20)30791-1.

58. United Nations, "UN System Task Team on the Post-2015 UN Development Agenda," January 2013, https://www.un.org/en/development/desa/policy/untaskteam_undf/thinkpieces/24_thinkpiece_global_governance.pdf.

Chapter 9

1. Anthony S. Fauci and David M. Morens, "The Perpetual Challenge of Infectious Diseases," *New England Journal of Medicine* 366, no. 5 (February 2, 2012): 454–61, https://doi.org/10.1056/NEJMra1108296.

2. Christian Drosten et al., "Identification of a Novel Coronavirus in Patients with Severe Acute Respiratory Syndrome," *New England Journal of Medicine* 348, no. 20 (May 15, 2003): 1967–76, https://doi.org/10.1056/NEJMoa030747; Kumnuan Ungchusak et al., "Probable Person-to-Person Transmission of Avian Influenza A (H5N1)," *New England Journal of Medicine* 352, no. 4 (January 27, 2005): 333–40, https://doi.org/10.1056/NEJMoa044021.

3. E. Delisle et al., "Chikungunya Outbreak in Montpellier, France, September to October 2014," *Euro Surveillance: Bulletin Europeen Sur Les Maladies Transmissibles = European Communicable Disease Bulletin* 20, no. 17 (April 30, 2015), https://doi.org/10.2807/1560-7917.es2015.20.17.21108; Maria Tseroni et al., "Prevention of Malaria Resurgence in Greece through the Association of Mass Drug Administration (MDA) to Immigrants from Malaria-Endemic Regions and Standard Control Measures," *PLoS Neglected Tropical Diseases* 9, no. 11 (November 2015): e0004215, https://doi.org/10.1371/journal.pntd.0004215; E. Marchand et al., "Autochthonous Case of Dengue in France, October 2013," *Euro Surveillance: Bulletin Europeen Sur Les Maladies Transmissibles = European Communicable Disease Bulletin* 18, no. 50 (December 12, 2013): 20661, https://doi.org/10.2807/1560-7917.es2013.18.50.20661.

4. M. A. Isler et al., "Screening Employees of Services for Homeless Individuals

in Montréal for Tuberculosis Infection," *Journal of Infection and Public Health* 6, no. 3 (June 2013): 209–15, https://doi.org/10.1016/j.jiph.2012.11.010.

5. María-Luisa Vázquez et al., "Was Access to Health Care Easy for Immigrants in Spain? The Perspectives of Health Personnel in Catalonia and Andalusia," *Health Policy (Amsterdam, Netherlands)* 120, no. 4 (April 2016): 396–405, https://doi.org /10.1016/j.healthpol.2016.01.011; Lilian Magalhaes, Christine Carrasco, and Denise Gastaldo, "Undocumented Migrants in Canada: A Scope Literature Review on Health, Access to Services, and Working Conditions," *Journal of Immigrant and Minority Health* 12, no. 1 (February 2010): 132–51, https://doi.org/10.1007/s10903-009 -9280-5; Nicolas Vignier et al., "Access to Health Insurance Coverage among Sub-Saharan African Migrants Living in France: Results of the ANRS-PARCOURS Study," *PloS One* 13, no. 2 (2018): e0192916, https://doi.org/10.1371/journal.pone .0192916.

6. Judit Simon et al., "Public Health Aspects of Migrant Health: A Review of the Evidence on Health Status for Labour Migrants in the European Region. (Health Evidence Network Synthesis Report 43)," WHO Regional Office for Europe, 2015; Elisabetta De Vito et al., *Public Health Aspects of Migrant Health: A Review of the Evidence on Health Status for Undocumented Migrants in the European Region* (Copenhagen: World Health Organisation Regional Office for Europe, 2015).

7. Bernd Rechel et al., "Migration and Health in an Increasingly Diverse Europe," *Lancet* 381, no. 9873 (April 6, 2013): 1235–45, https://doi.org/10.1016/S0140 -6736(12)62086-8; Emmanuel Scheppers et al., "Potential Barriers to the Use of Health Services among Ethnic Minorities: A Review," *Family Practice* 23, no. 3 (June 2006): 325–48, https://doi.org/10.1093/fampra/cmi113; Bradford H. Gray and Ewout van Ginneken, "Health Care for Undocumented Migrants: European Approaches," *Issue Brief (Commonwealth Fund)* 33 (December 2012): 1–12.

8. Michel Guillot et al., "Understanding Age Variations in the Migrant Mortality Advantage: An International Comparative Perspective," *PloS One* 13, no. 6 (2018): e0199669, https://doi.org/10.1371/journal.pone.0199669.

9. "Epidemiological Assessment of Hepatitis B and C among Migrants in the EU/EEA," European Centre for Disease Prevention and Control, July 27, 2016, https://www.ecdc.europa.eu/en/publications-data/epidemiological-assessment -hepatitis-b-and-c-among-migrants-eueea; Carmine Rossi et al., "Seroprevalence of Chronic Hepatitis B Virus Infection and Prior Immunity in Immigrants and Refugees: A Systematic Review and Meta-Analysis," *PloS One* 7, no. 9 (2012): e44611, https://doi.org/10.1371/journal.pone.0044611.

10. Adria Tassy Prosser, Tian Tang, and H. Irene Hall, "HIV in Persons Born Outside the United States, 2007–2010," *JAMA* 308, no. 6 (August 8, 2012): 601–7, https://doi.org/10.1001/jama.2012.9046.

11. Annabel Desgrees-du-Lou et al., "Is Hardship during Migration a Determinant of HIV Infection? Results from the ANRS PARCOURS Study of Sub-Saharan

African Migrants in France," *AIDS (London, England)* 30, no. 4 (February 20, 2016): 645–56, https://doi.org/10.1097/QAD.0000000000000957.

12. Anne Gosselin et al., "When and Why? Timing of Post-Migration HIV Acquisition among Sub-Saharan Migrants in France," *Sexually Transmitted Infections* 96, no. 3 (2020): 227–31, https://doi.org/10.1136/sextrans-2019-054080.

13. Csaba Ködmön, Phillip Zucs, and Marieke J. van der Werf, "Migration-Related Tuberculosis: Epidemiology and Characteristics of Tuberculosis Cases Originating Outside the European Union and European Economic Area, 2007 to 2013," *Euro Surveillance: Bulletin Europeen Sur Les Maladies Transmissibles = European Communicable Disease Bulletin* 21, no. 12 (2016), https://doi.org/10.2807/1560-7917 .ES.2016.21.12.30164.

14. K. Lönnroth et al., "Tuberculosis in Migrants in Low-Incidence Countries: Epidemiology and Intervention Entry Points," *The International Journal of Tuberculosis and Lung Disease: The Official Journal of the International Union Against Tuberculosis and Lung Disease* 21, no. 6 (June 1, 2017): 624–37, https://doi.org/10 .5588/ijtld.16.0845.

15. Eric Kendjo et al., "Epidemiologic Trends in Malaria Incidence among Travelers Returning to Metropolitan France, 1996–2016," *JAMA Network Open* 2, no. 4 (April 5, 2019): e191691, https://doi.org/10.1001/jamanetworkopen.2019.1691.

16. F. Deniaud et al., "Urogenital Schistosomiasis Detected in Sub-Saharan African Migrants Attending Primary Healthcare Consultations in Paris, France: A 14-Year Retrospective Cohort Study (2004–2017)," *European Journal of Clinical Microbiology and Infectious Diseases: Official Publication of the European Society of Clinical Microbiology* 39, no. 6 (June 2020): 1137–45, https://doi.org/10.1007 /s10096-020-03819-6.

17. Antoine Gessain and Olivier Cassar, "Epidemiological Aspects and World Distribution of HTLV-1 Infection," *Frontiers in Microbiology* 3 (2012): 388, https:// doi.org/10.3389/fmicb.2012.00388.

18. Yiting Lin, Ping Zhong, and Ting Chen, "Association Between Socioeconomic Factors and the COVID-19 Outbreak in the 39 Well-Developed Cities of China," *Frontiers in Public Health* 8 (October 30, 2020), https://doi.org/10.3389 /fpubh.2020.546637.

19. Monica Webb Hooper, Anna María Nápoles, and Eliseo J. Pérez-Stable, "COVID-19 and Racial/Ethnic Disparities," *JAMA*, May 11, 2020, https://doi.org /10.1001/jama.2020.8598; Eboni G. Price-Haywood et al., "Hospitalization and Mortality among Black Patients and White Patients with Covid-19," *New England Journal of Medicine* (May 27, 2020), https://doi.org/10.1056/NEJMsa2011686; Sylvain Papon and Isabelle Robert-Bobée, "An Increase in Deaths Twice as High for People Born Abroad than for Those Born in France in March-April 2020," *Insee Focus* (July 7, 2020).

20. Travis P. Baggett et al., "Prevalence of SARS-CoV-2 Infection in Residents of a Large Homeless Shelter in Boston," *JAMA* 323, no. 21 (June 2, 2020): 2191–92, https://doi.org/10.1001/jama.2020.6887.

21. Sven Drefahl et al., "A Population-Based Cohort Study of Socio-Demographic Risk Factors for COVID-19 Deaths in Sweden," *Nature Communications* 11, no. 1 (October 9, 2020): 5097, https://doi.org/10.1038/s41467-020-18926-3.

22. Eva Clark et al., "Disproportionate Impact of the COVID-19 Pandemic on Immigrant Communities in the United States," *PLoS Neglected Tropical Diseases* 14, no. 7 (2020): e0008484, https://doi.org/10.1371/journal.pntd.0008484.

Chapter 10

1. Jairo Acuña Alfaro and David Khoudour, "El Potencial de La Migración en America Latina y El Caribe," PNUD, January 31, 2020. Accessed May 9, 2021, https://www1.undp.org/content/undp/es/home/blog/2020/harnessing-the-potential -of-migration-in-latin-america-and-the-c.html.

2. Kenneth S. Kendler, "Toward a Philosophical Structure for Psychiatry," *American Journal of Psychiatry* 162, no. 3 (March 1, 2005): 433–40. https://doi.org/10.1176 /appi.ajp.162.3.433.

3. Joseba Achotegui, "La crisis como factor agravante del Síndrome de Ulises," *Temas de Psicoanálisis* 3 (January 2012): 1–16.

4. Sharon Schwartz and Ezra Susser, "Genome-wide Association Studies: Does Only Size Matter?" *American Journal of Psychiatry* 167, no. 7 (July 1, 2010): 741– 44. https://doi.org/10.1176/appi.ajp.2010.10030465.

5. Ezra Susser and Rebecca P. Smith, "Epidemiology in Public Mental Health." In *Population Mental Health: Evidence, Policy, and Public Health Practice*, edited by N. Cohen and S. Galea, 38–50. New York: Routledge, 2011.

6. Achotegui, "La crisis."

7. Steven F. Maier and Martin E. Seligman, "Learned Helplessness: Theory and Evidence," *Journal of Experimental Psychology: General* 105, no. 1 (March 1, 1976): 3–46. https://doi.org/10.1037/0096-3445.105.1.3.

8. Albert Bandura, "Recycling Misconceptions of Perceived Self-Efficacy," *Cognitive Therapy and Research* 8 (1984): 231–55. https://doi.org/10.1007/BF0117 2995.

9. James S. Colman, "Social Capital in the Creation of Human Capital," *American Journal of Sociology* 94 (1988): S95–S120. http://www.jstor.org/stable/2780 243.

10. Alfaro and Khoudour, "El Potencial de la Migración en America Latina y El Caribe."

11. Alfaro and Khoudour, "El Potencial de la Migración en America Latina y El Caribe."

12. Alicia Bárcena, "III Reunión Anual del Marco Integral Regional para la Protección y Soluciones al Desplazamiento Forzado (MIRPS)," *CEPAL* (December 8, 2020). https://www.cepal.org/es/comunicados/cepal-resalto-enfoque-innovador -plan-desarrollo-integral-norte-centroamerica-mexico.

13. J. Durand, "La Migración como amenaza ideológica, política y cultural." Conferencia impartida en el marco de la XXXIII Reunión Anual de Investigación, 2018. https://www.youtube.com/watch?v=qen9sdlurEk.

14. César Infante, Alvaro J. Idrovo, Mario S. Sánchez-Domínguez, Stéphane Vinhas, and Tonatiuh González-Vázquez, "Violence Committed against Migrants in Transit: Experiences of the Northern Mexican Border," *Journal of Immigrant and Minority Health* 14, no. 3 (June 2012): 449–59. http://doi 10.1007/s10903-011-9489-y.

15. Ricardo Orozco, Guilherme Borges, Maria Elena Medina-Mora, Sergio Aguilar-Gaxiola, and Joshua Breslau, "A Cross National Study on Prevalence of Mental Disorders, Service Use and Adequacy or Treatment among Mexican and Mexican American Populations," *American Journal of Public Health* 103, no. 9 (September 2013): 1610–18. https://doi.org/10.2105/AJPH.2012.301169.

16. Xiao Zhang, Ana P. Martinez-Donate, Jenna Nobles, Melbourne F. Hovell, Maria Gudelia Rangel, and Natalie M. Rhodes, "Substance Use across Different Phases of the Migration Process: A Survey of Mexican Migrants Flows," *Journal of Immigrant and Minority Health* 17, no. 6 (December 1, 2015): 1746–57. https://doi.org/10.1007/s10903-014-0109-5.

17. Miguel Pinedo, Yasmin Campos, Daniela Leal, Julio Fregoso, Shira M. Goldenberg, and María Luisa Zúñiga, "Alcohol Use Behaviors among Indigenous Migrants: A Transnational Study on Communities of Origin and Destination," *Journal of Immigrant and Minority Health* 16, no. 3 (June 1, 2014): 348–55. https://doi.org/10.1007/s10903-013-9964-8.

18. Guilherme Borges, Claudia Rafful, Daniel J. Tancredi, Naomi Saito, Sergio Aguilar-Gaxiola, Maria-Elena Medina Mora, and Joshua Breslau, "Mexican Immigration to the U.S., the Occurrence of Violence and the Impact of Mental Disorders," *Revista Brasileira de Psiquiatría* 35, no. 2 (September 16, 2014): 161–68. https://doi.org/10.1590/1516-4446-2012-0988.

19. Luz M. Garcini, Melanie M. Domenech Rodríguez, Alfonso Mercado, and Manuel Paris, "A Tale of Two Crises: The Compounded Effect of COVID-19 and Anti-Immigration Policy in the United States," *Psychological Trauma: Theory, Research, Practice, and Policy* 12, no. S1 (August 2020): S230–32. http://dx.doi.org/10.1037/tra0000775.

20. Erika Garcia, Sandrah P. Eckel, Zhanghua Chen, Kenan Li, and Frank D. Gilliland, "COVID-19 Mortality in California Based on Death Certificates: Disproportionate Impacts across Racial/Ethnic Groups and Nativity," *Annals of Epidemiology* 58 (June 2021): 69–75. https://doi.org/10.1016/j.annepidem.2021.03.006.

21. Olivia Willis, "Poor Air Quality Caused by Bushfire Smoke Posing Serious Risk for Healthy People Too, Health Experts Warn," *ABC Health and Wellbeing* (November 7, 2020). Accessed on October 13, 2020, https://www.abc.net.au/news/health/2020-01-07/prolonged-bushfire-smoke-creates-new-health-risks/11844934.

22. Matthew J. Townsend, Theodore K. Kyle, and Fatima C. Stanford, "Outcomes of COVID-19: Disparities in Obesity and by Ethnicity/Race," *International Journal of Obesity* 44 (July 9, 2020): 1807–9. https://doi.org/10.1038/s41366-020-0635-2.

23. William F. Owen, Richard Carmona, and Claire Pomeroy, "Failing Another National Stress Test on Health Disparities," *Journal of the American Medical Association* 323, no. 19 (April 15, 2020): 1905–6. https://doi.org/10.1001/jama.2020.6547.

24. Garcia et al., "COVID-19 Mortality."

25. International Fund for Agricultural Development (IFAD), "Remittances in Times of Crisis: Facing the Challenges of COVID-19," April 20, 2020.

26. IFAD, "Remittances in Times of Crisis."

27. International Labour Organization, "*ILO Global Estimates on International Migrant Workers—Results and Methodologies*," December 5, 2018.

28. IFAD, "Sending Money Home: Contributing to the SDGs, One Family at a Time," June 2017.

29. *New York Times*, "Even When They Lost Their Jobs, Immigrants Sent Money Home," September 24, 2020. Accessed October 13, 2020, https://www.nytimes.com/2020/09/24/us/coronavirus-immigrants-remittances.html.

30. Ann S. Masten, "Resilience in Children Threatened by Extreme Adversity: Frameworks for Research, Practice, and Translational Synergy," *Developmental and Psychopathology* 23, no. 2 (May 23, 2011): 493–506. https://doi.org/10.1017/S0954579411000198.

31. Carolina M. Lemus-Way and Helena Johansson, "Strengths and Resilience of Migrant Women in Transit: An Analysis of the Narratives of Central American Women in Irregular Transit Through Mexico Towards the USA," *Journal of International Migration and Integration* 21 (June 4, 2019): 745–63. https://doi.org/10.1007/s12134-019-00690-z.

32. Cassandra Kisiel, Faith Summersett-Ringgold, Lindsey E. G. Weil, and Gary McClelland, "Understanding Strengths in Relation to Complex Trauma and Mental Health Symptoms within Child Welfare," *Journal of Child and Family Studies* 26, no. 2 (October 14, 2017): 437–51. https://doi.org/10.1007/s10826-016-0569-4.

33. Paolo Stratta, Cristina Capanna, Liliana Dell'Osso, Claudia Carmassi, Sara Patricia, Gabriella Di Emidio, Ilaria Riccardi, Alberto Collazzoni, and Alessandro Rossi, "Resilience and Coping in Trauma Spectrum Symptoms Prediction: A Structural Equation Modeling Approach," *Personality Individual Differences* 77 (April 2015): 55–61. https://doi.org/10.1016/j.paid.2014.12.035.

34. Dante Cicchetti, "Annual Research Review: Resilient Functioning in Maltreated Children–Past, Present, and Future Perspectives," *Journal of Child Psychology and Psychiatry* 54, no. 4 (August 28, 2013): 402–22. https://doi.org/10.1111/j.1469-7610.2012.02608.x.

35. Karen Hughes, Bellis A. Mark, Hardcastle A. Katherine, Dinesh Sethi, Alexander Butchart, Mikton Christopher, Lisa Jones, and Michael P. Dunne, "The Effect of Multiple Adverse Childhood Experiences on Health: A Systematic Review and Meta-analysis," *Lancet Public Health* 2, no. 8 (July 31, 2017): e356–66. https://doi.org/10.1016/S2468-2667(17)30118-4.

36. Justine M. Gatt, Rebecca Alexander, Alan Emond, Kim Foster, Kristin Hadfield, Amanda Mason-Jones, Steve Reid, Linda Theron, Michael Ungar, Trecia A.

Wouldes, and Qiaobing Wu, "Trauma, Resilience, and Mental Health in Migrant and Non-Migrant Youth: An International Cross-Sectional Study Across Six Countries," *Frontiers in Psychiatry* 10, no. 997 (March 9, 2020): 1–15. https://doi.org/10 .3389/fpsyt.2019.00997.

37. Ralf Schwarzer and Lisa M. Warner, "Perceived Self-Efficacy and Its Relationship to Resilience," in *The Springer Series on Human Exceptionality: Resilience in Children, Adolescents, and Adults: Translating Research into Practice*, edited by S. Prince-Embury and D. H. Saklofske, 139–50. https://doi.org/10.1007/978-1-4614 -4939-3_10.

38. Charles C. Benight and Albert Bandura, "Social Cognitive Theory and Posttraumatic Recovery: The Role of Perceived Efficacy," *Behaviour Research and Therapy* 42, no. 10 (October 2004): 1129–48. https://doi.org/10.1016/j.brat.2003.08.008.

39. Urie Bronfenbrenner, "Toward an Experimental Ecology of Human Development," *American Psychologist* 32, no. 7 (1977): 513–31. https://doi.org/ 10.1037 /0003-066X.32.7.513.

40. Urie Bronfenbrenner, "Contexts of Child Rearing: Problems and Prospects," *American Psychologist* 34, no. 10 (1979): 844–50. https://doi.org/10.1037/0003-066X .34.10.844.

41. Anna Aizik-Reebs, Kim Yuval, Yuval Hadash, Solomon Gebreyohans Gebremariam, and Amit Bernstein, "Mindfulness-Based Trauma Recovery for Refugees (MBTR-R): Randomized Waitlist-Control Evidence of Efficacy and Safety," *MindRxiv* (May 15, 2020). https://doi.org/10.31231/osf.io/jyhwa.

42. Eric Lopez-Maya, Richard Olmstead, and Michael R. Irwin, "Mindfulness Meditation and Improvement in Depressive Symptoms Among Spanish- and English-Speaking Adults: A Randomized, Controlled, Comparative Efficacy Trial," *PloS One* 14, no. 7 (July 5, 2019): e0219425. https://doi.org/10.1371/journal.pone .0219425.

43. Alice Malpass, Kate Binnie, and Lauren Robson, "Medical Students' Experience of Mindfulness Training in the UK: Well-Being, Coping Reserve, and Professional Development," *Education Research International* (February 3, 2019). https:// doi10.1155/2019/4021729.

44. Naomi Breslau, Howard D. Chilcoat, Ronald C. Kessler, and Glenn C. Davis, "Previous Exposure to Trauma and PTSD Effects of Subsequent Trauma: Results from the Detroit Area Survey of Trauma," *American Journal of Psychiatry* 156, no. 6 (June 1, 1999): 902–7. https://doi.org/10.1176/ajp.156.6.902.

45. Jenna Boyd, Ruth A. Lanius, and Margaret C. McKinnon, "Mindfulness-based Treatments for Posttraumatic Stress Disorder: A Review of the Treatment Literature and Neurobiological Evidence," *Journal of Psychiatry and Neuroscience* 43, no. 1 (October 3, 2018): 7–25. https://doi.org/10.1503/jpn.170021.

46. Kristy Banks, Emily Newman, and Jannat Saleem, "An Overview of The Research on Mindfulness-based Interventions for Treating Symptoms of Posttraumatic Stress Disorder: A Systematic Review," *Journal of Clinical Psychology* 71, no.10 (July 20, 2015): 935–63. https://doi.org/ 10.1002/jclp.22200.

47. Sonia Nazario, *Enrique's Journey: The True Story of a Boy Determined to Reunite with His Mother*. New York: Random House Trade Paperbacks, 2014.

48. Joan Rosenbaum-Asarnow, "Promoting Stress Resistance in War-Exposed Children," *Journal of the American Academy of Child and Adolescent Psychiatry* 50, no. 4 (April 1, 2011): 320–22. https://doi.org/10.1016/j.jaac.2011.01.010.

49. *The Guardian*, "'Being Prepared for The Worst' Is Nothing New for Immigrants During COVID-19," April 15, 2020.

50. Fiona Charlson, Mark van Ommeren, Abraham Flaxman, Joseph Cornett, Harvey Whiteford, and Shekhar Saxena, "New WHO Prevalence Estimates of Mental Disorders in Conflict Settings: A Systemic Review and Meta-Analysis," *Lancet* 394, no. 10194 (July 20, 2019): 240–48. https://doi.org/10.1016/S0140-6736(19)30934-1.

Chapter 11

This work was supported by The National Social Science Fund of China [No. 19 BSH035].

1. Beine, Michel A. R., Pauline Bourgeon, and Jean Charles Bricongne. 2013. "Aggregate Fluctuations and International Migration." *SSRN Electronic Journal* 117, no. 1: 110–17.

2. Gushulak, Brian D., Jason Weekers, and Douglas W. MacPherson. 2009. "Migrants and Emerging Public Health Issues in a Globalized World: Threats, Risks and Challenges, an Evidence-Based Framework." *Emerging Health Threats Journal* 2, no. 1: 7091.

3. Black, Maureen M., and Ambika Krishnakumar. 1998. "Children in Low-Income, Urban Settings. Interventions to Promote Mental Health and Well-Being." *American Psychologist* 53, no. 6: 635–46.

4. Peen, Jaap, Jack Dekker, Robert A. Schoevers, Margreet Ten Have, Ron de Graaf, and Aartjan T. Beekman. 2007. "Is the Prevalence of Psychiatric Disorders Associated with Urbanization?" *Social Psychiatry and Psychiatric Epidemiology* 42, no. 12: 984–89.

5. World Health Organization (WHO). 2001. "The World Health Report 2001—Mental Health: New Understanding, New Hope."

6. Allen, Jessica, Reuben Balfour, and Ruth Bell. 2014. "Social Determinants of Mental Health." *International Review of Psychiatry* 4, no. 26: 392–407.

7. Hummer, Robert A., Daniel A. Powers, Starling G. Pullum, Ginger L. Gossman, and W. Parker Frisbie. 2007. "Paradox Found (Again): Infant Mortality among the Mexican-Origin Population in the United States." *Demography* 44, no. 3: 441–57.

8. Urquia, Marcelo L., Patricia J. O'Campo, and Maureen I. Heaman. 2012. "Revisiting the Immigrant Paradox in Reproductive Health: The Roles of Duration of Residence and Ethnicity." *Social Science and Medicine* 74, no. 10: 1610–21. https://doi.org/10.1016/j.socscimed.2012.02.013.

9. Abraído-Lanza, A. F., B. P. Dohrenwend, D. S. Ng-Mak, and J. B. Turner. 1999. "The Latino Mortality Paradox: A Test of the 'Salmon Bias' and Healthy Migrant Hypotheses." *American Journal of Public Health* 89, no. 10: 1543–48. https://doi .org/10.2105/AJPH.89.10.1543.

10. Palloni, Alberto, and Jeffrey D. Morenoff. 2001. "Interpreting the Paradoxi- cal in the Hispanic Paradox." *Population Health and Aging: Strengthening the Dia- logue Between Epidemiology and Demography* 954, no. 1: 140–74.

11. Bruce Newbold, K. 2005. "Self-Rated Health within the Canadian Immigrant Population: Risk and the Healthy Immigrant Effect." *Social Science and Medicine* 60, no. 6: 1359–70. https://doi.org/10.1016/j.socscimed.2004.06.048.

12. Lu, Yao, and Lijian Qin. 2014. "Healthy Migrant and Salmon Bias Hypoth- eses: A Study of Health and Internal Migration in China." *Social Science and Medi- cine* 102: 41–48. https://doi.org/10.1016/j.socscimed.2013.11.040.

13. Xiao, Yang, Siyu Miao, and Chinmoy Sarkar. 2020. "Social Ties, Spatial Mi- gration Paradigm, and Mental Health among Two Generations of Migrants in China." *Population, Space and Place* 27, no. 2: e2389. https://doi.org/doi:10.1002/psp.2389.

14. McKenzie, Kwame. 2008. "Urbanization, Social Capital and Mental Health." *Global Social Policy* 8, no. 3: 359–77.

15. Bhugra, D. 2004. "Migration and Mental Health." *Acta Psychiatrica Scandi- navica* 109, no. 4: 243–58.

16. Malmusi, Davide. 2014. "Immigrants' Health and Health Inequality by Type of Integration Policies in European Countries." *European Journal of Public Health* 25, no. 2: 293–99. https://doi.org/10.1093/eurpub/cku156.

17. Alegría, Margarita, Kiara Álvarez, and Karissa DiMarzio. 2017. "Immigra- tion and Mental Health." *Current Epidemiology Reports* 4, no. 2: 145–55. https:// doi.org/10.1007/s40471-017-0111-2.

18. Riger, Stephanie, and Paul J. Lavrakas. 1981. "Community Ties: Patterns of Attachment and Social Interaction in Urban Neighborhoods." *American Journal of Community Psychology* 9, no. 1: 55–66.

19. Kawachi, Ichiro, and Lisa Berkman. 2000. "Social Cohesion, Social Capital, and Health." *Social Epidemiology* 174: 190.

20. Ellen, Ingrid Gould, Tod Mijanovich, and Keri-Nicole Dillman. 2001. "Neigh- borhood Effects on Health: Exploring the Links and Assessing the Evidence." *Jour- nal of Urban Affairs* 23 (3–4): 391–408. https://doi.org/10.1111/0735-2166.00096.

21. Young, Anne F., Anne Russell, and Jennifer R. Powers. 2004. "The Sense of Belonging to a Neighbourhood: Can It Be Measured and Is It Related to Health and Well Being in Older Women?" *Social Science and Medicine* 59, no. 12: 2627–37. https://doi.org/https://doi.org/10.1016/j.socscimed.2004.05.001.

22. Gale, Sara L., Sheryl L. Magzamen, John D. Radke, and Ira B. Tager. 2011. "Crime, Neighborhood Deprivation, and Asthma: A GIS Approach to Define and Assess Neighborhoods." *Spatial and Spatio-temporal Epidemiology* 2, no. 2: 59–67. https://doi.org/10.1016/j.sste.2011.01.001.

23. Na, Ling, and Dale Hample. 2016. "Psychological Pathways from Social Integration to Health: An Examination of Different Demographic Groups in Canada." *Social Science and Medicine* 151: 196–205.

24. Lu, Yao. 2010. "Rural-Urban Migration and Health: Evidence from Longitudinal Data in Indonesia." *Social Science and Medicine* 70, no. 3: 412–19. https://doi.org/10.1016/j.socscimed.2009.10.028.

25. Zimmerman, C., L. Kiss, and M. Hossain. 2011. "Migration and Health: A Framework for 21st Century Policy-Making." *Plos Medicine* 8, no. 5: e1001034.

26. Shuval, Judith T. 1993. "Migration and Stress." In *Handbook of Stress: Theoretical and Clinical Aspects*, 2nd ed., 641–57. New York: Free Press.

27. Williams, Carolyn L., and John W. Berry. 1991. "Primary Prevention of Acculturative Stress among Refugees: Application of Psychological Theory and Practice." *American Psychologist* 46, no. 6: 632–41.

28. Ascher, Francois. 1985. *Tourism: Transnational Corporations and Cultural Identities*. Paris: UNESCO.

29. Zheng, Xue, and John W. Berry. 1991. "Psychological Adaptation of Chinese Sojourners in Canada." *International Journal of Psychology* 26, no. 4: 451–70.

30. Hurh, Won Moo, and Kwang Chung Kim. 1990. "Correlates of Korean Immigrants' Mental Health." *Journal of Nervous and Mental Disease* 178, no. 11: 703–11. https://journals.lww.com/jonmd/Fulltext/1990/11000/Correlates_of_Korean_Immigrants__Mental_Health.6.aspx.

31. Williams and Berry, "Primary Prevention of Acculturative Stress."

32. Bhugra, "Migration and Mental Health."

33. Hovey, J. D., and C. G. Magaña. 2002. "Exploring the Mental Health of Mexican Migrant Farm Workers in the Midwest: Psychosocial Predictors of Psychological Distress and Suggestions for Prevention and Treatment." *Journal of Psychology* 136, no. 5: 493–13. https://doi.org/10.1080/00223980209605546.

34. Rogler, Lloyd H., Dharma E. Cortes, and Robert G. Malgady. 1991. "Acculturation and Mental Health Status among Hispanics: Convergence and New Directions for Research." *American Psychologist* 46, no. 6.

35. Liebkind, Karmela, and Inga Jasinskajalahti. 2000. "Acculturation and Psychological Well-Being among Immigrant Adolescents in Finland: A Comparative Study of Adolescents from Different Cultural Backgrounds." *Journal of Adolescent Research* 15, no. 4: 446–69.

36. Valenciagarcia, Dellanira, Jane M. Simoni, Margarita Alegría, and David T. Takeuchi. 2012. "Social Capital, Acculturation, Mental Health, and Perceived Access to Services among Mexican American Women." *Journal of Consulting and Clinical Psychology* 80, no. 2: 177–85.

37. Hunt, L. M., S. Schneider, and B. Comer. 2004. "Should 'Acculturation' Be a Variable in Health Research? A Critical Review of Research on US Hispanics." *Soc Sci Med* 59, no. 5: 973–86. https://doi.org/10.1016/j.socscimed.2003.12.009.

38. Salabarría-Peña, Y., P. T. Trout, J. K. Gill, D. E. Morisky, A. A. Muralles, and

V. J. Ebin. 2001. "Effects of Acculturation and Psychosocial Factors in Latino Ado-lescents' TB-Related Behaviors." *Ethnicity and Disease* 11, no. 4: 661–75.

39. Cuellar, Israel, Lorwen C. Harris, and Ricardo Jasso. 1980. "An Accultura-tion Scale for Mexican American Normal and Clinical Populations." *Hispanic Jour-nal of Behavioral Sciences* 2: 199–217.

40. Cabassa, Leopoldo J. 2003. "Measuring Acculturation: Where We Are and Where We Need to Go." *Hispanic Journal of Behavioral Sciences* 25, no. 2: 127–46. https://doi.org/10.1177/0739986303025002001.

41. Berry, J. W. 1980. "Social and Cultural Change." *African Studies Review* 17, no. 2: 79–88.

42. Kim, Uichol. 1988. "Psychological Acculturation of Immigrants." In *Cross-Cultural Adaptation: Current Approaches*, edited by Y. Y. Kim, W. B. Gudykunst, 62–89. Newbury Park, CA: Sage.

43. Berry, "Social and Cultural Change."

44. Kim, "Psychological Acculturation of Immigrants."

45. Fassaert, T., A. E. Hesselink, and A. P. Verhoeff. 2009. "Acculturation and Use of Health Care Services by Turkish and Moroccan Migrants: A Cross-Sectional Population-Based Study." *Bmc Public Health* 9, no. 1: 1–9.

46. Berry, J. W., Uichol Kim, Thomas Minde, and Doris Mok. 1987. "Compara-tive Studies of Acculturative Stress." *International Migration Review* 21, no. 3: 491–511.

47. Yeh, Christine J. 2003. "Age, Acculturation, Cultural Adjustment, and Men-tal Health Symptoms of Chinese, Korean, and Japanese Immigrant Youths." *Cul-tural Diversity and Ethnic Minority Psychology* 9, no. 1: 34–48.

48. Zagefka, Hanna, and Rupert Brown. 2002. "The Relationship between Ac-culturation Strategies, Relative Fit and Intergroup Relations: Immigrant-Majority Relations in Germany." *European Journal of Social Psychology* 32, no. 2: 171–88.

49. Bourhis, Richard Y., Léna Céline Moïse, Stéphane Perreault, and Sacha Se-nécal. 1997. "Towards an Interactive Acculturation Model: A Social Psychological Approach." *International Journal of Psychology* 32, no. 6: 369–86.

50. Sodowsky, Gargi Roysircar, and Wai Ming Lai Edward. 1997. "Asian Im-migrant Variables and Structural Models of Cross-Cultural Distress." In *Immigra-tion and the Family: Research and Policy on U.S. Immigrants*, edited by A. Booth, A. C. Crouter, and N. S. Landale, 211–34. Mahwah, NJ: Lawrence Erlbaum.

51. Gaertner, Samuel L., and John F. Dovidio. 2000. "Reducing Intergroup Bias: The Common Ingroup Identity Model." *Psychology Press*.

52. Golding, Jacqueline M., M. Audrey Burnam. 1990. "Immigration, Stress, and Depressive Symptoms in a Mexican-American Community." *Journal of Nervous and Mental Disease* 178, no. 3: 161–71.

53. Kaplan, Mark S., and Gary Marks. 1990. "Adverse Effects of Acculturation: Psychological Distress among Mexican American Young Adults." *Social Science and Medicine* 31, no. 12: 1313–19.

54. Salant, Talya, and Diane S. Lauderdale. 2003. "Measuring Culture: A Critical Review of Acculturation and Health in Asian Immigrant Populations." *Social Science and Medicine* 57, no. 1: 71–90. https://doi.org/10.1016/S0277-9536(02)00300-3.

55. Cuellar, Israel, and Robert E. Roberts. 1997. "Relations of Depression, Acculturation, and Socioeconomic Status in a Latino Sample." *Hispanic Journal of Behavioral Sciences* 19, no. 2: 230–38.

56. Canabal, Maria E., and Jose A. Quiles. 1995. "Acculturation and Socioeconomic Factors as Determinants of Depression among Puerto Ricans in the United States." *Social Behavior and Personality: An International Journal* 23, no. 3: 235–46.

57. Lee, Mee Sook, Kathleen S. Crittenden, and Elena Yu. 1996. "Social Support and Depression among Elderly Korean Immigrants in the United States." *International Journal of Aging and Human Development* 42, no. 4: 313–27.

Chapter 12

1. UNDESA. "International Migrant Stock 2019." 2019. Accessed February 15, 2021. https://www.un.org/en/development/desa/population/migration/data/estimates2/estimates19.asp.

2. Davies, A.A., A. Basten, and C. J. E. Frattini. *Migration: A Social Determinant of the Health of Migrants* 16, no. 1 (2009): 10–12.

3. Abubakar, I., R. W. Aldridge, D. Devakumar et al. "The UCL–Lancet Commission on Migration and Health: The Health of a World on the Move." *Lancet Comission* 392, no. 10164 (2018): 2606–54.

4. Wickramage, K., J. Vearey, A. B. Zwi, C. Robinson, and M. Knipper. "Migration and Health: A Global Public Health Research Priority." *BMC Public Health* 18, no. 1 (2018): 1–9.

5. Shils, M. E., J. A. Olson, and M. Shike. *Modern Nutrition in Health and Disease*. Philadelphia: Lea & Febiger, 1994.

6. Thiele, S., G. B. Mensink, and R. Beitz. "Determinants of Diet Quality." *Public Health Nutrition* 7, no. 1 (2004): 29–37.

7. Nature. "Counting the Hidden $12 Trillion Cost of a Broken Food System." October 16, 2019.

8. World Health Organization. "Healthy Diet." Regional Office for the Eastern Mediterranean. 2019.

9. Black, R. E., L. H. Allen, Z. A. Bhutta et al. Maternal and Child Undernutrition: Global and Regional Exposures and Health Consequences. *Lancet* 371, no. 9608 (2008): 243–60.

10. Ramakrishnan, U. "Prevalence of Micronutrient Malnutrition Worldwide." *Nutrition Reviews* 60, no. 5 (2002): S46–S52.

11. Danaei, G., Y. Lu, G. M. Singh et al. "Cardiovascular Disease, Chronic Kidney Disease, and Diabetes Mortality Burden of Cardiometabolic Risk Factors from 1980

to 2010: A Comparative Risk Assessment." *Lancet Diabetes & Endocrinology* 2, no. 8 (2014): 634–47.

12. Afshin A., P. J. Sur, K. A. Fay et al. "Health Effects of Dietary Risks in 195 Countries, 1990–2017: A Systematic Analysis for the Global Burden of Disease Study 2017." *Lancet* 393, no. 10184 (2019): 1958–72.

13. Wickramage et al., "Migration and Health."

14. Sadiddin A., A. Cattaneo, M. Cirillo, and M. J. F. S. Miller. "Food Insecurity as a Determinant of International Migration: Evidence from Sub-Saharan Africa." *Food Security* 11, no. 3 (2019): 515–30.

15. Guerra, J. V. V., V. H. Alves, L. Rachedi et al. "Forced International Migration for Refugee Food: A Scoping Review." *Ciencia and Saude Coletiva* 24 (2019): 4499–508.

16. Vatanparast, H., C. Nisbet, and B. Gushulak. "Vitamin D Insufficiency and Bone Mineral Status in a Population of Newcomer Children in Canada." *Nutrients* 5, no. 5 (2013):1561–72.

17. Dharod, J. M., J. E. Croom, and C. G. Sady. "Food Insecurity: Its Relationship to Dietary Intake and Body Weight among Somali Refugee Women in the United States." *Journal of Nutrition Education and Behavior* 45, no. 1 (2013): 47–53.

18. Ghattas, H., A. J. Sassine, K. Seyfert, M. Nord, and N. R. Sahyoun. "Food Insecurity among Iraqi Refugees Living in Lebanon, 10 Years after the Invasion of Iraq: Data from a Household Survey." *British Journal of Nutrition* 112, no. 1 (2014): 70–79.

19. Ngongalah L., J. Rankin, T. Rapley, A. Odeniyi, Z. Akhter Z, and N. Heslehurst. "Dietary and Physical Activity Behaviours in African Migrant Women Living in High Income Countries: A Systematic Review and Framework Synthesis." *Nutrients* 10, no. 8 (2018): 1017.

20. Vangay, P., A. J. Johnson, T. L. Ward et al. "US Immigration Westernizes the Human Gut Microbiome." *Cell* 175, no. 4 (2018): 962–72.

21. Popkin, B. M., C. Corvalan, and L. M. Grummer-Strawn. "Dynamics of the Double Burden of Malnutrition and the Changing Nutrition Reality." *Lancet* 395, no. 10217 (2020): 65–74.

22. Akombi-Inyang, B., M. N. Huda, J. Byaruhanga, and A. Renzaho. "Double Burden of Malnutrition among Migrants and Refugees in Developed Countries." *Social Science Protocols* 4 (2021): 1–13.

23. Popkin et al., "Dynamics of the Double Burden."

24. WHO. "Children: Improving Survival and Well-Being." 2020.

25. Lake, A., T. Townshend. "Obesogenic Environments: Exploring the Built and Food Environments." *Journal of the Royal Society for the Promotion of Health* 126, no. 6 (2006): 262–67.

26. Saddidin, A., et al. "Food Insecurity as a Determinant of International Migration: Evidence from Sub-Saharan Africa." *Food Security* 11, no. 3 (2019): 515–30.

27. Zezza, A., C. Carletto, B. Davis, and P. Winters. "Assessing the Impact of Migration on Food and Nutrition Security." *Food Policy* 36, no. 1 (2011): 1–6.

28. Ujcic-Voortman, J. K., C. A. Baan, J. C. Seidell, and A. P. Verhoeff. "Obesity and Cardiovascular Disease Risk among Turkish and Moroccan Migrant Groups in Europe: A Systematic Review." *Obesity Reviews* 13, no. 1 (2012): 2–16.

29. Delavari, M., A. L. Sønderlund, D. Mellor, M. Mohebbi, and B. Swinburn. "Migration, Acculturation and Environment: Determinants of Obesity among Iranian Migrants in Australia." *International Journal of Environmental Research and Public Health* 12, no. 2 (2015): 1083–98.

30. Renzaho, A., C. Gibbons, B. Swinburn, D. Jolley, and C. Burns. "Obesity and Undernutrition in Sub-Saharan African Immigrant and Refugee Children in Victoria, Australia." *Healthy Eating Club* (2006).

31. Labree, L., H. Van De Mheen, F. Rutten, and M. Foets. "Differences in Overweight and Obesity among Children from Migrant and Native Origin: A Systematic Review of the European Literature." *Obesity Reviews* 12, no. 5 (2011): e535–47.

32. Zezza et al., "Assessing the Impact of Migration."

33. Terragni, L., L. M. Garnweidner, K. S. Pettersen, and A. Mosdøl. "Migration as a Turning Point in Food Habits: The Early Phase of Dietary Acculturation among Women from South Asian, African, and Middle Eastern Countries Living in Norway." *Ecology of Food and Nutrition* 53, no. 3 (2014): 273–91.

34. Guerra et al., "Forced International Migration."

35. Bhugra, D. "Migration, Distress and Cultural Identity." *British Medical Bulletin* 69, no. 1 (2004): 129–41.

36. Ore, H. J. F. "Culture, Society. Ambivalent Nostalgia: Jewish-Israeli Migrant Women 'Cooking' Ways to Return Home." *Food, Culture, & Society* 21, no. 4 (2018): 568–84.

37. Abbots, E-J, J. Klein, and J. Watson. "Approaches to Food and Migration: Rootedness, Being and Belonging." *The Handbook of Food and Anthropology* (2016): 115–32.

38. Hughes, M. "The Social and Cultural Role of Food for Myanmar Refugees in Regional Australia: Making Place and Building Networks." *Journal of Sociology* 55, no. 2 (2019): 290–305.

39. Gerodetti, N., and S. Foster. "Growing Foods from Home: Food Production, Migrants and the Changing Cultural Landscapes of Gardens and Allotments." *Landscape Research* 41, no. 7 (2016): 808–19.

40. Bailey, A. "The Migrant Suitcase: Food, Belonging and Commensality among Indian Migrants in the Netherlands." *Appetite* 110 (2017): 51–60.

41. Rissel, C. "The Development and Application of a Scale of Acculturation." *Australian and New Zealand Journal of Public Health* 21, no. 6 (1997): 606–13.

42. Cunningham, S. A., J. D. Ruben, and K. M. V. Narayan. "Health of Foreign-Born People in the United States: A Review." *Health Place* 14, no. 4 (2008): 623–35.

43. Popovic-Lipovac, A., and B. Strasser. "A Review on Changes in Food Habits among Immigrant Women and Implications for Health." *Journal of Immigration and Minority Health* 17, no. 2 (2015): 582–90.

44. Satia-Abouta, J. "Dietary Acculturation: Definition, Process, Assessment, and Implications." *International Journal of Human Ecology* 4, no. 1 (2003): 71–86.

45. Delavari, M., A. L. Sønderlund, B. Swinburn, D. Mellor, and A. Renzaho. "Acculturation and Obesity among Migrant Populations in High Income Countries—A Systematic Review." *BMC Public Health* 13, no. 1 (2013): 458.

46. Popovic-Lipovac and Strasser, "A Review on Changes in Food Habits."

47. Warner, K., and T Afifi. "Where the Rain Falls: Evidence from 8 Countries on How Vulnerable Households Use Migration to Manage the Risk of Rainfall Variability and Food Insecurity." *Climate and Development* 6, no. 1 (2014): 1–17.

48. Fennelly, K. "The 'Healthy Migrant' Effect." *Minnesota Medicine* 90, no. 3 (2007): 51–53.

49. Hunter, L. M., and D. H. Simon. "Might Climate Change the 'Healthy Migrant' Effect?" *Global Environmental Change* 47 (2017): 133–42.

50. Fanzo, J., C. Davis, R. McLaren, and J. Choufani. "The Effect of Climate Change across Food Systems: Implications for Nutrition Outcomes." *Global Food Security* 18 (2018): 12–19.

51. Willett, W., J. Rockström, B. Loken et al. "Food in the Anthropocene: The EAT–Lancet Commission on Healthy Diets from Sustainable Food Systems." *Lancet* 393, no. 10170 (2019): 447–92.

Chapter 13

1. UN, "Transforming Our World: The 2030 Agenda for Sustainable Development," Division for Sustainable Development Goals, 2015.

2. WHO, "Defining Sexual Health: Report of a Technical Consultation on Sexual Health," January 28–31, 2002, Geneva.

3. IOM, "Key Migration Terms," 2020. https://www.iom.int/key-migration-terms.

4. Brian Gushulak, Jason Weekers, and Douglas MacPherson, "Migrants and Emerging Public Health Issues in a Globalized World: Threats, Risks and Challenges, an Evidence-Based Framework," *Emerging Health Threats Journal* 2, no. 1 (2009): 7091.

5. Olena Ivanova, Masna Rai, and Elizabeth Kemigisha, "A Systematic Review of Sexual and Reproductive Health Knowledge, Experiences and Access to Services among Refugee, Migrant and Displaced Girls and Young Women in Africa," *International Journal of Environmental Research and Public Health* 15, no. 8 (2018): 1583.

6. Cristianne Rocha, Sónia Dias, and Ana Gama, "Knowledge of Contraceptive Methods and STD Prevention among Immigrant Women," *Cadernos de Saúde Pública* 26, no. 5 (2010): 1003–12.

7. Hongfei Du and Xiaoming Li, "Acculturation and HIV-Related Sexual Behaviours among International Migrants: A Systematic Review and Meta-Analysis,"

Health Psychology Review 9, no. 1 (2015): 103–22; Marielena Lara, Cristina Gamboa, Kahramanian, Leo S. Morales, and David E. Hayes Bautista, "Acculturation and Latino Health in the United States: A Review of the Literature and Its Sociopolitical Context," *Annual Review Public Health* 26 (2005): 367–97.

8. Charlotte Oliveira, Ines Keygnaert, Maria do Rosário Oliveira Martins, and Sónia Dias, "Assessing Reported Cases of Sexual and Gender-Based Violence, Causes and Preventive Strategies, in European Asylum Reception Facilities," *Globalization and Health* 14, no. 1 (2018): 1–12.

9. Government of Germany, "Health, Well-Being and Personal Safety of Women in Germany," 2004.

10. Charlotte Oliveira, Maria do Rosário Oliveira Martins, Sónia Dias, and Ines Keygnaert, "Conceptualizing Sexual and Gender-Based Violence in European Asylum Reception Centers," *Archives of Public Health* 77, no. 1 (2019): 27.

11. Ines Keygnaert, Koen Dedoncker, Kathia Van Egmond, Marleen Temmerman, Christiana Nostlinger, Jasna Loos, Patricia Kennedy, Sonia F. Dias, Luis T. Tavira, Isabel Craveiro, Elisabeth Ioannidi, Eirini Kampriani, Najla Wassie, Dorota Sienkiewicz, and Erick Vloeberghs, *Sexual and Reproductive Health and Rights of Refugees, Asylum Seekers and Undocumented Migrants* (Ghent, Belgium: Academia, 2009).

12. Y. Joon Choi, Jennifer Elkins, and Lindsey Disney, "A Literature Review of Intimate Partner Violence among Immigrant Populations: Engaging the Faith Community," *Aggression and Violent Behavior* 29 (2016): 1–9.

13. TAMPEP, "Sex Work in Europe: A Mapping of the Prostitution Scene Europe and Central Asia. Progress Report," Amsterdam, 2009.

14. Kathleen Deering, Avni Amin, Jean Shoveller, Ariel Nesbitt, Claudia Garcia-Moreno, Putu Duff, Elena Argento, and Kate Shannon, "A Systematic Review of the Correlates of Violence against Sex Workers," *American Journal of Public Health* 104, no. 5 (2014): e42–54.

15. Lucy Platt, Pippa Grenfell, Adam Fletcher, Annik Sorhaindo, Emma Jolley, Tim Rhodes, and Chris Bonell, "Systematic Review Examining Differences in HIV, Sexually Transmitted Infections and Health-Related Harms between Migrant and Non-Migrant Female Sex Workers," *Sexually Transmitted Infections* 89, no. 4 (2013): 311–19; Sónia Dias, Ana Gama, Marta Pingarilho, Daniel Simões, and Luís Mendão, "Health Services Use and HIV Prevalence Among Migrant and National Female Sex Workers in Portugal: Are We Providing the Services Needed?," *AIDS and Behaviour* 21, no. 8 (2016): 2316–21; Sónia Dias, Ana Gama, Ricardo Fuertes, Luís Mendão, and Henrique Barros, "Risk-Taking Behaviours and HIV Infection among Sex Workers in Portugal: Results from a Cross-Sectional Survey," *Sexually Transmitted Infections* 91, no. 5 (2015): 346–52.

16. Sónia Dias, Ana Gama, Ana Maria Tavares, Vera Reigado, Daniel Simões, Emília Carreiras, Cristina Mora, and Andreia Pinto Ferreira, "Are Opportunities Being Missed? Burden of HIV, STI and TB, and Unawareness of HIV among

African Migrants," *International Journal of Environmental Research and Public Health* 16, no. 15 (2019): 2610.

17. Gry Omland, Sabine Ruths, and Esperanza Díaz, "Use of Hormonal Contraceptives among Immigrant and Native Women in Norway: Data from the Norwegian Prescription Database," *BJOG: An International Journal of Obstetrics and Gynecology* 121, no. 10 (2014): 1221–28.

18. Radilaite Cammock, Patricia Priest, Sarah Lovell, and Peter Herbison, "Awareness and Use of Family Planning Methods among ITaukei Women in Fiji and New Zealand," *Australian and New Zealand Journal of Public Health* 42, no. 4 (2018): 365–71.

19. Alyna Smith, "The Sexual and Reproductive Health Rights of Undocumented Migrants: Narrowing the Gap between Their Rights and the Reality in the EU," PICUM, 2016.

20. Ines Keygnaert, Olena Ivanova, Aurore Guieu, An-Sofie Van Parys, Els Leye, and Kristien Roelens, "What Is the Evidence on the Reduction of Inequalities in Accessibility and Quality of Maternal Health Care Delivery for Migrants? A Review of the Existing Evidence in the WHO European Region," WHO Regional Office for Europe, Copenhagen, 2016.

21. Nicola Heslehurst, Heather Brown, Augustina Pemu, Hayley Coleman, and Judith Rankin, "Perinatal Health Outcomes and Care among Asylum Seekers and Refugees: A Systematic Review of Systematic Reviews," *BMC Medicine* 16 (2018), 1–25.

22. Lígia Moreira Almeida, José Caldas, Diogo Ayres-de-Campos, Dora Salcedo-Barrientos, and Sónia Dias, "Maternal Healthcare in Migrants: A Systematic Review," *Maternal and Child Health Journal* 17 (2013): 1346–54.

23. Heslehurst et al., "Perinatal Health Outcomes."

24. Ibidun Fakoya, Débora Álvarez-del Arco, Melvina Woode-Owusu, Susana Monge, Yaiza Rivero-Montesdeoca, Valerie Delpech, Brian Rice, Teymur Noori, Anastasia Pharris, Andrew J. Amato-Gauci, Julia del Amo, and Fiona M. Burns, "A Systematic Review of Post-Migration Acquisition of HIV among Migrants from Countries with Generalised HIV Epidemics Living in Europe: Implications for Effectively Managing HIV Prevention Programmes and Policy," *BMC Public Health* 15, no. 1 (2015): 561; Sónia Dias, Ana Gama, Jasna Loos, Luis Roxo, Daniel Simões, and Christiana Nöstlinger., "The Role of Mobility in Sexual Risk Behaviour and HIV Acquisition among Sub-Saharan African Migrants Residing in Two European Cities," *PLoS ONE* 15, no. 2 (2020): 1–17.

25. Sónia Dias, Adilson Marques, Ana Gama, and Maria O Martins, "HIV Risky Sexual Behaviors and HIV Infection among Immigrants: A Cross-Sectional Study in Lisbon, Portugal," *International Journal of Environmental Research and Public Health* 11, no. 8 (2014): 8552–66.

26. Keygnaert et al., *Sexual and Reproductive Health.*

27. Marian Knight, Jennifer J. Kurinczuk, Patsy Spark, and Peter Brocklehurst, "Inequalities in Maternal Health: National Cohort Study of Ethnic Variation in

Severe Maternal Morbidities," *BMJ* 338 (2009): b542; Almeida et al., "Maternal Healthcare in Migrants."

28. Aldo Rosano, Marie Dauvrin, Sandra C. Buttigieg, Elena Ronda, Jean Tafforeau, and Sonia Dias, "Migrant's Access to Preventive Health Services in Five EU Countries," *BMC Health Services Research* 17, no. 1 (2017): 1–11; Mariana Nunes, Andreia Leite, and Sónia Dias, "Inequalities in Adherence to Cervical Cancer Screening in Portugal," *European Journal of Cancer Prevention: The Official Journal of the European Cancer Prevention Organization (ECP)*, 2020.

29. Dias et al., "Health Services Use."

30. Birgitta Essén, Veronica Costea, Luce Mosselmans, and Talia Salzmann, "Improving the Health Care of Pregnant Refugee and Migrant Women and Newborn Children: Technical Guidance on Refugee and Migrant Health," WHO Regional Office for Europe, Copenhagen, 2018.

31. Sónia Dias, Ana Gama, and Cristianne Rocha, "Immigrant Women's Perceptions and Experiences of Health Care Services: Insights from a Focus Group Study," *Journal of Public Health* 18, no. 5 (2010): 489–96.

32. Zelalem Mengesha, Janette Perz, Tinashe Dune, and Jane Ussher, "Challenges in the Provision of Sexual and Reproductive Health Care to Refugee and Migrant Women: A Q Methodological Study of Health Professional Perspectives," *Journal of Immigrant and Minority Health* 20, no. 2 (2018): 307–16.

33. Patrícia Marques, Mariana Nunes, Maria da Luz Antunes, Bruno Heleno, and Sónia Dias, "Factors Associated with Cervical Cancer Screening Participation among Migrant Women in Europe: A Scoping Review," *International Journal for Equity in Health* 19, no. 1 (2020): 1–15.

34. Birgitta Essén et al., "Improving the Health Care of Pregnant Refugee and Migrant Women and Newborn Children: Technical Guidance on Refugee and Migrant Health," WHO Regional Office for Europe, Copenhagen, 2018.

35. Smith, "The Sexual and Reproductive Health Rights of Undocumented Migrants."

36. Keygnaert et al., *Sexual and Reproductive Health.*

37. Alba González-Timoneda, Vicente Ruiz Ros, Marta González-Timoneda, and Antonio Cano Sánchez, "Knowledge, Attitudes and Practices of Primary Healthcare Professionals to Female Genital Mutilation in Valencia, Spain: Are We Ready for This Challenge?," *BMC Health Services Research* 18, no. 1 (2018): 579.

38. Martine Collumbien, Joanne Busza, John G Cleland, Oöna Campbell, World Health Organization, and UNDP/UNFPA/WHO/World Bank Special Programme of Research, Development and Research Training in Human Reproduction, "Social Science Methods for Research on Sexual and Reproductive Health," WHO, 2012.

39. Sónia Dias, Ana Gama, Daniel Simões, and Luís Mendão, "Implementation Process and Impacts of a Participatory HIV Research Project with Key Populations," *BioMed Research International* 2018 (2018).

Chapter 14

1. UNHCR, the UN Refugee Agency, "Global Trends Forced Displacement in 2019," 2019.

2. UNHCR, the UN Refugee Agency, "What Is a Refugee?," 2020, https://www.unrefugees.org/refugee-facts/what-is-a-refugee/.

3. UNHCR, "Global Trends."

4. UNHCR, the UN Refugee Agency.

5. UNHCR, the UN Refugee Agency; Sarah Opitz-Stapleton et al., "Climate Change, Migration and Displacement: The Need for a Risk-Informed and Coherent Approach," *ODI*, 2017, https://www.odi.org/publications/10977-climate-change -migration-and-displacement-need-risk-informed-and-coherent-approach; Ashwini Virgincar, Shannon Doherty, and Chesmal Siriwardhana, "The Impact of Forced Migration on the Mental Health of the Elderly: A Scoping Review," *International Psychogeriatrics* 28, no. 6 (2016): 889–96, https://doi.org/10.1017/S1041610216000193; Michaela Hynie, "The Social Determinants of Refugee Mental Health in the Post-Migration Context: A Critical Review," *Canadian Journal of Psychiatry* 63, no. 5 (2017), https://journals.sagepub.com/doi/10.1177/0706743717746666; Wai Kai Hou, Huinan Liu, Li Liang, Jeffery Ho, Hyojin Kim, Eunice Seong, George A. Bonanno, Stevan E. Hobfoll, and Brian J. Hall, "Everyday Life Experiences and Mental Health among Conflict-Affected Forced Migrants: A Meta-Analysis," *Journal of Affective Disorders* 264 (March 1, 2020): 50–68, https://doi.org/10.1016/j.jad.2019 .11.165; Martha von Werthern, Georgios Grigorakis, and Eileen Vizard, "The Mental Health and Wellbeing of Unaccompanied Refugee Minors (URMs)," *Child Abuse and Neglect* 98 (December 1, 2019): 104146, https://doi.org/10.1016/j.chiabu .2019.104146; Tarissa Mitchell, Michelle Weinberg, Drew L. Posey, and Martin Cetron, "Immigrant and Refugee Health: A Centers for Disease Control and Prevention Perspective on Protecting the Health and Health Security of Individuals and Communities during Planned Migrations," *Pediatric Clinics of North America* 66, no. 3 (2019): 549–60, https://doi.org/10.1016/j.pcl.2019.02.004.

6. David Keen, *Complex Emergencies*, vol. 21 (Cambridge, UK: Polity, 2008).

7. UNHCR, "Global Trends."

8. United Nations Development Programme, "Human Development Report 2019," 2019.

9. Martin Müller, Dana Khamis, David Srivastava, Aristomenis K. Exadaktylos, and Carmen Andrea Pfortmueller, "Understanding Refugees' Health," *Seminars in Neurology* 38, no. 2 (2018): 152–62, https://doi.org/10.1055/s-0038-1649337; World Health Organization, "World Health Statistics 2020: Monitoring Health for the SDGs, Sustainable Development Goals," 2020.

10. United Nations, "Refugees and Migrants with Disabilities," 2020, https://www .un.org/development/desa/disabilities/refugees_migrants_with_disabilities.html.

11. Women's Refugee Commission, "Refugees with Disabilities Fact Sheet," 2014, https://www.womensrefugeecommission.org/disabilities/disabilities-fact-sheet; World

Health Organization, "Disability and Health," 2015, http://www.who.int/mediacen tre/factsheets/fs352/en; Human Rights Watch, "Leave No One Behind," May 19, 2016, https://www.hrw.org/news/2016/05/19/leave-no-one-behind.

12. Human Rights Watch, "Leave No One Behind."

13. Jovana Arsenijević, Erin Schillberg, Aurelie Ponthieu, Lucio Malvisi, Waeil A. Elrahman Ahmed, Stefano Argenziano, Federica Zamatto, Simon Burroughs, Natalie Severy, Christophe Hebting, Brice de Vingne, Anthony D. Harries, and Rony Zachariah, "A Crisis of Protection and Safe Passage: Violence Experienced by Migrants/Refugees Travelling along the Western Balkan Corridor to Northern Europe," *Conflict and Health* 11, no. 1 (April 16, 2017): 6, https://doi.org/10.1186/s130 31-017-0107-z.

14. Müller et al., "Understanding Refugees' Health"; Arsenijević et al., "A Crisis of Protection and Safe Passage."

15. Arsenijević et al., "A Crisis of Protection and Safe Passage"; Müller et al., "Understanding Refugees' Health."

16. Caterina La Cascia, Giulia Cossu, Jutta Lindert, Anita Holzinger, Thurayya Zreik, Antonio Ventriglio, and Dinesh Bhugra, "Migrant Women-Experiences from the Mediterranean Region," *Clinical Practice and Epidemiology in Mental Health* 16, no. 1 (July 30, 2020): 101–8, https://doi.org/10.2174/1745017902016010101; UNICEF, "A Deadly Journey for Children: The Central Mediterranean Migration Route," Child Alert, February 2017, https://www.unicef.org/publications/files/EN_UNICEF _Central_Mediterranean_Migration.pdf; Amnesty International, "Female Refugees Face Physical Assault, Exploitation and Sexual Harassment on Their Journey through Europe," January 18, 2016.

17. La Cascia et al., "Migrant Women-Experiences from the Mediterranean Region"; Amnesty International, "Lives Adrift: Refugees and Migrants at Peril in the Central Mediterranean," September 30, 2014; Mauro Giovanni Carta, Maria Francesca Moro, and Judith Bass, "War Traumas in the Mediterranean Area," *International Journal of Social Psychiatry* 61, no. 1 (February 2015): 33–38, https://doi .org/10.1177/0020764014535754.

18. UNHCR, "Global Trends."

19. UNHCR, the UN Refugee Agency.

20. UNHCR, the UN Refugee Agency.

21. UNHCR, the UN Refugee Agency; David Miliband and Mesfin Teklu Tessema, "The Unmet Needs of Refugees and Internally Displaced People," *Lancet* 392, no. 10164 (December 5, 2018): 2530–32, https://doi.org/10.1016/S0140-6736(18) 32780-6.

22. Lindsay Stark and Alastair Ager, "A Systematic Review of Prevalence Studies of Gender-Based Violence in Complex Emergencies," *Trauma, Violence and Abuse* 12, no. 3 (July 2011): 127–34, https://doi.org/10.1177/1524838011404252; S. R. Meyer et al., "Latent Class Analysis of Violence against Adolescents and Psychosocial Outcomes in Refugee Settings in Uganda and Rwanda," *Global Mental Health* 4 (October 16, 2017), https://doi.org/10.1017/gmh.2017.17.

23. UNHCR, "Global Trends."

24. Alastair Ager, Courtney Blake, Lindsay Stark, and Tsufit Daniel, "Child Protection Assessment in Humanitarian Emergencies: Case Studies from Georgia, Gaza, Haiti and Yemen," *Child Abuse and Neglect*, Convention on the Rights of the Child Special Issue 35, no. 12 (December 1, 2011): 1045–52, https://doi.org/10.1016/j.chiabu.2011.08.004; Sabrina Hermosilla, Janna Metzler, Kevin Savage, Miriam Musa, and Alastair Ager, "Child Friendly Spaces Impact across Five Humanitarian Settings: A Meta-Analysis," *BMC Public Health* 19, no. 1 (2019): 1–11.

25. Alliance for Child Protection in Humanitarian Action, "Minimum Standards for Child Protection in Humanitarian Action," 2019, https://alliancecpha.org/en/CPMS_home.

26. UNICEF, "Emergency Mine Risk Education Toolkit: Emergency MRE Handbook," 2008; Alliance for Child Protection in Humanitarian Action, "Minimum Standards for Child Protection."

27. UNHCR, "Global Trends."

28. UNHCR, "Protracted Refugee Situations Explained," accessed September 5, 2020, https://www.unrefugees.org/news/protracted-refugee-situations-explained/.

29. Sarah R. Meyer, Gary Yu, Sabrina Hermosilla, and Lindsay Stark, "Latent Class Analysis of Violence"; Hermosilla et al., "Child Friendly Spaces"; C. Panter-Brick, Rana Dajani, Mark Eggerman, Sabrina Hermosilla, Amelia Sancilio, and Alastair Ager, "Insecurity, Distress and Mental Health: Experimental and Randomized Controlled Trials of a Psychosocial Intervention for Youth Affected by the Syrian Crisis," *Journal of Child Psychology and Psychiatry* (October 2, 2017), https://doi.org/10.1111/jcpp.12832; Fiona Charlson, Mark van Ommeren, Abraham Flaxman, Joseph Cornett, Harvey Whiteford, and Shekhar Saxena, "New WHO Prevalence Estimates of Mental Disorders in Conflict Settings: A Systematic Review and Meta-Analysis," *Lancet* 394, no. 10194 (July 20, 2019): 240–48, https://doi.org/10.1016/S0140-6736(19)30934-1.

30. United Nations, "Refugees and Migrants with Disabilities."

31. UNHCR, "Global Trends."

32. Mina Fazel, Ruth V Reed, Chatherine Panter-Brick, and Alan Stein, "Mental Health of Displaced and Refugee Children Resettled in High-Income Countries: Risk and Protective Factors," *Lancet* 379, no. 9812 (January 21, 2012): 266–82, https://doi.org/10.1016/S0140-6736(11)60051-2; Hynie, "The Social Determinants of Refugee Mental Health"; B. Heidi Ellis, Emily W. Lankau Trong Ao, Molly A. Benson, Alisa B. Miller, Sharmila Shetty, Barbara Lopes Cardozo, Paul L. Geltman, and Jennifer Cochran, "Understanding Bhutanese Refugee Suicide Through the Interpersonal-Psychological Theory of Suicidal Behavior," *American Journal of Orthopsychiatry* 85, no. 1 (January 2015): 43–55, https://doi.org/10.1037/ort0000028.

33. Ellis et al., "Understanding Bhutanese Refugee Suicide"; Jonah Meyerhoff, Kelly J. Rohan, and Karen M. Fondacaro, "Suicide and Suicide-Related Behavior

among Bhutanese Refugees Resettled in the United States," *Asian American Journal of Psychology* 9, no. 4 (December 2018): 270–83, https://doi.org/10.1037/aap0000125.

34. Ellis et al., "Understanding Bhutanese Refugee Suicide."

35. J. Schlecht et al., *Community Preparedness: Reproductive Health and Gender* (New York: Women's Refugee Commission, 2015).

36. Stephanie Leutert, "Migrant Protection Protocols: Implementation and Consequences for Asylum Seekers in Mexico, PRP 218," LBJ School of Public Affairs, 2020.

37. T. Brofft, "Migrant and Refugee Caravans: Failed Responses to Women and Children in Need of International Protection and Humanitarian Aid," 2019, https://s33660.pcdn.co/wp-content/uploads/2020/04/Migrant-and-Refugee-Caravans-Failed-Responses-to-Women-Children-in-Need-of-International-Protection-Humanitarian-Aid.pdf.

38. Women's Refugee Commission, "Statement from the Women's Refugee Commission on the Election of Joseph R. Biden, Jr., as the 46th President of the United States," 2020, https://www.womensrefugeecommission.org/press-releases/election-of-joseph-biden-as-46th-president-of-united-states/.

39. Hermosilla et al., "Child Friendly Spaces"; Ager et al., "Child Protection Assessment"; Alliance for Child Protection in Humanitarian Action, "Minimum Standards for Child Protection."

40. J. Leigh Prativa Baral, Alexa Edmier, Janna Metzler, Courtland Robinson, Thakshayeni Skanthakumar, Kate Paik, and Katherine Gambir, "Child Marriage in Humanitarian Settings in South Asia: Study Results from Bangladesh and Nepal," UNFPA APRO and UNICEF ROSA, 2020, https://reliefweb.int/report/bangladesh/child-marriage-humanitarian-settings-south-asia-study-results-bangladesh-and-nepal; K. Hunersen, W. C. Robinson, N. Krishnapalan, and J. Metzler, "Child Marriage in Humanitarian Settings in the Arab States Region: Study Results from Djibouti, Egypt, Kurdistan Region of Iraq, and Yemen," Women's Refugee Commission, 2020; Lindsay Stark et al., "Effects of a Social Empowerment Intervention on Economic Vulnerability for Adolescent Refugee Girls in Ethiopia," *Journal of Adolescent Health, Economic Strengthening and Adolescent Health* 62, no. 1 (January 1, 2018): S15–20, https://doi.org/10.1016/j.jadohealth.2017.06.014; Ann M. Starrs et al., "Accelerate Progress—Sexual and Reproductive Health and Rights for All: Report of the Guttmacher–Lancet Commission," *Lancet* 391, no. 10140 (June 30, 2018): 2642–92, https://doi.org/10.1016/S0140-6736(18)30293-9.

41. United Nations High Commissioner for Refugees, "Afghan Sports Coach Helps Young Refugees Find a Path to School in Iran," UNHCR, accessed November 8, 2020, https://www.unhcr.org/news/stories/2020/9/5f61e9504/afghan-sports-coach-helps-young-refugees-find-path-school-iran.html.

42. The Center, "History of The Center, Resettling Refugees Since 1981," accessed November 8, 2020, https://www.thecenterutica.org/about/our-history/.

Chapter 15

1. C. M. Law and A. M. Warnes, "The Movement of Retired People to Seaside Resorts: A Study of Morecambe and Llandudno," *Town Planning Review* 44, no. 4 (1973): 373–90.

2. Russell King, Tony Warnes, and Allan Williams, *Sunset Lives: British Retirement to the Mediterranean* (Oxford: Berg, 2000). The study was funded by the UK Economic and Social Research Council.

3. Anthony Warnes, Klaus Friedrich, Leonie Kellaher, and Sandra Torres, "The Diversity of Older Migrants in Europe," *Ageing and Society* 24, no. 3 (2004): 307–26.

4. Maria Angele Casado-Díaz, Claudia Kaiser, and Anthony M. Warnes, "Northern European Retired Residents in Eight Southern European Areas: Characteristics, Motivations and Adjustment," *Ageing and Society* 24, no. 3 (2004): 353–81.

5. World Health Organization (WHO), "Migration and Health," accessed December 7, 2021, https://www.euro.who.int/en/health-topics/health-determinants/migration-and-health.

6. Michel Poulain, Nicolas Perrin, and Ann Singleton, *Towards Harmonised European Statistics on International Migration* (Louvain-la-Neuve, Belgium: Presses Universitaires de Louvain, 2006).

7. Veronica Montes de Oca, Telésforo Ramírez García, Rogelio Sáenz, and Jennifer Guillén, "The Linkage of Life Course, Migration, Health, and Aging: Health in Adults and Elderly Mexican Migrants," *Journal of Aging and Health* 23, no. 7 (2011): 1116–40.

8. A. Rogers and J. Watkins, "General versus Elderly Interstate Migration and Population Redistribution in the United States," *Research on Aging* 9, no. 4 (1987), 483–529.

9. Charles F. Longino, Don E. Bradley, Eleanor P. Stoller, and William H. Haas III, "Predictors of Non-Local Moves among Older Adults: A Prospective Study," *Journal of Gerontology: Social Sciences* 63B, no. 1 (2008): S7–S14.

10. Four academic journals feature migration studies: *International Migration Review*, *Migration Letters*, *International Migration*, and *Journal of Ethnic and Migration Studies*.

11. A. M. Warnes, "International Retirement Migration," In *International Handbook of Population Aging*, edited by P. Uhlenberg (New York: Springer Science, 2009): 341–63.

12. L. Ackers and P. Dwyer, *Senior Citizenship? Retirement, Migration and Welfare in the European Union* (Bristol, UK: Policy, 2002).

13. Irene Hardill, Jacqui Spradbery, Judy Arnold-Boakes, and Maria Luisa Arruga, "Severe Health and Social Care Issues among British Migrants Who Retire to Spain," *Ageing and Society* 25, no. 5 (2005): 769–84.

14. Maria Evandrou, Jane Falkingham, and Marcus Green, "ISER, British Household Panel Survey," accessed December 7, 2021, https://www.iser.essex.ac.uk/bhps/.

15. K. Conway and J. Rork, "The Changing Roles of Disability, Veteran and Socioeconomic Status in Elderly Interstate Migration," *Research on Aging* 33, no. 3 (2011): 256–85.

16. F. Bastian, "Defoe's *Journal of the Plague Year* reconsidered," *Review of English Studies* 16, no. 62 (1965): 151–73.

Chapter 16

1. Masten, A. S. 2014. "Global Perspectives on Resilience in Children and Youth." *Child Dev* 85, no. 1: 6–20. https://doi.org/10.1111/cdev.12205.

2. United Nations. 1989. "Convention on the Rights of the Child."

3. UNICEF. 2021. "Child Migration" (April). Accessed January 15, 2022. https://data.unicef.org/topic/child-migration-and-displacement/migration/.

4. UNHCR. 2020. *Global Trends: Forced Displacement in 2019* (June 18). https://www.unhcr.org/uk/statistics/unhcrstats/5ee200e37/unhcr-global-trends-2019.html; UNHCR. 2021. *Global Trends: Forced Displacement in 2020* (June 18). https://www.unhcr.org/60b638e37/unhcr-global-trends-2020.

5. Fellmeth, Gracia, et al. 2018. "Health Impacts of Parental Migration on Left-Behind Children and Adolescents: A Systematic Review and Meta-Analysis." *Lancet* 392, no. 10164: 2567–82. https://doi.org/10.1016/S0140-6736(18)32558-3.

6. Tong, Lian, et al. 2019. "The Factors Associated with Being Left-Behind Children in China: Multilevel Analysis with Nationally Representative Data." *PLoS One* 14, no. 11: e0224205. https://doi.org/10.1371/journal.pone.0224205.

7. ISSOP Migration Working Group. 2017. "ISSOP Position Statement on Migrant Child Health." *Child Care Health Dev* 44, no. 1: 161–70. https://doi.org/10.1111/cch.12485.

8. Hughes, K., et al. 2017. "The Effect of Multiple Adverse Childhood Experiences on Health: A Systematic Review and Meta-Analysis." *Lancet Public Health* 2, no. 8: e356–66. https://doi.org/10.1016/s2468-2667(17)30118-4.

9. UNICEF, "Child Migration."

10. UNHCR, *Global Trends*.

11. Kadir, A., et al. 2019. "Children on the Move in Europe: A Narrative Review of the Evidence on the Health Risks, Health Needs and Health Policy for Asylum Seeking, Refugee and Undocumented Children." *BMJ Paediatr Open* 3, no. 1. https://doi.org/10.1136/bmjpo-2018-000364.

12. Kadir et al., "Children on the Move in Europe."

13. ISSOP, "ISSOP Position Statement."

14. Kadir et al., "Children on the Move in Europe."

15. International Organization for Migration (IOM). 2020. "Missing Migrants: Tracking Deaths Along Migratory Routes." Accessed October 3, 2020. https://missingmigrants.iom.int/.

16. Hjern, Anders, and Ayesha Kadir. 2018. *Health of Refugee and Migrant Children.* WHO Regional Office for Europe (Copenhagen).

17. ISSOP, "ISSOP Position Statement."

18. Kadir et al., "Children on the Move in Europe."

19. Baauw, A., et al. 2019. "Health Needs of Refugee Children Identified on Arrival in Reception Countries: A Systematic Review and Meta-Analysis." *BMJ Paediatr Open* 3, no. 1: e000516. https://doi.org/10.1136/bmjpo-2019-000516.

20. Kadir et al., "Children on the Move in Europe."

21. ISSOP, "ISSOP Position Statement."

22. Kadir et al., "Children on the Move in Europe."

23. Hjern and Kadir, *Health of Refugee and Migrant Children.*

24. Kadir et al., "Children on the Move in Europe."

25. ISSOP, "ISSOP Position Statement."

26. ISSOP, "ISSOP Position Statement."

27. Bryant, R. A., et al. 2018. "The Effect of Post-Traumatic Stress Disorder on Refugees' Parenting and Their Children's Mental Health: A Cohort Study." *Lancet Public Health* 3, no. 5: e249–58. https://doi.org/10.1016/s2468-2667(18)30051-3.

28. LeBrun, Annie, et al. 2015. "Review of Child Maltreatment in Immigrant and Refugee Families." *Canadian Journal of Public Health* 106, no. 7: eS45–56. https://doi.org/10.17269/CJPH.106.4838.

29. ISSOP, "ISSOP Position Statement."

30. Hughes et al., "The Effect of Multiple Adverse Childhood Experiences on Health."

31. Bryant et al., "The Effect of Post-Traumatic Stress Disorder on Refugees' Parenting."

32. Sara, Grant, and Peter Brann. 2018. "Understanding the Mechanisms of Trans-generational Mental Health Impacts in Refugees." *Lancet Public Health* 3, no. 5: e211–12. https://doi.org/10.1016/S2468-2667(18)30067-7.

33. Fazel, M., et al. 2012. "Mental Health of Displaced and Refugee Children Resettled in High-Income Countries: Risk and Protective Factors." *Lancet* 379, no. 9812: 266–82. https://doi.org/10.1016/s0140-6736(11)60051-2.

34. Hjern and Kadir, *Health of Refugee and Migrant Children.*

35. Montgomery, E. 2011. "Trauma, Exile and Mental Health in Young Refugees." *Acta Psychiatrica Scandinavica* 124, no. s440: 1–46. https://doi.org/10.1111/j.1600-0447.2011.01740.x.

36. UNHCR, *Global Trends.*

37. Eurostat. 2018. "Asylum Statistics Explained." http://ec.europa.eu/eurostat/statistics-explained/index.php/Asylum_statistics.

38. Eide, Ketil, and Anders Hjern. 2013. "Unaccompanied Refugee Children—Vulnerability and Agency." *Acta Paediatrica, International Journal of Paediatrics* 102: 666–68. https://doi.org/10.1111/apa.12258.

39. Eide and Hjern, "Unaccompanied Refugee Children."

40. Eide and Hjern, "Unaccompanied Refugee Children."

41. Eide and Hjern, "Unaccompanied Refugee Children."

42. Jensen, T. K., et al. 2014. "Development of Mental Health Problems—A Follow-Up Study of Unaccompanied Refugee Minors." *Child Adolesc Psychiatry Ment Health* 8: 29. https://doi.org/10.1186/1753-2000-8-29.

43. Aynsley-Green, A., et al. 2012. "Medical, Statistical, Ethical and Human Rights Considerations in the Assessment of Age in Children and Young People Subject to Immigration Control." *Br Med Bull* 102: 17–42. https://doi.org/10.1093/bmb/lds014.

44. Cole, T. J. 2015. "The Evidential Value of Developmental Age Imaging for Assessing Age of Majority." *Ann Hum Biol* 42, no. 4: 379–88. https://doi.org/10.3109/03014460.2015.1031826.

45. European Asylum Support Office. 2018. *Age Assessment Practice in Europe*, 2nd ed. European Asylum Support Office. https://www.easo.europa.eu/sites/default/files/public/EASO-Age-assessment-practice-in-Europe1.pdf.

46. United Nations, "Convention on the Rights of the Child."

47. Masten, "Global Perspectives."

48. Fazel et al., "Mental Health of Displaced and Refugee Children."

49. ISSOP, "ISSOP Position Statement."

50. Fazel et al., "Mental Health of Displaced and Refugee Children."

51. Fazel et al., "Mental Health of Displaced and Refugee Children."

52. Kadir, A., et al. 2019. "Effects of Armed Conflict on Child Health and Development: A Systematic Review." *PLoS One* 14, no. 1: e0210071. https://doi.org/10.1371/journal.pone.0210071.

53. ISSOP, "ISSOP Position Statement."

54. ISSOP, "ISSOP Position Statement."

Chapter 17

1. International Organization for Migration (IOM). *World Migration Report 2020.* 2020.

2. United Nations Department of Economic and Social Affairs, Population Division. "International Migrant Stock 2019." https://www.un.org/en/development/desa/population/migration/data/estimates2/docs/MigrationStockDocumentation_2019.pdf.

3. Jud, A., E. Pfeiffer, and M. Jarczok. "Epidemiology of Violence against Children in Migration: A Systematic Literature Review." *Child Abuse and Neglect* 108 (October 2020): 104634. https://doi.org/10.1016/j.chiabu.2020.104634.

4. Chandan, J. S. "Improving Global Surveillance of Gender-Based Violence." *Lancet* 396, no. 10262 (2020): 1562. https://doi.org/10.1016/S0140-6736(20)32319-9.

5. World Health Organization (WHO). *World Report on Violence and Health.* 2002.

6. WHO. "Constitution of the World Health Organization." *American Journal of Public Health* 36, no. 11 (1946): 1315–23. https://doi.org/10.2105/ajph.36.11.1315.

7. Bronfenbrenner, U. "Ecological Systems Theory." In *Six Theories of Child Development: Revised Formulations and Current Issues*, edited by R. Vasta, 187–249. London: Jessica Kingsley Publishers, 1992.

8. Jiménez-Lasserrotte, M. D. M., E. López-Domene, J. M. Hernández-Padilla, I. M. Fernández-Medina, and J. Granero-Molina. "Understanding Violence against Women Irregular Migrants Who Arrive in Spain in Small Boats." *Healthcare* 8, no. 3 (2020): 299.

9. Bouhenia, M., J. B. Farhat, M. E. Coldiron, S. Abdallah, D. Visentin, M. Neuman, M. Berthelot, K. Porten, and S. Cohuet. "Quantitative Survey on Health and Violence Endured by Refugees during Their Journey and in Calais, France." *International Health* 9, no. 6 (2017): 335–42. https://doi.org/10.1093/inthealth/ihx040.

10. Timshel, I., E. Montgomery, and N. T. Dalgaard. "A Systematic Review of Risk and Protective Factors Associated with Family Related Violence in Refugee Families." *Child Abuse and Neglect* 70 (August 2017): 315–30. https://doi.org/10.1016/j.chiabu.2017.06.023.

11. Cook, T. L., P. J. Shannon, G. A. Vinson, J. P. Letts, and E. Dwee. "War Trauma and Torture Experiences Reported during Public Health Screening of Newly Resettled Karen Refugees: A Qualitative Study." *BMC International Health and Human Rights* 15, no. 1 (April 8, 2015): 8. https://doi.org/10.1186/s12914-015-0046-y.

12. Brown, C. "Rape as a Weapon of War in the Democratic Republic of the Congo." *Torture* 22, no. 1 (2012): 24–37.

13. Deps, P., S. M. Collin, H. P. Aborghetti, and P. Charlier. "Evidence of Physical Violence and Torture in Refugees and Migrants Seeking Asylum in France." *Journal of Forensic and Legal Medicine* 77 (December 13, 2020): 102104. https://doi.org/10.1016/j.jflm.2020.102104.

14. Ba, I., and R. S. Bhopal. "Physical, Mental and Social Consequences in Civilians Who Have Experienced War-Related Sexual Violence: A Systematic Review (1981–2014)." *Public Health* 142 (January 1, 2017): 121–35. https://doi.org/10.1016/j.puhe.2016.07.019.

15. Ainamani, H. E., T. Elbert, D. K. Olema, and T. Hecker. "Gender Differences in Response to War-Related Trauma and Posttraumatic Stress Disorder—A Study among the Congolese Refugees in Uganda." *BMC Psychiatry* 20, no. 1 (January 10, 2020): 17. https://doi.org/10.1186/s12888-019-2420-0.

16. Tausch, A. "Multivariate Analyses of the Global Acceptability Rates of Male Intimate Partner Violence (IPV) against Women Based on World Values Survey Data." *International Journal of Health Planning and Management* 34, no. 4 (2019): 1155–94. https://doi.org/10.1002/hpm.2781.

17. Elghossain, T., S. Bott, C. Akik, and C. M. Obermeyer. "Prevalence of Intimate Partner Violence against Women in the Arab World: A Systematic Review." *BMC International Health and Human Rights* 19, no. 1 (October 22, 2019): 29. https://doi.org/10.1186/s12914-019-0215-5.

18. Ellsberg, M., J. Ovince, M. Murphy, A. Blackwell, D. Reddy, J. Stennes, T. Hess, and M. Contreras. "No Safe Place: Prevalence and Correlates of Violence against Conflict-Affected Women and Girls in South Sudan." *PLoS One* 15, no. 10 (2020): e0237965. https://doi.org/10.1371/journal.pone.0237965.

19. Stark, L., K. Asghar, G. Yu, C. Bora, A. A. Baysa, and K. L. Falb. "Prevalence and Associated Risk Factors of Violence against Conflict-Affected Female Adolescents: A Multi-Country, Cross-Sectional Study." *Journal of Global Health* 7, no. 1 (June 2017): 010416. https://doi.org/10.7189/jogh.07.010416.

20. Moody, G., R. Cannings-John, K. Hood, A. Kemp, and M. Robling. "Establishing the International Prevalence of Self-Reported Child Maltreatment: A Systematic Review by Maltreatment Type and Gender." *BMC Public Health* 18, no. 1 (October 10, 2018): 1164. https://doi.org/10.1186/s12889-018-6044-y.

21. Lindert, J., O. S. von Ehrenstein, R. Grashow, G. Gal, E. Braehler, and M. G. Weisskopf. "Sexual and Physical Abuse in Childhood Is Associated with Depression and Anxiety over the Life Course: Systematic Review and Meta-Analysis." *International Journal of Public Health* 59, no. 2 (April 2014): 359–72. https://doi.org/10.1007/s00038-013-0519-5.

22. Moody et al., "Establishing the International Prevalence."

23. Devries, K. M., J. Y. Mak, C. Garcia-Moreno, M. Petzold, J. C. Child, G. Falder, S. Lim, L. J. Bacchus, R. E. Engell, and C. H. Watts. "Global Health: The Global Prevalence of Intimate Partner Violence against Women." *Science* 340, no. 6140 (June 28, 2013): 1527–28. https://doi.org/10.1126/science.1240937.

24. Infante, C., A. J. Idrovo, M. S. Sánchez-Domínguez, S. Vinhas, and T. González-Vázquez. "Violence Committed Against Migrants in Transit: Experiences on the Northern Mexican Border." *Journal of Immigrant and Minority Health* 14, no. 3 (June 1, 2012): 449–59. https://doi.org/10.1007/s10903-011-9489-y.

25. Borumandnia, N., N. Khadembashi, M. Tabatabaei, and H. Alavi Majd. "The Prevalence Rate of Sexual Violence Worldwide: A Trend Analysis." *BMC Public Health* 20, no. 1 (November 30, 2020): 1835. https://doi.org/10.1186/s12889-020-09926-5.

26. Chynoweth, S. K., D. Buscher, S. Martin, and A. B. Zwi. "Characteristics and Impacts of Sexual Violence against Men and Boys in Conflict and Displacement: A Multicountry Exploratory Study." *Journal of Interpersonal Violence* (October 2020). https://doi.org/10.1177/0886260520967132.

27. De Schrijver, L., T. Vander Beken, B. Krahé, and I. Keygnaert. "Prevalence of Sexual Violence in Migrants, Applicants for International Protection, and Refugees in Europe: A Critical Interpretive Synthesis of the Evidence." *International Journal of Environmental Research and Public Health* 15, no. 9 (2018): 1979.

28. Reques, L., E. Aranda-Fernandez, C. Rolland, A. Grippon, N. Fallet, C. Reboul, N. Godard, and N. Luhmann. "Episodes of Violence Suffered by Migrants Transiting through Libya: A Cross-Sectional Study in 'Medecins du Monde's' Reception and Healthcare Centre in Seine-Saint-Denis, France." *Conflict and Health* 14 (2020): 12. https://doi.org/10.1186/s13031-020-0256-3.

29. Ottisova, L., P. Smith, and S. Oram. "Psychological Consequences of Human Trafficking: Complex Posttraumatic Stress Disorder in Trafficked Children." *Behavioral Medicine* 44, no. 3 (July 3, 2018): 234–41. https://doi.org/10.1080/08964 289.2018.1432555.

30. Gezie, L. D., A. Worku, Y. Kebede, and A. Gebeyehu. "Sexual Violence at Each Stage of Human Trafficking Cycle and Associated Factors: A Retrospective Cohort Study on Ethiopian Female Returnees via Three Major Trafficking Corridors." *BMJ Open* 9, no. 7 (2019): e024515. https://doi.org/10.1136/bmjopen-2018 -024515.

31. Beiser, M., F. Hou, I. Hyman, and M. Tousignant. "Poverty, Family Process, and the Mental Health of Immigrant Children in Canada." *American Journal of Public Health* 92, no. 2 (2002): 220–27. https://doi.org/10.2105/ajph.92.2.220.

32. WHO, "Constitution."

33. Abubakar, I., R. W. Aldridge, D. Devakumar, M. Orcutt, R. Burns, M. L. Narreto, P. Dhavan, M. Fouad, N. Goce, Y. Guo et al. "The UCL-Lancet Commission on Migration and Health: The Health of a World on the Move." *Lancet* 392, no. 10164 (December 15, 2018): 2606–54. https://doi.org/10.1016/S0140-6736(18)32114-7.

34. Bogic, M., A. Njoku, and S. Priebe. "Long-Term Mental Health of War-Refugees: A Systematic Literature Review." *BMC International Health and Human Rights* 15, no. 1 (October 28, 2015): 29. https://doi.org/10.1186/s12914-015-0064-9.

35. Lindert, J., M. G. Carta, I. Schäfer, and R. F. Mollica. "Refugees Mental Health—A Public Mental Health Challenge." *European Journal of Public Health* 26, no. 3 (2016): 374–75. https://doi.org/10.1093/eurpub/ckw010.

36. Amone-P'Olak, K., and B. Omech. "Coping with Post-War Mental Health Problems among Survivors of Violence in Northern Uganda: Findings from the WAYS Study." *Journal of Health Psychology* 25, no. 12 (2020): 1857–70. https://doi .org/10.1177/1359105318775185.

37. Bogic, M., A. Njolu, and S. Priebe. "Long-Term Mental Health of War Refugees: A Systematic Literature Review." *BMC International Health and Human Rights* 29 (2015).

38. Blackmore, R., J. A. Boyle, M. Fazel, S. Ranasinha, K. M Gray, G. Fitzgerald, M. Misso, and M. Gibson-Helm. "The Prevalence of Mental Illness in Refugees and Asylum Seekers: A Systematic Review and Meta-Analysis." *PLOS Medicine* 17, no. 9 (2020): e1003337. https://doi.org/10.1371/journal.pmed.1003337.

39. Curtis, P., J. Thompson, and H. Fairbrother. "Migrant Children within Europe: A Systematic Review of Children's Perspectives on Their Health Experiences." *Public Health* 158 (May 2018): 71–85. https://doi.org/10.1016/j.puhe.2018.01 .038.

40. Jud et al., "Epidemiology of Violence."

41. Wickramage, K., J. Vearey, A. B. Zwi, C. Robinson, and M. Knipper. "Migration and Health: A Global Public Health Research Priority." *BMC Public Health* 18, no. 1 (August 8, 2018): 987. https://doi.org/10.1186/s12889-018-5932-5.

Chapter 18

1. World Bank, "Resilience: Covid-19 Crisis Through a Migration Lens," *Migration and Development Brief* 34 (May 2021).

2. World Bank, "Resilience."

3. Luis Miguel Tovar Cuevas, María Teresa Victoria Paredes, Camilo Zarama, and Matheo Arellano Morales, "International Migration and Health in the Countries of Origin: The Effect on Households with Migrants and/or Recipients of Remittances, and on Returned Migrants; A Systematic Review," *Gerencia y Políticas de Salud* 18, no. 37 (November 5, 2019): 1–33, https://doi.org/10.11144/Javeriana.rgps18-37.imhc.

4. Fernando Riosmena, Reanne Frank, Ilana Redstone Akresh, and Rhiannon A. Kroeger, "U.S. Migration, Translocality, and the Acceleration of the Nutrition Transition in Mexico," *Annals of the Association of American Geographers* 102, no. 5 (September 1, 2012): 1209–18, https://doi.org/10.1080/00045608.2012.659629.

5. Reanne Frank, "International Migration and Infant Health in Mexico," *Journal of Immigrant Health* 7, no. 1 (January 1, 2005): 11–22, https://doi.org/10.1007/s10903-005-1386-9.

6. José-Ignacio Antón, "The Impact of Remittances on Nutritional Status of Children in Ecuador," *International Migration Review* 44, no. 2 (2010): 269–99.

7. T. S. Sunil, M. Flores, and G. E. Garcia, "New Evidence on the Effects of International Migration on the Risk of Low Birthweight in Mexico," *Maternal and Child Nutrition* 8, no. 2 (2012): 185–98.

8. J. L. Castillo Hernández, M. M. Álvarez Ramírez, E. Y. Romero Hernández, S. C. Cortés, R. Zenteno-Cuevas, and L. N. Berrún-Castañón, "Asociación de las remesas con el estado nutricio y la adecuación de la dieta en habitantes de la localidad El Espinal, municipio de Naolinco, Veracruz, México," *Revista Avances en Seguridad Alimentaria y Nutricional* 1, no. 1 (2009): 77–87.

9. Erin R. Hamilton and Kate H. Choi, "The Mixed Effects of Migration: Community-Level Migration and Birthweight in Mexico," *Social Science and Medicine* 132 (May 2015): 278–86, https://doi.org/10.1016/j.socscimed.2014.08.031.

10. Anne Marie Thow, Jessica Fanzo, and Joel Negin, "A Systematic Review of the Effect of Remittances on Diet and Nutrition," *Food and Nutrition Bulletin* (February 25, 2016), https://doi.org/10.1177/0379572116631651.

11. Carlo Azzarri and Alberto Zezza, "International Migration and Nutritional Outcomes in Tajikistan," *Food Policy*, 36, no. 1 (February 1, 2011): 54–70, https://doi.org/10.1016/j.foodpol.2010.11.004.

12. M. H. Böhme, R. Persian, and T. Stöhr, "Alone but Better Off? Adult Child Migration and Health of Elderly Parents in Moldova," *Journal of Health Economics* 39 (2015): 211–27.

13. Antje Kroeger and Kathryn H. Anderson, "Remittances and the Human Capital of Children: New Evidence from Kyrgyzstan during Revolution and Financial

Crisis, 2005–2009," *Journal of Comparative Economics* 42, no. 3 (August 1, 2014): 770–85, https://doi.org/10.1016/j.jce.2013.06.001.

14. Yao Lu, "Household Migration, Remittances and Their Impact on Health in Indonesia1," *International Migration* 51, no. s1 (2013): e202–15, https://doi.org/10.1111 /j.1468-2435.2012.00761.x.

15. Sophia C. Terrelonge, "For Health, Strength, and Daily Food: The Dual Impact of Remittances and Public Health Expenditure on Household Health Spending and Child Health Outcomes," *Journal of Development Studies* 50, no. 10 (October 3, 2014): 1397–1410, https://doi.org/10.1080/00220388.2014.940911.

16. Larry L. Howard and Denise L. Stanley, "Remittances Channels and the Physical Growth of Honduran Children," *International Review of Applied Economics* 31, no. 3 (November 21, 2016): 376–96.

17. Ricardo Bebczuk and Diego Battistón, "Remittances and Life Cycle Deficits in Latin America," CEDLAS, Working Papers (Universidad Nacional de La Plata, February 2010), https://ideas.repec.org/p/dls/wpaper/0094.html.

18. Alan de Brauw, "Migration and Child Development during the Food Price Crisis in El Salvador," *Food Policy* 36, no. 1 (February 1, 2011): 28–40, https://doi .org/10.1016/j.foodpol.2010.11.002.

19. Calogero Carletto, Katia Covarrubias, and John A. Maluccio, "Migration and Child Growth in Rural Guatemala," *Food Policy* 36, no. 1 (February 1, 2011): 16–27, https://doi.org/10.1016/j.foodpol.2010.08.002.

20. L. D. Acosta and I. Vizcarra-Bordi, "Desnutrición infantil en comunidades mazahuas con migración masculina internacional en México Central," *Poblac y Salud en Mesoamérica* 6, no. 2 (2009): 118.

21. Uzochukwu Amakom and Chukwunonso Gerald Iheoma, "Impact of Migrant Remittances on Health and Education Outcomes in Sub-Saharan Africa," *IOSR Journal of Humanities and Social Science* 19, no. 8 (2014): 33–44, https://doi .org/10.9790/0837-19813344.

22. Terrelonge, "For Health, Strength, and Daily Food."

23. Maria Cristina Zhunio, Sharmila Vishwasrao, and Eric P. Chiang, "The Influence of Remittances on Education and Health Outcomes: A Cross Country Study," *Applied Economics* 44, no. 35 (December 1, 2012): 4605–16, https://doi.org /10.1080/00036846.2011.593499.

24. Lisa Chauvet, Flore Gubert, and Sandrine Mesplé-Somps, "Aid, Remittances, Medical Brain Drain and Child Mortality: Evidence Using Inter and Intra-Country Data," *Journal of Development Studies* 49, no. 6 (June 1, 2013): 801–18, https://doi.org/10.1080/00220388.2012.742508.

25. Komla Amega, "Remittances, Education and Health in Sub-Saharan Africa," ed. Francesco Tajani, *Cogent Economics and Finance* 6, no. 1 (January 1, 2018): 1516488, https://doi.org/10.1080/23322039.2018.1516488.

26. Theodore P. Gerber and Karine Torosyan, "Remittances in the Republic of Georgia: Correlates, Economic Impact, and Social Capital Formation," *Demog-*

raphy 50, no. 4 (August 1, 2013): 1279–1301, https://doi.org/10.1007/s13524-013-01 95-3.

27. Awojobi Oladayo Nathaniel, "Impact of Remittances on Healthcare Utilisation and Expenditure in Developing Countries: A Systematic Review," *Rwanda Journal of Medicine and Health Sciences* 2, no. 3 (2019): 304–10, https://doi.org/10 .4314/rjmhs.v2i3.15.

28. Juan Ponce, Iliana Olivié, and Mercedes Onofa, "The Role of International Remittances in Health Outcomes in Ecuador: Prevention and Response to Shocks," *International Migration Review*, July 19, 2018, http://journals.sagepub.com/doi/10 .1111/j.1747-7379.2011.00864.x.

29. Edmundo Murrugarra, "Public Transfers and Migrants' Remittances: Evidence from the Recent Armenian Experience," vol. 2, World Bank Economists' Forum, 2002.

30. Alassane Drabo and Christian Ebeke, "Remittances, Public Health Spending and Foreign Aid in the Access to Health Care Services in Developing Countries," Etudes et Documents Du CERDI (1 Centre d'Etudes et de Recherches sur le Développement International, 2011).

31. John D. Piette et al., "Report on Honduras: Ripples in the Pond—The Financial Crisis and Remittances to Chronically ILL Patients in Honduras," *International Journal of Health Services* 42, no. 2 (April 1, 2012): 197–212, https://doi .org/10.2190/HS.42.2.c.

32. Cuong Viet Nguyen and Hoa Quynh Nguyen, "Do Internal and International Remittances Matter to Health, Education and Labor of Children and Adolescents? The Case of Vietnam," *Children and Youth Services Review* 58 (November 1, 2015): 28–34, https://doi.org/10.1016/j.childyouth.2015.09.002.

33. Shujaat Farooq and Nasir Iqbal, "Migration and Health Outcomes: The Case of a High Migration District in South Punjab" (Islamabad: Pakistan Institute Of Development Economics, 2015).

34. Catalina Amuedo-Dorantes, Tania Sainz, and Susan Pozo, "Remittances and Healthcare Expenditure Patterns of Populations in Origin Communities: Evidence from Mexico" (Buenos Aires: Inter-American Development Bank, 2007).

35. Reanne Frank et al., "The Relationship Between Remittances and Health Care Provision in Mexico," *American Journal of Public Health* 99, no. 7 (July 1, 2009): 1227–31, https://doi.org/10.2105/AJPH.2008.144980.

36. Daniel F. López-Cevallos and Chunhuei Chi, "Migration, Remittances, and Health Care Utilization in Ecuador," *Revista Panamericana de Salud Pública* 31 (January 2012): 9–16, https://doi.org/10.1590/S1020-49892012000100002.

37. Jennifer J. Salinas, "Tapping Healthcare Resource by Older Mexicans with Diabetes: How Migration to the United States Facilitates Access," *Journal of Cross-Cultural Gerontology* 23, no. 3 (September 1, 2008): 301–12, https://doi.org/10.1007 /s10823-008-9076-4.

38. Farooq and Iqbal, "Migration and Health Outcomes."

Chapter 19

1. *Merriam-Webster*, s.v. "technology," accessed October 29, 2020, https://www
.merriam-webster.com/dictionary/technology.

2. "Global Indicator Framework for the Sustainable Development Goals and
Targets of the 2030 Agenda for Sustainable Development" (New York: United Nations, 2020), https://doi.org/10.1891/9780826190123.0013.

3. Ibrahim Abubakar, Robert W, Aldridge, Devan Devakumar, Miriam Orcutt,
Rachel Burns, Mauricio L Barreto et al., "The UCL–Lancet Commission on Mi-
gration and Health: The Health of a World on the Move," *Lancet* 392, no. 10164
(December 15, 2018): 2606–54, https://doi.org/10.1016/S0140-6736(18)32114-7; Marie
McAuliffe, Binod Khadria, and International Organization for Migration, *World
Migration Report 2020* (2019), https://publications.iom.int/system/files/pdf/wmr_2020
.pdf.

4. United Nations, "The Sustainable Development Goals Report," 2020, https://
sdgs.un.org/sites/default/files/2020-09/The-Sustainable-Development-Goals-Report
-2020.pdf.

5. Meghan D. Morris, Steve T. Popper, Timothy C. Rodwell, Stephanie K. Brodine,
and Kimberly C. Brouwer, "Healthcare Barriers of Refugees Post-Resettlement,"
Journal of Community Health 34, no. 6 (December 2009): 529–38, https://doi.org
/10.1007/s10900-009-9175-3; Bertha M. N. Ochieng, "Black African Migrants: The
Barriers with Accessing and Utilizing Health Promotion Services in the UK," *European Journal of Public Health* 23, no. 2 (April 1, 2013): 265–69, https://doi.org/10
.1093/eurpub/cks063.

6. Luke Robertshaw, Surindar Dhesi, and Laura L. Jones, "Challenges and Facilitators for Health Professionals Providing Primary Healthcare for Refugees and
Asylum Seekers in High-Income Countries: A Systematic Review and Thematic
Synthesis of Qualitative Research," *BMJ Open* 7, no. 8 (August 1, 2017): e015981,
https://doi.org/10.1136/bmjopen-2017-015981; Frank Müller, Shivani Chandra, Ghe-
far Furaijat, Stefan Kruse, Alexandra Waligorski, Anne Simmenroth, and Evelyn
Kleinert, "A Digital Communication Assistance Tool (DCAT) to Obtain Medical History from Foreign-Language Patients: Development and Pilot Testing in a
Primary Health Care Center for Refugees," *International Journal of Environmental Research and Public Health* 17, no. 4 (February 2020), https://doi.org/10.3390
/ijerph17041368.

7. Tarjimly, "Tarjimly," 2019, https://tarjimly.org.

8. WHO, "Health Resources and Services Availability Monitoring System
(HeRAMS)," 2020, https://www.who.int/initiatives/herams.

9. Ghada Ballout, Najeeb Al-Shorbaji, Nada Abu-Kishk, Yassir Turki, Wafaa
Zeidan, and Akihiro Seita, "UNRWA's Innovative e-Health for 5 Million Palestine
Refugees in the Near East," *BMJ Innovations* 4, no. 3 (July 1, 2018), https://doi
.org/10.1136/bmjinnov-2017-000262.

10. United Nations High Commissioner for Refugees, "UNHCR Wins €1m Prize for Novel Water Tech in Refugee Camps," 2020, https://www.unhcr.org/news /latest/2020/9/5f6c5a424/unhcr-wins-1m-prize-novel-water-tech-refugee-camps.html.

11. United Nations High Commissioner for Refugees, "Innovation, Green Tech and Sunlight Help Secure Safe Water for Rohingya Refugees," 2019, https://www .unhcr.org/news/briefing/2019/1/5c2f239b4/innovation-green-tech-sunlight-help -secure-safe-water-rohingya-refugees.html.

12. Marija Bogic, Anthony Njoku, and Stefan Priebe, "Long-Term Mental Health of War-Refugees: A Systematic Literature Review," *BMC International Health and Human Rights* 15 (October 28, 2015): 29, https://doi.org/10.1186/s12914-015-0064-9; Adeel Ashfaq, Shawn Esmaili, Mona Najjar, Farva Batool, Tariq Mukatash, Hadeer Akram Al-Ani, and Patrick Marius Koga, "Utilization of Mobile Mental Health Services among Syrian Refugees and Other Vulnerable Arab Populations-A Systematic Review," *International Journal of Environmental Research and Public Health* 17, no. 4 (February 18, 2020), https://doi.org/10.3390/ijerph17041295; Nour El Arnaout, Spenser Rutherford, Thurayya Zreik, Dana Nabulsi, Nasser Yassin, and Shadi Saleh, "Assessment of the Health Needs of Syrian Refugees in Lebanon and Syria's Neighboring Countries," *Conflict and Health* 13, no. 1 (June 27, 2019): 31, https:// doi.org/10.1186/s13031-019-0211-3.

13. Melissa Joanne Harper Shehadeh, Jinane Abi Ramia, Pim Cuijpers, Rabih El Chammay, Eva Heim, Wissam Kheir, Khalid Saeed, Mark van Ommeren, Edith van't Hof, Sarah Watts, Andreas Wenger, Edwina Zoghbi, and Kenneth Carswell, "Step-by-Step, an E-Mental Health Intervention for Depression: A Mixed Methods Pilot Study From Lebanon," *Frontiers in Psychiatry* 10 (February 12, 2020), https://doi.org/10.3389/fpsyt.2019.00986.

14. Sebastian Burchert, Mohammed Salem Alkneme, Martha Bird, Kenneth Carswell, Pim Cuijpers, Pernille Hansen, Eva Heim, Melissa Harper Shehadeh, Marit Sijbrandij, Edith van't Hof, and Christine Knaevelsrud, "User-Centered App Adaptation of a Low-Intensity E-Mental Health Intervention for Syrian Refugees," *Frontiers in Psychiatry* 9 (January 25, 2019): 663, https://doi.org/10.3389/fpsyt.2018.00663.

15. Naser Morina, Simon M. Ewers, Sandra Passardi, Ulrich Schnyder, Christine Knaevelsrud, Julia Müller, Richard A. Bryant, Angela Nickerson, and Matthis Schick, "Mental Health Assessments in Refugees and Asylum Seekers: Evaluation of a Tablet-Assisted Screening Software," *Conflict and Health* 11, no. 1 (December 2017): 18, https://doi.org/10.1186/s13031-017-0120-2.

16. Bahar Hashemi, Sara Ali, Rania Awaad, Laila Soudi, Lawrence Housel, and Stephen J. Sosebee, "Facilitating Mental Health Screening of War-Torn Populations Using Mobile Applications," *Social Psychiatry and Psychiatric Epidemiology* 52, no. 1 (January 2017): 27–33, https://doi.org/10.1007/s00127-016-1303-7.

17. Ashley Gulden et al., "HADStress Screen for Posttraumatic Stress: Replication in Ethiopian Refugees," *Journal of Nervous and Mental Disease* 198, no. 10 (October 2010): 762–67, https://doi.org/10.1097/NMD.0b013e3181f49c0a.

18. Hospital and Healthcare, "How AI Is Helping Rohingya Refugee Health," February 25, 2019, accessed October 23, 2020, http://hospitalhealth.com.au/content/technology/article/how-ai-is-helping-rohingya-refugee-health-1250125458; Polyfins Technology, "Free Skin Consultation Online," Tibot.ai, 2020, https://tibot.ai/.

19. Devika Nadkarni, Imad Elhajj, Zaher Dawy, Hala Ghattas, and Muhammad H Zaman, "Examining the Need and Potential for Biomedical Engineering to Strengthen Health Care Delivery for Displaced Populations and Victims of Conflict," *Conflict and Health* 11 (November 1, 2017), https://doi.org/10.1186/s13031-017-0122-0.

20. Nadkarni et al., "Examining the Need and Potential."

21. Bria Mitchell-Gillespie, Hiba Hashim, Megan Griffin, and Rawan AlHeresh, "Sustainable Support Solutions for Community-Based Rehabilitation Workers in Refugee Camps: Piloting Telehealth Acceptability and Implementation," *Globalization and Health* 16, no. 1 (September 15, 2020): 82, https://doi.org/10.1186/s12992-020-00614-y; Fatema Khatun et al., "Community Readiness for Adopting MHealth in Rural Bangladesh: A Qualitative Exploration," *International Journal of Medical Informatics* 93 (September 2016): 49–56, https://doi.org/10.1016/j.ijmedinf.2016.05.010; Shelly Culbertson, James Dimarogonas, Katherine Costello, and Serafina Lanna, *Crossing the Digital Divide: Applying Technology to the Global Refugee Crisis* (Santa Monica, CA: RAND Corporation, 2019), https://doi.org/10.7249/RR4322.

22. UNHCR, "Is Your App the Best Way to Help Refugees? Improving the Collaboration between Humanitarian Actors and the Tech Industry," *UNHCR Innovation* (blog), October 14, 2016, https://www.unhcr.org/innovation/app-best-way-help-refugees-improving-collaboration-humanitarian-actors-tech-industry/.

23. GSMA, "The Digital Lives of Refugees: How Displaced Populations Use Mobile Phones and What Gets in the Way," 2019, https://www.gsma.com/mobilefordevelopment/wp-content/uploads/2019/07/The-Digital-Lives-of-Refugees.pdf.

24. Alison Fox, Sally Baker, Koula Charitonos, Victoria Jack, and Barbara Moser-Mercer, "Ethics-in-Practice in Fragile Contexts: Research in Education for Displaced Persons, Refugees and Asylum Seekers," *British Educational Research Journal* 46, no. 4 (August 2020): 829–47, https://doi.org/10.1002/berj.3618; Kristin Bergtora Sandvik, Katja Lindskov Jacobsen, and Sean Martin McDonald, "Do No Harm: A Taxonomy of the Challenges of Humanitarian Experimentation," *International Review of the Red Cross* 99, no. 904 (2017): 319–44; Ulrike Krause, "Researching Forced Migration: Critical Reflections on Research Ethics during Fieldwork," *Refugee Studies Centre*, Working Paper Series, no. 123 (2017).

25. United Nations Office for the Coordination of Humanitarian Affairs, "Rohingya Refugee Crisis," 2020, https://www.unocha.org/rohingya-refugee-crisis.

26. Human Rights Watch, "Bangladesh: Internet Ban Risks Rohingya Lives," March 26, 2020, accessed October 5, 2020, https://www.hrw.org/news/2020/03/26/bangladesh-internet-ban-risks-rohingya-lives#; Star Online Report, "No Mobile Phone Services for Rohingya Refugees: BTRC | Daily Star," September 2, 2019,

https://www.thedailystar.net/rohingya-crisis/no-mobile-phone-services-for-rohingya
-refugees-1794367.

27. *Star* Online Report, "Mobile Internet Use Drops after Facebook Bar," *Daily Star*, December 25, 2015, https://www.thedailystar.net/country/drastic-drop-mobile
-internet-users-after-facebook-bar-190993.

28. Human Rights Watch, "Bangladesh."

29. Kamran Reza Chowdury and Sunil Barua, "Bangladesh Restores Internet to Rohingya Camps," *BenarNews*, August 28, 2020, https://www.benarnews.org/en
glish/news/bengali/internet-restored-08282020174831.html.

30. UNHCR, "UNHCR Welcomes Uganda Communications Commission Directive to Improve Refugees' Access to SIM Cards," accessed October 5, 2020, https://
www.unhcr.org/afr/news/press/2019/8/5d5ba4274/unhcr-welcomes-uganda-commu
nications-commission-directive-to-improve-refugees.html.

31. Petra Molnar, "New Technologies in Migration: Human Rights Impacts," *Forced Migration Review* (June 2019), https://www.fmreview.org/ethics/molnar.

32. Ed Pilkington, "Dreamers' New Risk after Daca: US Could Use Their Personal Data to Target Them," *The Guardian*, September 5, 2017, https://www.the
guardian.com/us-news/2017/sep/05/daca-dreamers-personal-data-undocumented
-immigrants; Kaurin Dragana, "Data Protection and Digital Agency for Refugees," Centre for International Governance Innovation, May 15, 2019, https://www.cigi
online.org/publications/data-protection-and-digital-agency-refugees.

33. Harvard Humanitarian Initiative and Signal, "The Signal Code—A Human Rights Approach to Information during Crisis," 2020, https://signalcode.org/.

34. Nadkarni et al., "Examining the Need and Potential."

35. Mateusz J. Filipski, Ernesto Tiburcio, Paul A Dorosh, John F Hoddinott, and Gracie Rosenbach, "Modelling the Economic Impact of the Rohingya Influx in Southern Bangladesh" (Washington, DC: International Food Policy Research Institute, 2019), https://doi.org/10.2499/p15738coll2.133397.

Chapter 20

1. World Health Organization, "Health of Migrants World Health Assembly," 2008.

2. Michael Flynn and Kolitha Wickramage, "Leveraging the Domain of Work to Improve Migrant Health," *International Journal of Environmental Research and Public Health* (2017): 14.

3. Flynn and Wickramage, "Leveraging the Domain of Work."

4. Kimberlé Crenshaw, "Demarginalising the Intersection of Race and Sex: A Black Feminist Critique of Anti-Discrimination Doctrine, Feminist Theory, and Anti-Racist Politics." In *Framing Intersectionality: Debates on a Multi-Faceted Concept in Gender Studies*, edited by H. Lutz, M. Vivar, and L. Supik. London: Routledge, 2016.

5. Anju Kapilashrami and Olena Hankivsky, "Intersectionality and Why It Matters to Global Health," *Lancet* (June 30, 2018): 2589–91.

6. Val Morrison, "Health Inequalities and Intersectionality," 2016, Montréal, National Collaborating Centre for Healthy Public Policy.

7. Denise L. Spitzer, "Engendered Movements: Migration, Gender, and Health in a Globalized World." In *The Handbook of Gender and Health*, edited by J. Gideon. Cheltenham, UK: E. Elgar, 2016.

8. Helma Lutz, Maria Vivar, and Linda Supik, "Framing Intersectionality: An Introduction." In *Framing Intersectionality: Debates on a Multi-Faceted Concept in Gender Studies*, edited by Lutz, Vivar, and Supik. London: Routledge, 2016.

9. Olena Hankivsky. "Women's Health, Men's Health, and Gender and Health: Implications of Intersectionality," *Social Science and Medicine* 74 (2012): 1712–20.

10. Spitzer, "Engendered Movements."

11. Heide Castañeda, Seth Holmes, Daniel Madrigal, Maria-Elena De Trinidad Young, Namoi Beyeler, and James Quesada, "Immigration as a Social Determinant of Health," *Annual Review of Public Health* 36 (2015): 375–92.

12. Denise L. Spitzer et al., "Towards Inclusive Migrant Health Care," *BMJ* 366 (2019): l4256, https://doi.org/10.1136/bmj.l4256.

13. Spitzer, "Engendered Movements."

14. Aihwa Ong, "Ecologies of Expertise: Assembling Flow, Managing Citizenship." In *Global Assemblages: Technology, Politics, and Ethics as Anthropological Problems*, edited by A. Ong and S. Collier. Malden, MA: Blackwell, 2005.

15. Denise L. Spitzer and Sara Torres, "Oppression and Im/migrant Health in Canada." In *Oppression as a Determinant of Health* (2nd ed.), edited by E. McGibbon. Halifax, Brunswick: Fernwood, 2021.

16. Castañeda et al., "Immigration as a Social Determinant of Health."

17. Ursula Trummer and Allan Krasnik, "Migrant Integration Policies and Health Inequalities in Europe," *European Journal of Public Health* 27, no. 4 (2017): 590–91.

18. Spitzer et al., "Towards Inclusive Migrant Care."

19. Spitzer and Torres, "Oppression and Im/migrant Health in Canada."

20. Denise L. Spitzer, "Migration and Health Through an Intersectional Lens." In *The Handbook of Migration and Health*, edited by F. Thomas. Cheltenham, UK: Edward Elgar, 2016.

21. Salim Ahmed, Nusrat Shommu, Nahid Rumana, Gary Barron, Sonja Wicklum, and Tanvir Turin, "Barriers to Access of Primary Healthcare by Immigrant Populations in Canada: A Literature Review," *Journal of Immigrant and Minority Health* 18 (2016):1522–40.

22. Antonio Chianrenza, Marie Dauvrin, Valentina Chiesa, Sonia Baatout, and Hans Verrept, "Supporting Access to Healthcare for Refugees and Migrants in European Countries Under Particular Migratory Pressure," *BMC Health Services Research* 19 (2019).

23. Helena Legido-Quigley, Nicola Pocock, Sok Teng Tan, Repeepong Suphan-

chamat, Kolita Wiskramage, Martin McKee, and Kevin Pottie, "Health Care Is Not Universal If Undocumented Migrants Are Excluded," *BMJ* 366 (2019): 14160.

24. Flynn and Wickramage, "Leveraging the Domain of Work."

25. Migration Integration Policy Index, "Health," 2015, accessed August 18, 2018, http://www.mipex.eu/health.

26. Trummer and Krasnik, "Migration Integration Policies."

27. Kolitha Wickramage, Paul Simpson, and Kamran Abbasi, "Improving the Health of Migrants: Toxic Narratives Complicate Rational Debates and Hinder Workable Solutions," *BMJ* 366 (2019): 15324.

28. Migration Integration Policy Index, "Health."

29. Tali Filler, Bishmah Jameel, and Anna Gagliardi, "Barriers and Facilitators of Patient-Centered Care for Immigrant and Refugee Women: A Scoping Review," *BMC Public Health* (2020): 20, https://doi.org/10.1186/s12889-020-09159-6.

30. Chianrenza et al., "Supporting Access to Healthcare."

31. Chianrenza et al., "Supporting Access to Healthcare."

32. Migration Integration Policy Index, "Health."

33. Spitzer et al., "Towards Inclusive Migrant Care."

34. Legido-Quigley et al., "Health Care Is Not Universal."

35. Chianrenza et al., "Supporting Access to Healthcare."

36. Wickramage et al., "Improving the Health of Migrants."

37. Spitzer et al., "Towards Inclusive Migrant Care."

38. Migration Integration Policy Index, "Health."

39. Jaime Calderon, Barbara Rijks, and Dovelyn Rannveig Aguinas, *Asian Labour Migrants and Health: Exploring Policy Routes.* Bangkok: IOM/MPI, 2012.

40. Spitzer and Torres, "Oppression and Im/migrant Health in Canada."

41. Philippe Bourgois, Seth Holmes, Kime Sue, and James Quesada, "Structural Vulnerability: Operationalizing the Concept to Address Health Disparities in Clinical Care," *Academic Medicine* 92, no. 3, (2017): 299–307.

42. Spitzer et al., "Towards Inclusive Migrant Care."

43. Ahmed et al., "Barriers to Access of Primary Healthcare."

44. Spitzer and Torres, "Oppression and Im/migrant Health in Canada."

45. Spitzer, "Migration and Health Through an Intersectional Lens."

46. Migration Integration Policy Index, "Health."

47. Ahmed et al., "Barriers to Access of Primary Healthcare."

48. Spitzer, "Migration and Health Through an Intersectional Lens."

49. Spitzer and Torres, "Oppression and Im/migrant Health in Canada."

50. Spitzer, "Migration and Health Through an Intersectional Lens."

51. Wickramage et al., "Improving the Health of Migrants."

52. Spitzer et al., "Towards Inclusive Migrant Care."

53. Denise L. Spitzer, "In Visible Bodies: Minority Women, Nurses, Time, and the New Economy of Care," *Medical Anthropology Quarterly* 18, no. 4, (2004): 490–508.

54. Morrison, "Health Inequalities and Intersectionality."

55. Hankivsky, "Women's Health, Men's Health, and Gender and Health."

56. Spitzer et al., "Towards Inclusive Migrant Care."

57. Lynn Weber and Deborah Parra-Medina, "Intersectionality and Women's Health: Charting a Path to Eliminating Health Disparities," *Advances in Gender Research* 7 (2003): 181–230.

58. Kapilashrami and Hankivsky, "Intersectionality and Why It Matters to Global Health."

59. Spitzer et al., "Towards Inclusive Migrant Care."

60. Weber and Parra-Medina, "Intersectionality and Women's Health."

61. Filler et al., "Barriers and Facilitators of Patient-Centered Care."

62. Elena Riza et al., "Community-Based Healthcare for Migrants and Refugees: A Scoping Literature Review of Best Practices," *Healthcare* 8 (2020): 115.

63. Fillier et al., "Barriers and Facilitators of Patient-Centered Care."

64. Bourgois et al., "Structural Vulnerability."

65. Fillier et al., "Barriers and Facilitators of Patient-Centered Care."

66. Bourgois et al., "Structural Vulnerability."

67. Ahmed et al., "Barriers to Access of Primary Healthcare."

68. Fillier et al., "Barriers and Facilitators of Patient-Centered Care."

69. Bourgois., "Structural Vulnerability."

70. Spitzer et al., "Towards Inclusive Migrant Care."

71. Chianrenza et al., "Supporting Access to Healthcare."

72. Spitzer et al., "Towards Inclusive Migrant Care."

73. Sol Pia Juárez et al., "Effects of Non-Health-Targeted Policies on Migrant Health: A Systematic Review and Meta-Analysis," *Lancet Global Health* 7 (2019): e420–35.

74. Margherita Gionnoni, Luisa Franzini, and Giuliano Masiero, "Migrant Integration Policies and Health Inequalities in Europe," *BMC Public Health* 16 (2016): 463.

75. Denise L. Spitzer, "Work, Worries, and Weariness: Towards an Embodied and Engendered Migrant Health." In *Engendering Migrant Health; Canadian Perspectives*, edited by Spitzer. Toronto: University of Toronto Press, 2011.

76. Nancy Krieger, Jarvis Chen, and Joe Selby, "Class inequalities in Women's Health: Combined Impact of Childhood and Adult Social Class—A Study of 630 US Women," *Public Health* (2001): 115: 175–85.

77. Spitzer, "Work, Worries, and Weariness."

78. Spitzer, "Work, Worries, and Weariness."

79. Juárez et al. "Effects of Non-Health-Targeted Policies on Migrant Health."

80. Gionnoni et al., "Migrant Integration Policies and Health Inequalities in Europe."

81. Calderon, Rijks, and Rannveig Aguinas, *Asian Labour Migrants and Health.*

82. Trummer and Krasnik, "Migration Integration Policies."

83. Calderon, Rijks, and Rannveig Aguinas, *Asian Labour Migrants and Health.*

84. Castañeda et al., "Immigration as a Social Determinant of Health."

85. Chianrenza et al., "Supporting Access to Healthcare."

86. Chianrenza et al., "Supporting Access to Healthcare."

87. Weber and Parra-Medina, "Intersectionality and Women's Health."

Chapter 21

1. Parmet, Wendy E. "Immigration Law's Adverse Impact on COVID-19." *Assessing Legal Responses to COVID-19.* Boston: Public Health Law Watch, 2020. https://static1.squarespace.com/static/5956e16e6b8f5b8c45f1c216/t/5f4d657822570 5285562d0f0/1598908033901/COVID19PolicyPlaybook_Aug2020+Full.pdf.

2. OECD. "Country Policy Tracker—Tackling Coronavirus (COVID-19): Contributing to a Global Effort." Updated October 23, 2020. https://oecd.github.io /OECD-covid-action-map/.

3. Tsouros, Agis D. "Global Governance and the Health of Migrants." In *Migration and Health*, edited by Sandro Galea, Catherine K. Ettman, and Muhammad H. Zaman. Chicago: University of Chicago Press, 2022.

4. Gusterson, Hugh. "From Brexit to Trump: Anthropology and the Rise of Nationalist Populism." *Journal of the American Ethnological Society* 40, no. 2 (2017): 209–14. Accessed October 25, 2020. https://doi.org/10.1111/amet.12469.

5. Fabi, Rachel. "Public Health in the Context of Migration: Ethics Issues Related to Immigrants and Refugees." *Oxford Handbook of Public Health Ethics.* Oxford: Oxford University Press, 2019. https://doi.org/10.1093/oxfordhb/9780190245 191.001.0001.

6. Illingsworth, Patricia, and Wendy E. Parmet. *The Health of Newcomers: Immigration, Health Policy, and the Case for Global Solidarity.* New York: New York University Press, 2017, 169.

7. Chacón, Jennifer M. "Citizenship Matters: Conceptualizing Belonging in an Era of Fragile Inclusion." *U.C. Davis Law Review* 32, no. 1 (2018): 1–80.

8. Marshall, T. H. *Citizenship and Social Class.* London: Cambridge at the University Press, 1950.

9. Illingworth and Parmet, *Health of Newcomers,* 169.

10. Walzer, Michael. *Spheres of Justice: A Defense of Pluralism and Equality.* New York: Basic Books, 1983.

11. Ibid, 15.

12. Song, Yaoxi. "The Relationship between Citizenship and Solidarity." *International Journal of Law and Interdisciplinary Studies* 6 (2018): 4–10.

13. Makhlouf, Medha D. "Health Justice for Immigrants." *University of Pennsylvania Journal of Law. and Public Affairs* 4, no. 2 (2019): 235–11.

14. Song, "The Relationship," 7.

15. Illingsworth and Parmet, *Health of Newcomers*, 176.

16. Koning, Edward Anthony. *Immigration and the Politics of Welfare Exclusion: Selective Solidarity in Western Democracies*. Toronto: University of Toronto Press, 2019, 174.

17. West-Oram, Peter G. N. "From Self-Interest to Solidarity: One Path towards Delivering Refugee Health." *Bioethics* 32, no. 6 (2018): 343–52, 345. Accessed October 25, 2020. http://doi.org/10.1111/bioe.12472.

18. Ibid.

19. Ibid, 345.

20. Landolt, Patricia. "Assembling the Politics of Noncitizenship: Local Struggles to Enforce and Extend Access to Health Care." *University of Toronto Sociology Working Paper* 2019-01 (2019): 1–33, 2.

21. Artiga, Samantha, and Matthew Rae. "Health and Financial Risks for Noncitizen Immigrants Due to the COVID-19 Pandemic." Kaiser Family Foundation. Accessed January 23, 2021. https://www.kff.org/report-section/health-and-financial-risks-for-noncitizen-immigrants-due-to-the-covid-19-pandemic-issue-brief/.

22. Illingworth and Parmet, *Health of Newcomers*, 170.

23. Hardcastle, Gary. "Every Night, New York City Salutes Its Health Care Workers." NPR. Accessed November 3, 2020. https://www.npr.org/2020/04/10/832131816/every-night-new-york-city-salutes-its-health-care-workers.

24. Parmet, Wendy E. "The COVID Cases: A Preliminary Assessment of Judicial Review of Public Health Powers During a Partisan and Polarized Pandemic." *San Diego Law Review* 57, no. 4 (2020): 999–1048.

25. Illingsworth and Parmet, *Health of Newcomers*, 106.

26. Ibid, 76.

27. Daniels, Norman. *Just Health: Meeting Health Needs Fairly*. Cambridge: Cambridge University Press, 2007, 2. https://doi.org/10.1017/CBO9780511809514.

28. G.A. Res. 217 (III) A, Universal Declaration of Human Rights (December 10, 1948).

29. G.A. Res. 2200A (XXI), International Covenant on Economic, Social and Cultural Rights (December 16, 1966).

30. Illingworth and Parmet, *Health of Newcomers*, 100.

31. Ibid.

32. Rawls, John. *A Theory of Justice*. Cambridge: Harvard University Press, 1971.

33. Daniels, *Just Health*, 21.

34. Ibid, 97.

35. Nussbaum, Martha. "Human Rights and Human Capabilities." *Harvard Human Rights Journal* 20 (2007): 21–24, 23.

36. Sen, Amartya. "Why Health Equity?" *Health Economics* 11 (2002): 659–66, 659. Accessed October 25, 2020. https://doi.org/10.1002/hec.762.

37. *The Stanford Encyclopedia of Philosophy* (2017), s.v. "Justice and Individual Claims."

38. Bhatnagar, Prashasti. "Children in Cages: A Legal and Public Health Crisis." *Georgetown Immigration Law Journal* 34 (2019): 181–85.

39. Erfani, Parsa, Nishant Uppal, and Caroline H. Lee. "COVID-19 Testing and Cases in Immigration Detention Centers, April–August 2020." *JAMA* (2020). Accessed November 3, 2020. https://jamanetwork.com/journals/jama/fullarticle/2772627.

40. Castañeda, Heide, Seth M. Holmes, Daniel S. Madrigal, Maria-Elena De-Trinidad Young, Naomi Beyeler, and James Quesada. "Immigration as a Social Determinant of Health." *Annual Review of Public Health* 36 (2015): 375–92. Accessed October 25, 2020. https://doi-org.ezproxy.neu.edu/10.1146/annurev-publhealth -032013-182419.

41. Braveman, Paula, and Laura Gottlieb. "The Social Determinants of Health: It's Time to Consider the Causes of the Causes." *Public Health Rep.* 129, no. 1 (2014): 19–31.

42. Gelatt, Julia. "Immigrant Workers: Vital to the U.S. COVID-19 Response, Disproportionately Vulnerable." Migration Policy Institute. Accessed November 3, 2020. https://www.migrationpolicy.org/research/immigrant-workers-us-covid-19-response.

43. Bahar, Dany. "Don't Forget to Thank Immigrants, Too." Brookings. Accessed November 3, 2020. https://www.brookings.edu/blog/up-front/2020/04/01/dont-forget -to-thank-immigrants-too/.

44. Hartmann, Heidi, Jeffrey Hayes, Rebecca Huber, Kelly Rolfes-Haase, and Jooyeoun Suh. *The Shifting Supply and Demand of Care Work: The Growing Role of People of Color and Immigrants*. Washington, DC: Institute for Women's Policy Research, 2018. https://iwpr.org/wp-content/uploads/2020/08/C470_Shifting-Supply -of-Care-Work-Immigrants-and-POC.pdf.

45. Alderwick, Hugh, and Lucinda Allen. "Immigration and the NHS: The Evidence." The Health Foundation (blog). https://www.health.org.uk/news-and-com ment/blogs/immigration-and-the-nhs-the-evidence.

46. Illingworth and Parmet, *Health of Newcomers*, 173.

47. Duncan, Whitney L., and Sarah B. Horton. "Serious Challenges and Potential Solutions for Immigrant Health During COVID-19." Health Affairs (blog), April 18, 2020. https://www.healthaffairs.org/do/10.1377/hblog20200416.887086/full/.

48. Fatinocci-Fernós, Jorge M. "Looking Beyond the Negative-Positive Rights Distinction: Analyzing Constitutional Rights According to their Nature, Effect, and Reach." *Hastings International and Comparative Law Rev.* 41, no. 1 (2018): 31–51, 39.

49. Parmet, "Immigration Law's Adverse Impact on COVID-19," 243.

Chapter 22

1. Göktürk, D., D. Gramling, and A. Kaes. *Germany in Transit: Nation and Migration, 1955–2005*. Berkeley: University of California Press, 2007.

2. Bade, Klaus J., Pieter C. Emmer, Leo Lucassen, Jochen Oltmer, and Corrie

van Eijl, eds. *The Encyclopedia of Migration and Minorities in Europe: From the 17th Century to the Present.* Cambridge: Cambridge University Press, 2011.

3. Lanz, T. "Turkish Immigrants in Germany: Behind the Fantasy Screen of Multiculturalism." In *Turks in Europe: Culture, Identity and Integration,* edited by Talip Kucukcan and Veyis Gungor. Amsterdam: Turkevi Research Center, 2009.

4. Hoskins, Bryony, and Sallah Momodou. "Developing Intercultural Competence in Europe: The Challenges," *Language and Intercultural Communication* 11, no. 2 (2011): 113–25. https://doi.org/10.1080/14708477.2011.556739.

5. Rivers, W. H. R. *Medicine, Magic and Religion.* London: Kegan, Paul, Trench, Turner, 1924.

6. Scheper-Hughes, N., and M. Lock. "The Mindful Body: A Prolegomenon to Future Work in Medical Anthropology," *Medical Anthropology Quarterly* 1 (1987): 6–41.

7. Csordas, T. J. "Embodiment as a Paradigm for Anthropology," *Ethos* 18, no. 1 (1990): 5–47.

8. van der Geest, S., and K. W. van der Veen, eds. *In Search of Health: Essays in Medical Anthropology,* Amsterdam: Vakgroep Culturele Anthropologie en Niet-westerse Sociologie Algemeen, Univ. Amsterdam, 1979.

9. Kleinman, A. "Concepts and a Model for the Comparison of Medical Systems as Cultural Systems," *Social Science and Medicine* B12 (1978): 85–93.

10. Kleinman, A. "Clinical Relevance of Anthropological and Cross-Cultural Research: Concepts and Strategies," *American Journal of Psychiatry* 135 (1978): 427–31.

11. Wood, C. S. *Human Sickness and Health: A Biocultural View.* Palo Alto: Mayfield, 1979.

12. Molly, G. "Language Barriers and Health of Syrian Refugees in Germany," *American Journal of Public Health* 107 (2017): 486.

13. Jacobs, Elizabeth A., and Lisa Diamond, eds. *Providing Health Care in the Context of Language Barriers: International Perspectives.* Bristol: Multilingual Matters, 2017.

14. Fassin, D. *L'éspace politique de la santé.* Paris: Presses Universitaires de France, 1996.

15. Farmer, Paul. *AIDS and Accusation: Haiti and the Geography of Blame.* Berkeley: University of California Press, 1992.

16. Augé, M., and C. Herlich. *Le sens du mal. Anthropologie, histoire, sociologie de la maladie.* Paris: Des archives contemporaines, 1983.

17. Helman, Cecil. *Culture, Health, and Illness,* 5th ed. London: Hodder Arnold, 2007.

18. Kumar, Bernadette N., and Esperanza Diaz, eds. *Migrant Health: A Primary Care Perspective.* Boca Raton: CRC Press, 2019.

19. Sargent, Carolyn, and Stéphanie Larchanché. "Transnational Migration and Global Health: The Production and Management of Risk, Illness, and Access to Care," *Annual Review of Anthropology* 40 (2011): 345–61.

20. Hadley, C. "The Complex Interactions between Migration and Health: An Introduction," *NAPA Bulletin* 34 (2010): 1–5.

21. Napier, David, Michael Depledge, Michael Knipper, Rebecca Lovell, Eduard Ponarin, Emilia Sanabria, and Felicity Thomas. *Culture Matters: Using a Cultural Contexts of Health Approach to Enhance Policy-Making.* WHO Policy Brief. Geneva: Regional Office for Europe, 2017.

22. Quaranta, I. "Anthropology, Health Care and the Transformation of Experience." In *Culture and Wellbeing: New Pathologies and Emerging Challenges*, edited by A. D. Napier, A. Hobart, and R. Muller. Canon Pyon: Sean Kingston, 2017.

23. Urquia, Marcelo, and Anita Gagnon. "Glossary: Migration and Health," *Journal of Epidemiology and Community Health* 65, no. 5 (2011): 467–72.

24. De Pisanie, Lourens, and Christie Caldwell. "Cultural Competency in Global Health." In *Radiology in Global Health*, edited by Daniel Mollura, Melissa Culp, and Matthew Lungren. Cham, Switzerland: Springer Nature, 2019, 49–59. https://doi.org/10.1007/978-3-319-98485-8_5.

25. Fadiman, A. *The Spirit Catches You and You Fall Down.* New York: Farrar, Straus and Giroux, 2012.

26. Fuller, J. "Multicultural Health Care: Reconciling Universalism and Particularism," *Nurs Inq* 4, no. 3 (1997): 153–59.

27. Adams, V., N. J. Burke, and I. Whitmarsh. "Slow Research: Thoughts for a Movement in Global Health," *Medical Anthropology* 33, no. 3 (2014): 179–97. https://doi.org/10.1080/01459740.2013.858335.

28. Biehl, J., and A. Petryna. *When People Come First: Critical Studies in Global Health.* Princeton, Princeton University Press, 2013.

29. Farmer, Paul, Jim Yong Kim, Arthur Kleinman, and Matthew Basilico. *Reimagining Global Health.* Berkeley: University of California Press, 2013.

30. Huang, Shu-Ling, and Anne Spurgeon. "The Mental Health of Chinese Immigrants in Birmingham, UK," *Ethnicity and Health* 11, no. 4 (2006): 365–87. https://doi.org/10.1080/13557850600824161.

31. Hecker, T., and F. Neuner. "Mental Health Enables Integration: Re-thinking Treatment Approaches for Refugees." In *Refugee Migration and Health. Migration, Minorities and Modernity*, vol. 4, edited by A. Krämer and F. Fischer F. Cham, Switzerland: Springer, 2019. https://doi-org.proxy-ub.rug.nl/10.1007/978-3-030-03155-8_5.

32. Sargent, Carolyn, and Stephanie Larchanché. "Transnational Health Care Circuits: Managing Therapy among Immigrants in France and Kinship Networks in West Africa." In *Affective Circuits: Transnational Migration and Intimacies of Care*, edited by Jennifer Cole and Christian Groes. Chicago: University of Chicago Press, 2016.

33. Reis, R., M. R. Crone, and L. H. Berckmoes. "Unpacking Context and Culture in Mental Health Pathways of Child and Adolescent Refugees." In *Child, Adolescent and Family Refugee Mental Health*, edited by S. Song and P. Ventevogel. Cham, Switzerland: Springer, 2020. https://doi-org.proxy-ub.rug.nl/10.1007/978-3-030-45278-0_3.

34. Glick Schiller, N., and G. E. Fouron. *Georges Woke Up Laughing: Long-Distance Nationalism and the Search for Home*. Durham: Duke University Press, 2001.

35. Andits, P. "Rethinking Home, Belonging, and the Potentials of Transnationalism: Australian Hungarians After the Fall of the Berlin Wall," *Ethos* 43, no. 4 (2015): 313–31. https://doi.org/10.1111/etho.12101.

36. Lanz, T., E. J. Daussà, and R. Pera-Ros. "Two-way Integration of Migrants and Minoritized Speakers: Voices from Catalonia," in *The Impact of Migration on Linguistic and Cultural Areas*, edited by Ulrich Hoinkes and Matthias Meyer. Berlin: Peter Lang, 2021, 179–206.

37. Iarmolenko, S., P. F. Titzmann, and R. K. Silbereisen. "Bonds to the Homeland: Patterns and Determinants of Women's Transnational Travel Frequency among Three Immigrant Groups in Germany," *International Journal of Psychology* 51, no. 2 (2016): 130–38. https://doi.org/10.1002/ijop.12141.

38. Fouron, G., and N. Glick Schiller. "All in the Family: Gender, Transnational Migration, and the Nation-State," *Identities* 7, no. 4 (2001): 539–82.

39. Elias, N., and D. Lemish. "Spinning the Web of Identity: The Roles of the Internet in the Lives of Immigrant Adolescents," *New Media and Society* 11, no. 4 (2009): 533–51.

40. Modood, T. *Post-immigration "Difference" and Integration: The Case of Muslims in Western Europe*. London: British Academy, 2012.

41. King, R., T. Warnes, and A. Williams. *Sunset Lives — British Retirement Migration to the Mediterranean*. New York: Berg, 2000.

42. Escandon, S. "Cross-Cultural Caregiving and the Temporal Dimension," *Issues in Mental Health Nursing* 34, no. 11 (2013): 820–26. https://doi.org/10.3109/01612840.2013.830664.

43. Kou, Lirong, Honggang Xu, and Mei-Po Kwan. "Seasonal Mobility and Well-Being of Older People: The Case of 'Snowbirds' to Sanya, China," *Health and Place* 54 (2018): 155–63. https://doi.org/10.1016/j.healthplace.2018.08.008.

Chapter 23

1. United Nations (UN), Department of Economic and Social Affairs, "The Number of International Migrants Reaches 272 Million, Continuing an Upward Trend in All World Regions, Says UN," September 17, 2019. https://bit.ly/Migration2019.

2. UN, "The Number of International Migrants Reaches 272 Million."

3. American Sociological Association (ASA), "What Is Sociology?," 2014. https://www.asanet.org/about-asa/asa-story/what-sociology.

4. Rubén G. Rumbaut, "Paradoxes (and Orthodoxies) of Assimilation," *Sociological Perspectives* 40, no. 3 (1997): 483–511. http://www.jstor.com/stable/1389453.

5. Edna A. Viruell-Fuentes, "Beyond Acculturation: Immigration, Discrimina-

tion, and Health Research among Mexicans in the United States," *Social Science and Medicine* 65 (2007): 1524–35.

6. Alan M. Kraut, "Bodies from Abroad: Immigration, Health and Disease," in *A Companion to American Immigration*, edited by Reed Ueda, 110. Malden, MA: Blackwell, 2006.

7. Alexandre I. R. White and Katrina Quisumbing King, "The US Has an Ugly History of Blaming 'Foreigners' for Disease," *Washington Post*, March 24, 2020.

8. Carolyn Sargent and Stéphanie Larchanché, "Transnational Migration and Global Health: The Production and Management of Risk, Illness, and Access to Care," *Annual Review of Anthropology* 40 (2011): 345–61.

9. Sargent and Larchanché, "Transnational Migration and Global Health."

10. Angela R. Gover, Shannon B. Harper, and Lynn Langston, "Anti-Asian Hate Crime During the COVID-19 Pandemic: Exploring the Reproduction of Inequality," *American Journal of Criminal Justice* (July 7, 2020). https://doi.org/10.1007/s12103-020-09545-1.

11. Katherine Fennelly, "The Healthy Migrant Effect," *Healthy Generations: Immigrant and Refugee Health* 5, no. 3 (February 2005): 1.

12. Fennelly, "The Healthy Migrant Effect."

13. National Academies of Sciences, Engineering, and Medicine (NASEM), *The Integration of Immigrants into American Society*. Washington, DC: The National Academies Press, 2015, 387. https://doi.org/10.17226/21746.

14. NASEM, *The Integration of Immigrants into American Society*.

15. NASEM, *The Integration of Immigrants into American Society*.

16. NASEM, *The Integration of Immigrants into American Society*.

17. NASEM, *The Integration of Immigrants into American Society*.

18. NASEM, *The Integration of Immigrants into American Society*.

19. Mark Vandingham and Mengxi Zhang, "Migration and Health," in *The Blackwell Encyclopedia of Sociology*, edited by George Ritzer. Hoboken, NJ: John Wiley & Sons, 2016. https://doi.org/10.1002/9781405165518.wbeos0769.

20. Rumbaut, "Paradoxes (and Orthodoxies) of Assimilation."

21. Fennelly, "The Healthy Migrant Effect."

22. Sargent and Larchanché, "Transnational Migration and Global Health."

23. Vandingham and Zhang, "Migration and Health."

24. Sargent and Larchanché, "Transnational Migration and Global Health."

25. Viruell-Fuentes, "Beyond Acculturation."

26. Bernd Rechel, Philipa Mladovsky, David Ingleby, Johan P. Mackenbach, and Martin McKee, "Migration and Health in an Increasingly Diverse Europe," *Lancet* (2013): 1235–45. https://doi.org/10.1016/S0140-6736(12)62086-8.

27. Davide Malmusi, Carme Borrell, and Joan Benach, "Migration-Related Health Inequalities: Showing the Complex Interactions between Gender, Social Class and Place of Origin," *Social Science and Medicine* 71 (2010): 1610–19.

28. Viruell-Fuentes, "Beyond Acculturation."

29. World Bank, "COVID-19 Crisis through a Migration Lens." *Migration and Development Brief*, no. 32. Washington, DC: World Bank, 2020. https://openknowl edge.worldbank.org/handle/10986/33634.

30. Viruell-Fuentes, "Beyond Acculturation."

31. NASEM, *The Integration of Immigrants into American Society*.

32. NASEM, *The Integration of Immigrants into American Society*.

33. Cathy Zimmerman, Ligia Kiss, and Mazeda Hossain, "Migration and Health: A Framework for 21st Century Policy Making." *PLoS Med* 8, no. 5 (2011): e1001034. https://doi.org/10.1371/journal.pmed.1001034.

34. Samantha Artiga and Maria Diaz, "Health Coverage and Care of Undocumented Immigrants," *Issue Brief*. Washington, DC: Kaiser Family Foundation, 2019.

35. Sargent and Larchanché, "Transnational Migration and Global Health."

36. Rechel et al., "Migration and Health."

37. Rechel at al., "Migration and Health."

38. Matthew Stutz and Arshiya Baig, "International Examples of Undocumented Immigration and the Affordable Care Act," *Journal Immigrant Minor Health* 16, no. 4 (August 2014): 765–68. https://doi.org/10.1007/s10903-013-9790-z.

39. Sargent and Larchanché, "Transnational Migration and Global Health."

40. Sergio D. Cristancho, Marcela Garces, Karen E. Peters, and Benjamin C. Mueller, "Listening to Rural Hispanic Immigrants in the Midwest: A Community-Based Participatory Assessment of Major Barriers to Health Care Access and Use," *Qualitative Health Research* 18, no. 5 (2008).

41. Cristancho et al., "Listening to Rural Hispanic Immigrants in the Midwest."

42. Kathryn Pitkin Derose, José J. Escarce, and Nicole Lurie, "Immigrants and Health Care: Sources of Vulnerability," *Health Affairs* 26, no. 5 (2007): 1258–68. https://doi.org/10.1377/hlthaff.26.5.1258.

43. Jennifer Asanin and Kathi Wilson, "'I Spent Nine Years Looking for a Doctor': Exploring Access to Health Care among Immigrants in Mississauga, Ontario, Canada," *Social Science and Medicine* 66 (2008): 1271–83. http://www.elsevier.com /locate/socscimed.

44. Phillip Connor, Jeffrey S. Passel, and Jens Manuel Krogstad, "How European and US Unauthorized Immigrant Populations Compare," *Pew Research Center* (2019). https://pewrsr.ch/2p7kj59.

45. Sargent and Larchanché, "Transnational Migration and Global Health."

46. Robert C. Smith, *Mexican New York*. Berkeley: University of California Press, 2006.

47. NASEM, *The Integration of Immigrants into American Society*.

48. Stutz and Baig, "International Examples of Undocumented Immigration."

49. Stutz and Baig, "International Examples of Undocumented Immigration."

50. UCLA Health, "The True Healthcare Costs of Undocumented Immigrants," *U Magazine* 34, no. 4 (2014): 10.

Chapter 24

1. Organisation for Economic Co-operation and Development (OECD). "Is Migration Good for the Economy? Migration Policy Debates," May 2014, https://www.oecd.org/migration/migration-policy-debates.htm.

2. OECD. *International Migration Outlook 2020*. Paris: OECD, 2020, https://read.oecd-ilibrary.org/social-issues-migration-health/international-migration-out look-2020_ec98f531-en#page1.

3. Paola Pace, ed. "Migration and the Right to Health: A Review of European Community Law and Council of Europe Instruments," International Organization for Migration (IOM), Migration Health Division, Research and Epidemiology Unit, 2007, https://publications.iom.int/system/files/pdf/iml_12_en.pdf.

4. Ursula Trummer and Allan Krasnik. "Migrant Health: The Economic Argument," *European Journal of Public Health* 27, no. 4 (2017): 590–91, https://doi.org/10.1093/eurpub/ckx087.

5. Nora Gottlieb, Ursula Trummer, Nadav Davidovitch, Alan Krasnik, Sol P. Juárez, Mikael Rostila, Louise Biddle, and Kayvan Bozorgmehr. "Economic Arguments in Migrant Health Policymaking: Proposing a Research Agenda," Manuscript Submitted for Publication, *Globalization and Health* 16, no. 113 (2020), https://doi.org/10.1186/s12992-020-00642-8.

6. European Agency for Fundamental Rights/FRA. "The Cost of Exclusion from Healthcare to Migrants in an Irregular Situation in the EU, Vienna," September 3, 2015, https://fra.europa.eu/en/publication/2015/cost-exclusion-healthcare -case-migrants-irregular-situation-summary.

7. Kayvan Bozorgmehr and Oliver Razum. "Effect of Restricting Access to Health Care on Health Expenditures among Asylum-Seekers and Refugees: A Quasi-Experimental Study in Germany, 1994–2013," *PLoS ONE* 10, no. 7 (2015), https://doi.org/10.1371/journal.pone.0131483.

8. Ursula Trummer, Sonja Novak-Zezula, Anna-Theresa Renner, and Ina Wilcze-wska. "Cost Savings through Timely Treatment for Irregular Migrants and EU Citizens without Insurance," *European Journal of Public Health* 28, no. 1 (April 17, 2018).

9. Lika Nusbaum, Brenda Douglas, Karla Damus, Michael Paasche-Orlow, and Neenah Estrella-Luna. "Communicating Risks and Benefits in Informed Consent for Research: A Qualitative Study," *Global Qualitative Nursing Research* 4 (2017), https://doi.org/10.1177/2333393617732017.

10. Nusbaum et al., "Communicating Risks and Benefits."

11. Haran Ratna. "The Importance of Effective Communication in Health-care Practice," *Harvard Public Health Review* 23 (2019): 1–6, http://harvardpublic healthreview.org/wp-content/uploads/2019/09/Vol-23_Effective-Communication-in -Healthcare_HPHR.pdf.

12. Ursula Trummer, Ulrich Otto Mueller, Peter Nowak, Thomas Stidl, and Jürgen M. Pelikan. "Does Physician–Patient Communication That Aims at Empowering

Patients Improve Clinical Outcome?," *Patient Education and Counseling* 61, no. 2 (2006): 299–306, https://doi.org/10.1016/j.pec.2005.04.009.

13. Ratna, "The Importance of Effective Communication in Healthcare Practice"

14. Birgitta Essén, Birgit Bödker, N.-O. Sjöberg, Jens Langhoff-Roos, Gorm Greisen, Saemundur Gudmundsson, and P.-O. Ostergren. "Are Some Perinatal Deaths in Immigrant Groups Linked to Suboptimal Perinatal Care Services?" *International Journal of Obstetrics and Gynaecology* 109, no. 6 (June 2002): 677–82, https://pubmed.ncbi.nlm.nih.gov/12118647/.

15. Chandrika Divi, Richard G. Koss, Stephen P. Schmaltz, and Jerod M. Loeb. "Language Proficiency and Adverse Events in US Hospitals: A Pilot Study," *Journal of the International Society for Quality in Health Care* 19, no. 2 (April 2007): 60–67, https://doi.org/mzl069.

16. Essén et al., "Are Some Perinatal Deaths in Immigrant Groups Linked to Suboptimal Perinatal Care Services?"

17. Divi et al., "Language Proficiency and Adverse Events in US Hospitals."

18. Gregory Juckett and Kendra Unger. "Appropriate Use of Medical Interpreters," *American Family Physician* 90, no. 7 (October 1, 2014): 476–80, https://doi.org/11499.

19. Corey Joseph, Marie Garruba, and Angela Melder. "Patient Satisfaction of Telephone or Video Interpreter Services Compared with In-Person Services: A Systematic Review," *Australian Hospital Association* 42, no. 2 (April 2018): 168–77, https://doi.org/10.1071/AH16195.

20. Ann D. Bagchi, Stacy Dale, Natalya Verbitsky-Savitz, Sky Andrecheck, Kathleen Zavotsky, and Robert Eisenstein. "Costs and Benefits of Providing In-Person Professional Medical Interpreters in the Emergency Department: Results of a Randomized Controlled Study," *Mathematica Policy Research* (2010).

21. Juckett and Unger, "Appropriate Use of Medical Interpreters."

22. Milagros D. Silva, Margaux Genoff, Alexandra Zaballa, Sarah Jewell, Stacy Stabler, Francesca M. Gany, and Lisa C. Diamond. "Interpreting at the End of Life: A Systematic Review of the Impact of Interpreters on the Delivery of Palliative Care Services to Cancer Patients with Limited English Proficiency," *Journal of Pain and Symptom Management* 51, no. 3 (March 2016): 569–80, https://pubmed.ncbi.nlm.nih.gov/26549596/.

23. Erik Teunissen, Katja Gravenhorst, Chris Dowrick, E. Van Weel-Baumgarten, Francine Van den Driessen Mareeuw, Tomas de Brún, Nicola Burns et al. "Implementing Guidelines and Training Initiatives to Improve Cross-Cultural Communication in Primary Care Consultations: A Qualitative Participatory European Study," *International Journal for Equity in Health* 16, no. 1 (February 10, 2017), https://doi.org/10.1186/s12939-017-0525-y.

24. Silva et al., "Interpreting at the End of Life."

25. Ursula Trummer and Sonja Novak-Zezula. "Management of Doctor-Patient-Relationships: The Issue of Language Barriers in Codes of Conduct for Medical Doctors," Center for Health and Migration, Vienna, Austria, 2016.

26. Medical Board of Australia. "Good Medical Practice: A Code of Conduct for Doctors in Australia," 2016, https://www.medicalboard.gov.au/codes-guide lines-policies/code-of-conduct.aspx.

27. Sonja Novak-Zezula, Beate Schulze, Ursula Karl-Trummer, Karl Krajic, and Jürgen Pelikan. "Improving Interpreting in Clinical Communication: Models of Feasible Practice from the European Project 'Migrant-Friendly Hospitals,'" *Diversity in Health and Social Care* 2 (2005): 223–32.

28. IOM. "Summary Report on the MIPEX Health Strand and Country Reports. IOM Migration Research Series No. 52.," International Organization for Migration, 2016, https://publications.iom.int/system/files/mrs_52.pdf.

29. Antonio Chiarenza, Marie Dauvrin, Valentina Chiesa, Sonia Baatout, and Hans Verrept. "Supporting Access to Healthcare for Refugees and Migrants in European Countries under Particular Migratory Pressure," *BMC Health Services Research* 19, no. 513 (2019), https://doi.org/10.1186/s12913-019-4353-1.

30. Ursula Trummer and Sonja Novak-Zezula. "Diversitätsmanagement in Ambulanzen," *Aktuelle Herausforderungen und Lösungen aus Mitarbeitersicht, ZFPG* 3, no. 2 (2017): 19–27, http://c-hm.com/wp-content/uploads/2019/07/ZFPG_2017_J3_N2_04-1.pdf.

31. Teunissen, "Implementing Guidelines and Training Initiatives."

32. Fabienne N. Jaeger, Nicole Pellaud, Bénédicte Laville, and Pierre Klauser. "The Migration-Related Language Barrier and Professional Interpreter Use in Primary Health Care in Switzerland," *BMC Health Services Research* 19, no. 429 (2019), https://doi.org/10.1186/s12913-019-4164-4.

33. Mary Phelan. "Medical Interpreting and the Law in the European Union," *European Journal of Health Law*, 19, no. 4 (2012): 333–53, https://doi.org/10.1163/157180912X650681.

34. Louis Hampers and Jennifer E. McNulty. "Professional Interpreters and Bilingual Physicians in a Pediatric Emergency Department: Effect on Resource Utilization," *Archives of Pediatrics and Adolescent Medicine* 156, no. 11 (November 2002): 1108–13, https://doi.org/poa20135.

35. Judith Bernstein, Edward Bernstein, Ami Dave, Eric Hardt, Thea James, Judith Linden, P. Mitchell, Tokiko Oishi, and Clara Safi. "Trained Medical Interpreters in the Emergency Department: Effects on Services, Subsequent Charges, and Follow-Up," *Journal of Immigrant Health* 4, no. 4 (October 2002): 171–76, https://doi.org/10.1023/A:1020125425820.

36. Elizabeth A. Jacobs, Diane S. Lauderdale, David Meltzer, Jeanette M. Shorey, Wendy Levinson, and Ronald A. Thisted. "Impact of Interpreter Services on Delivery of Health Care to Limited-English-Proficient Patients," *Journal of General Internal Medicine* 16, no. 7 (July 2001): 468–74, https://doi.org/jgi00525.

37. Leah Karliner, Eliseo Pérez-Stable, and Steven E. Gregorich. "Convenient Access to Professional Interpreters in the Hospital Decreases Readmission Rates and Estimated Hospital Expenditures for Patients with Limited English Proficiency," *Medical Care* 55, no. 3 (2017): 199–206, https://doi.org/10.1097/MLR.0000000000000643.

38. Phelan, "Medical Interpreting and the Law in the European Union."

39. Alexander Bischoff and Kris Denhaerynck. "What Do Language Barriers Cost? An Exploratory Study among Asylum Seekers in Switzerland," *BMC Health Services Research* 10 (August 23, 2010). https://doi.org/10.1186/1472-6963-10-248.

40. Hampers and McNulty, "Professional Interpreters and Bilingual Physicians."

41. Kelvin Quan and Jessica Lynch. "The High Cost of Language Barriers in Medical Malpractice," University of California, Berkeley, National Health Law Program, 2010, https://9kqpw4dcaw91s37kozm5jx17-wpengine.netdna-ssl.com/wp-content/uploads/2018/09/Language-Access-and-Malpractice.pdf.

42. Bischoff and Denhaerynck, "What Do Language Barriers Cost?"

Chapter 25

1. Institute for Social Research, University of Michigan. "Resource Guide: Project on Human Development in Chicago Neighborhoods (PHDCN)." Accessed May 13, 2022, https://www.icpsr.umich.edu/pages/NACJD/guides/phdcn/index.html.

2. Faris, R. E. L., and H. W. Dunham. *Mental Disorders in Urban Areas*. Chicago: University of Chicago Press, 1939.

3. Rodriguez, D., H. A. Carlos, A. M. Adachi-Mejia, E. M. Berke, and J. D. Sargent. "Predictors of Tobacco Outlet Density Nationwide: A Geographic Analysis," *Tobacco Control* 22, no. 5 (2013): 349–55.

4. Marco, M., B. Freisthler, E. Gracia, A. Lopez-Quilez, and M. Lila. "Neighborhood Characteristics, Alcohol Outlet Density, and Alcohol-Related Calls-for-Service: A Spatiotemporal Analysis in a Wet Drinking Country," *International Journal of Geo-Information* 6, no. 12 (2017).

5. Schneider, S., and J. Gruber. "Neighbourhood Deprivation and Outlet Density for Tobacco, Alcohol and Fast Food: First Hints of Obesogenic and Addictive Environments in Germany," *Public Health Nutrition* 16, no. 7 (2013): 1168–77.

6. Ford, P. B., and D. A. Dzewaltowski. "Neighborhood Deprivation, Supermarket Availability, and BMI in Low-Income Women: A Multilevel Analysis," *Journal of Community Health* 36, no. 5 (2011): 785–96.

7. Astell-Burt, T., X. Feng, and G. S. Kolt. "Is Neighborhood Green Space Associated With a Lower Risk of Type 2 Diabetes? Evidence From 267,072 Australians," *Diabetes Care* 37, no. 1 (2014): 197.

8. Clair, A., A. Reeves, R. Loopstra, M. McKee, D. Dorling, and D. Stuckler. "The Impact of the Housing Crisis on Self-Reported Health in Europe: Multilevel Longitudinal Modelling of 27 EU Countries," *European Journal of Public Health* 26, no. 5 (2016): 788–93.

9. Logan, J. R., R. D. Alba, and W. Q. Zhang. "Immigrant Enclaves and Ethnic Communities in New York and Los Angeles," *American Sociological Review* 67, no. 2 (2002): 299–322.

10. Osypuk, T.L., A. V. Diez Roux, C. Hadley, and N. R. Kandula. "Are Immigrant Enclaves Healthy Places to Live? The Multi-ethnic Study of Atherosclerosis," *Social Science and Medicine* 69, no. 1 (2009): 110–20.

11. Lobo, J., and C. Mellander. "Let's Stick Together: Labor Market Effects from Immigrant Neighborhood Clustering," *Environment and Planning A: Economy and Space* 52, no. 5 (2020): 953–80.

12. Roosa, M. W., S. R. Weaver, R. M. B. White et al. "Family and Neighborhood Fit or Misfit and the Adaptation of Mexican Americans," *American Journal of Community Psychology* 44, no. 1–2 (2009): 15–27.

13. Osypuk et al., "Are Immigrant Enclaves Healthy Places to Live?"

14. Bell, S., K. Wilson, L. Bissonnette, and T. Shah. "Access to Primary Health Care: Does Neighborhood of Residence Matter?," *Annals of the American Association of Geographers* 103, no. 1 (2013): 85–105.

15. Castaneda, H., S. M. Holmes, D. S. Madrigal, M. E. D. Young, N. Beyeler, and J. Quesada. "Immigration as a Social Determinant of Health," *Annual Review of Public Health* 36 (2015): 375–92.

16. Institute for Social Research, "Resource Guide."

17. Garson, G. D. "Fundamentals of Hierarchical Linear and Multilevel Modeling." In *Hierarchical Linear Modeling: Guide and Applications*, edited by G. D. Garson, 3–25. Los Angeles: SAGE, 2013.

18. Blakely, T.A., and A. J. Woodward. "Ecological Effects in Multi-level Studies," *Journal of Epidemiology and Community Health* 54, no. 5 (2000): 367.

19. Diez Roux, A. V. "Ecological Variables, Ecological Studies, and Multilevel Studies in Public Health Research." In *Oxford Textbook of Global Public Health*, 6th ed., edited by R. Detels, M. Gulliford, Q. A. Karim, and C. C. Tan. Oxford, UK: Oxford University Press, 2015.

20. Diez Roux, A. V. "A Glossary for Multilevel Analysis," *Journal of Epidemiology and Community Health* 56, no. 8 (2002): 588.

21. Hedman, L., and M. van Ham. "Understanding Neighbourhood Effects: Selection Bias and Residential Mobility." In *Neighbourhood Effects Research: New Perspectives*, edited by M. van Ham, D. Manley, N. Bailey, L. Simpson, and D. Maclennan, 79–99. Dordrecht: Springer, 2012.

22. James, P., J. E. Hart, M. C. Arcaya, D. Feskanich, F. Laden, and S. V. Subramanian. "Neighborhood Self-Selection: The Role of Pre-Move Health Factors on the Built and Socioeconomic Environment," *International Journal of Environmental Research and Public Health* 12, no. 10 (2015): 12489–504.

23. Xue, Y., T. Leventhal, J. Brooks-Gunn, and F. J. Earls. "Neighborhood Residence and Mental Health Problems of 5- to 11-Year-Olds," *Archives of General Psychiatry* 62, no. 5 (2005): 554–63.

24. Fagan, A. A., E. M. Wright, and G. M. Pinchevsky. "A Multi-level Analysis of the Impact of Neighborhood Structural and Social Factors on Adolescent Substance Use," *Drug and Alcohol Dependence* 153 (2015): 180–86.

25. Lorant, V., V. E. Soto, J. Alves et al. "Smoking in School-Aged Adolescents:

Design of a Social Network Survey in Six European Countries," *BMC Research Notes* 8, no. 1 (2015): 91.

26. Lorant, V., V. S. Rojas, L. Becares et al. "A Social Network Analysis of Substance Use among Immigrant Adolescents in Six European Cities," *Social Science and Medicine* 169 (2016): 58–65.

27. Lorant et al., "A Social Network Analysis."

28. Tariq, S., and J. Woodman. "Using Mixed Methods in Health Research," *Journal of the Royal Society of Medicine Short Reports* 4, no. 6 (2013): 2042533313479197.

29. Ojeda, V. D., C. Magana, J. L. Burgos, and A. C. Vargas-Ojeda. "Deported Men's and Father's Perspective: The Impacts of Family Separation on Children and Families in the US," *Frontiers in Psychiatry* 11 (2020): 148.

30. Horvath, K., and R. Latcheva. "Mixing Methods in the Age of Migration Politics: A Commentary on Validity and Reflexivity in Current Migration Research," *Journal of Mixed Methods Research* 13, no. 2 (2019): 127–31.

31. Fetters, M. D., L. A. Curry, and J. W. Creswell. "Achieving Integration in Mixed Methods Designs—Principles and Practices," *Health Services Research* 48, no. 6 pt. 2 (2013): 2134–56.

32. Bergman, M. M. "The Century of Migration and the Contribution of Mixed Methods Research," *Journal of Mixed Methods Research* 12, no. 4 (2018): 371–73.

33. Fauser, M. "Mixed Methods and Multisited Migration Research: Innovations From a Transnational Perspective," *Journal of Mixed Methods Research* 12, no. 4 (2018): 394–412.

34. Massey, D. S., and K. E. Espinosa. "What's Driving Mexico-US Migration? A Theoretical, Empirical, and Policy Analysis," *American Journal of Sociology* 102, no. 4 (1997): 939–99.

35. Massey, D. S. "The Ethnosurvey in Theory and Practice," *International Migration Review* 21, no. 4 (1987): 1498–1522.

36. Massey, D. S., and R. Zenteno. "A Validation of the Ethnosurvey: The Case of Mexico-US Migration," *International Migration Review* 34, no. 3 (2000): 766–93.

37. Massey and Zenteno, "A Validation of the Ethnosurvey."

38. Kaczmarczyk, P., and D. S. Massey. "The Ethnosurvey Revisited: New Migrations, New Methodologies?," *Central and Eastern European Migration Review* 8, no. 2 (2019): 9–38.

39. Massey, D. S., J. Durand, and K. A. Pren. "The Precarious Position of Latino Immigrants in the United States: A Comparative Analysis of Ethnosurvey Data," *Annals of the American Academy of Political and Social Science* 666, no. 1 (2016): 91–109.

40. Ullmann, S. H., N. Goldman, and D. S. Massey. "Healthier Before They Migrate, Less Healthy When They Return? The Health of Returned Migrants in Mexico," *Social Science and Medicine* 73, no. 3 (2011): 421–28.

41. Ortmeyer, D. L., and M. A. Quinn. "Untangling the Health Impacts of Mexico–US Migration," *Review of Economic Analysis* 10, no. 2 (2018): 151–79.

42. Cheong, A. R., and D. S. Massey. "Undocumented and Unwell: Legal Status and Health among Mexican Migrants," *International Migration Review* 53, no. 2 (2019): 571–601.

43. Waldman, K., J. S.-H. Wang, and H. Oh. "Psychiatric Problems among Returned Migrants in Mexico: Updated Findings from the Mexican Migration Project," *Social Psychiatry and Psychiatric Epidemiology* 54, no. 10 (2019): 1285–94.

44. Donato, K. M., E. R. Hamilton, and A. Bernard-Sasges. "Gender and Health in Mexico: Differences between Returned Migrants and Nonmigrants," *Annals of the American Academy of Political and Social Science* 684, no. 1 (2019): 165–87.

45. Ullmann, S. H. "The Health Impacts of International Migration on Mexican Women," *Global Public Health* 7, no. 9 (2012): 946–60.

46. Graham, E., L. P. Jordan, and B. S. A. Yeoh. "Parental Migration and the Mental Health of Those Who Stay Behind to Care for Children in South-East Asia," *Social Science and Medicine* 132 (2015): 225–35.

47. Islam, F., and M. Oremus. "Mixed Methods Immigrant Mental Health Research in Canada: A Systematic Review," *Journal of Immigrant and Minority Health* 16, no. 6 (2014): 1284–89.

48. Weine, S. M., A. Durrani, and C. Polutnik. "Using Mixed Methods to Build Knowledge of Refugee Mental Health," *Intervention: Journal of Mental Health and Psychosocial Support in Conflict Affected Areas* 12, no. 4 (2014): 61–77.

49. Markova, V., and G. M. Sandal. "Lay Explanatory Models of Depression and Preferred Coping Strategies among Somali Refugees in Norway. A Mixed-Method Study," *Frontiers in Psychology* 7, no. 1435 (2016).

50. Simich, L., H. Hamilton, and B. K. Baya. "Mental Distress, Economic Hardship and Expectations of Life in Canada among Sudanese Newcomers," *Transcultural Psychiatry* 43, no. 3 (2006): 418–44.

Chapter 26

1. Ann Aschengrau and George R. Seage, *Essentials of Epidemiology in Public Health* (Burlington: Jones & Bartlett, 2013).

2. Aschengrau and Seage, *Essentials of Epidemiology*.

3. Aschengrau and Seage, *Essentials of Epidemiology*.

4. Robert William Sanson-Fisher, Billie Bonevski, Lawrence W. Green, and Cate D'Este, "Limitations of the Randomized Controlled Trial in Evaluating Population-Based Health Interventions," *American Journal of Preventive Medicine* 33, no. 2 (August 1, 2007): 155–61, https://doi.org/10.1016/j.amepre.2007.04.007.

5. Manning Feinleib, "Invited Commentary on 'Health Effects of Westernization and Migration among Chamorros,'" *American Journal of Epidemiology* 142, no. 7 (1995): 671–72.

6. Robert Friis, Agneta Yngve, and Viveka Persson, "Review of Social

Epidemiologic Research on Migrants' Health: Findings, Methodological Cautions, and Theoretical Perspectives," *Scandinavian Journal of Social Medicine* 26, no. 3 (1998): 173–80.

7. Friis, Yngve, and Persson, "Review of Social Epidemiologic Research."

8. Eric Kliewer, "Epidemiology of Diseases among Migrants," *International Migration* 30 (1992): 141–65.

9. Brian D. Gushulak and Douglas W. MacPherson, "The Basic Principles of Migration Health: Population Mobility and Gaps in Disease Prevalence," *Emerging Themes in Epidemiology* 3, no. 1 (2006): 3.

10. Stanislav V. Kasl and Lisa Berkman, "Health Consequences of the Experience of Migration," *Annual Review of Public Health* 4, no. 1 (1983): 69–90.

11. Gushulak and MacPherson, "The Basic Principles of Migration Health."

12. Gushulak and MacPherson, "The Basic Principles of Migration Health."

13. Brian Karl Finch and William A. Vega, "Acculturation Stress, Social Support, and Self-Rated Health among Latinos in California," *Journal of Immigrant Health* 5, no. 3 (2003): 109–17; Chantal A. Vella, Diana Ontiveros, Raul Y. Zubia, and Julia O. Bader, "Acculturation and Metabolic Syndrome Risk Factors in Young Mexican and Mexican–American Women," *Journal of Immigrant and Minority Health* 13, no. 1 (February 1, 2011): 119–26, https://doi.org/10.1007/s10903-009-9299-7.

14. J. V. Deporte, "Life Tables for the Population of New York State According to Nativity," *American Journal of Epidemiology* 4, no. 4 (July 1, 1924): 302–26, https://doi.org/10.1093/oxfordjournals.aje.a119314; Hsien W. Kung, "Life Tables for Various Racial Groups in Hawaii," *American Journal of Epidemiology* 6, no. 1 (January 1, 1926): 74–118, https://doi.org/10.1093/oxfordjournals.aje.a120008.

15. Howard Markel and Alexandra Minna Stern, "The Foreignness of Germs: The Persistent Association of Immigrants and Disease in American Society," *Milbank Quarterly* 80, no. 4 (December 2002): 757–88, https://doi.org/10.1111/1468-0009.00030.

16. Markel and Stern, "The Foreignness of Germs."

17. C.-E. A. Winslow and Z. W. Koh, "The Mortality of the Chinese in the United States, Hawaii, and the Philippines," *American Journal of Epidemiology* 4, no. 4 (July 1, 1924): 330–55, https://doi.org/10.1093/oxfordjournals.aje.a119316; Deporte, "Life Tables for the Population of New York State."

18. K Lönnroth, Z. Mor, C. Erkens, J. Burchfeld, R. R. Nathavitharana, M. J. van der Werf, and C. Lange, "Tuberculosis in Migrants in Low-Incidence Countries: Epidemiology and Intervention Entry Points," *International Journal of Tuberculosis and Lung Disease* 21, no. 6 (2017): 624–36; Laura B. Nellums, Hayley Thompson, Alison Holmes, Enrique Castro-Sanchez, Jonathan A. Otter, Marie Norredam, Jon S. Friedland, and Sally Hargreaves, "Antimicrobial Resistance among Migrants in Europe: A Systematic Review and Meta-Analysis," *Lancet Infectious Diseases* 18, no. 7 (2018): 796–811.

19. Félice Lê-Scherban, Sandra S. Albrecht, Alain Bertoni, Namratha Kandula, Neil Mehta, and Ana V. Diez Roux, "Immigrant Status and Cardiovascular Risk

over Time: Results from the Multi-Ethnic Study of Atherosclerosis," *Annals of Epidemiology* 26, no. 6 (2016): 429–35.

20. Jordan Edwards, Malini Hu, Amardeep Thind, Saverio Stranges, Maria Chiu, and Kelly K. Anderson, "Gaps in Understanding of the Epidemiology of Mood and Anxiety Disorders among Migrant Groups in Canada: A Systematic Review," *Canadian Journal of Psychiatry* 64, no. 9 (2019): 595–606.

21. Sally Hargreaves, Kieran Rustage, Laura B. Nellums, Alys McAlpine, Nicola Pocock, Delan Devakumar, Robert W. Aldridge, I. Abubakar, K. L. Kristensen, J. W. Himmels, and Jon S. Friedland, "Occupational Health Outcomes among International Migrant Workers: A Systematic Review and Meta-Analysis," *Lancet Global Health* 7, no. 7 (2019): e872–82; Danielle Horyniak, Jason S. Melo, Risa M. Farrell, Victoria D. Ojeda, and Steffanie A. Strathdee, "Epidemiology of Substance Use among Forced Migrants: A Global Systematic Review," *PLoS One* 11, no. 7 (2016): e0159134.

22. Robert W. Aldridge, Laura B. Nellums, Sean Bartlett, Anna Louise Barr, Parth Patel, Rachel Burns, Sally Hargreaves, J. J. Miranda, S. Tollman, Jon S. Friedland, and I Abubaker, "Global Patterns of Mortality in International Migrants: A Systematic Review and Meta-Analysis," *Lancet* 392, no. 10164 (2018): 2553–66.

23. Sol Pía Juárez, Helena Honkaniemi, Andrea C. Dunlavy, Robert W. Aldridge, Mauricio L. Barreto, Srinivasa Vittal Katikireddi, and Mikael Rostila, "Effects of Non-Health-Targeted Policies on Migrant Health: A Systematic Review and Meta-Analysis," *Lancet Global Health* 7, no. 4 (2019): e420–35.

24. Horyniak et al., "Epidemiology of Substance Use among Forced Migrants."

25. Hargreaves et al., "Occupational Health Outcomes among International Migrant Workers."

26. Nellums et al., "Antimicrobial Resistance among Migrants in Europe."

27. Whitney Duncan, "Serious Challenges And Potential Solutions For Immigrant Health During COVID-19," *Health Affairs*, n.d., 10; Ferdinand C. Mukumbang, Anthony N. Ambe, and Babatope O. Adebiyi, "Unspoken Inequality: How COVID-19 Has Exacerbated Existing Vulnerabilities of Asylum-Seekers, Refugees, and Undocumented Migrants in South Africa," *International Journal for Equity in Health* 19, no. 1 (August 20, 2020): 141, https://doi.org/10.1186/s12939-020-01259-4; "COVID-19 and Immigrants' Access to Sexual and Reproductive Health Services in the United States," accessed October 29, 2020, https://www-ncbi-nlm-nih-gov.proxy.bc.edu/pmc/articles/PMC7307065/.

28. Finch and Vega, "Acculturation Stress, Social Support, and Self-Rated Health"; Ada C. Mui and Suk-Young Kang, "Acculturation Stress and Depression among Asian Immigrant Elders," *Social Work* 51, no. 3 (2006): 243–55; Maria-Theresa C. Okafor, Olivia D. Carter-Pokras, and Min Zhan, "Greater Dietary Acculturation (Dietary Change) Is Associated with Poorer Current Self-Rated Health among African Immigrant Adults," *Journal of Nutrition Education and Behavior* 46, no. 4 (2014): 226–35; David L. Sam, Paul Vedder, Karmela Liebkind, Felix Neto, and

Erkki Virta, "Immigration, Acculturation and the Paradox of Adaptation in Europe," *European Journal of Developmental Psychology* 5, no. 2 (2008): 138–58.

29. Chaelin Karen Ra, Youngtae Cho, and Robert A. Hummer, "Is Acculturation Always Adverse to Korean Immigrant Health in the United States?," *Journal of Immigrant and Minority Health* 15, no. 3 (2013): 510–16; Nadia N. Abuelezam, Abdulrahman M. El-Sayed, and Sandro Galea, "Relevance of the 'Immigrant Health Paradox' for the Health of Arab Americans in California," *American Journal of Public Health* 109, no. 12 (2019): 1733–38.

30. Briana Mezuk, Xinjun Li, Klas Cederin, Jeannie Concha, Kenneth S. Kendler, Jan Sundquist, and Kristina Sundquist, "Ethnic Enclaves and Risk of Psychiatric Disorders among First-and Second-Generation Immigrants in Sweden," *Social Psychiatry and Psychiatric Epidemiology* 50, no. 11 (2015): 1713–22; Brittany N. Morey et al., "Ethnic Enclaves, Discrimination, and Stress among Asian American Women: Differences by Nativity and Time in the United States," *Cultural Diversity and Ethnic Minority Psychology* (2020); Tabashir Z. Nobari et al., "Immigrant Enclaves and Obesity in Preschool-Aged Children in Los Angeles County," *Social Science and Medicine* 92 (2013): 1–8.

31. Wendy D. Roth, "Establishing the Denominator: The Challenges of Measuring Multiracial, Hispanic, and Native American Populations," *Annals of the American Academy of Political and Social Science* 677, no. 1 (May 1, 2018): 48–56, https://doi.org/10.1177/0002716218756818; Brian Duncan and Stephen J. Trejo, "Identifying the Later-Generation Descendants of US Immigrants: Issues Arising from Selective Ethnic Attrition," *Annals of the American Academy of Political and Social Science* 677, no. 1 (2018): 131–38.

32. Karen Hacker, Maria Anies, Barbara L. Folb, and Leah Zallman, "Barriers to Health Care for Undocumented Immigrants: A Literature Review," *Risk Management and Healthcare Policy* 8 (October 30, 2015): 175–83, https://doi.org/10.2147/RMHP.S70173; Karen Hacker, Jocelyn Chu, Carolyn Leung, Robert Marra, Alex Pirie, Mohamed Brahimi, Margaret English, Joshua Beckmann, Dolores Acevedo-Garcia, and Robert P. Marlin, "The Impact of Immigration and Customs Enforcement on Immigrant Health: Perceptions of Immigrants in Everett, Massachusetts, USA," *Social Science and Medicine* 73, no. 4 (August 1, 2011): 586–94, https://doi.org/10.1016/j.socscimed.2011.06.007.

33. Eunsuk Choi, Grace Jeongim Heo, Youngshin Song, and Hae-Ra Han, "Community Health Worker Perspectives on Recruitment and Retention of Recent Immigrant Women in a Randomized Clinical Trial," *Family and Community Health* 39, no. 1 (2016): 53–61, https://doi.org/10.1097/FCH.0000000000000089; Jennifer S. Lin, Alyssa Finlay, Angela Tu, and Francesca M. Gany, "Understanding Immigrant Chinese Americans' Participation in Cancer Screening and Clinical Trials," *Journal of Community Health* 30, no. 6 (December 1, 2005): 451–66, https://doi.org/10.1007/s10900-005-7280-5; Sherrie Flynt Wallington, Gheorghe Luta, Anne-Michelle Noone, Larisa Caicedo, Maria Lopez-Class, Vanessa Sheppard, Cherie Spencer, and Jeanne

Mandelblatt, "Assessing the Awareness of and Willingness to Participate in Cancer Clinical Trials Among Immigrant Latinos," *Journal of Community Health* 37, no. 2 (April 1, 2012): 335–43, https://doi.org/10.1007/s10900-011-9450-y.

34. Kliewer, "Epidemiology of Diseases among Migrants."

35. Kliewer, "Epidemiology of Diseases among Migrants."

36. Lê-Scherban et al., "Immigrant Status and Cardiovascular Risk over Time."

37. Ana F. Abraido-Lanza, Bruce P. Dohrenwend, Daisy S. Ng-Mak, and J. Blake Turner, "The Latino Mortality Paradox: A Test of the 'Salmon Bias' and Healthy Migrant Hypotheses," *American Journal of Public Health* 89, no. 10 (1999): 1543–48; Kyriakos S. Markides and Jeannine Coreil, "The Health of Hispanics in the Southwestern United States: An Epidemiologic Paradox," *Public Health Reports* 101, no. 3 (1986): 253; Alberto Palloni and Jeffrey D. Morenoff, "Interpreting the Paradoxical in the Hispanic Paradox: Demographic and Epidemiologic Approaches," *Annals of the New York Academy of Sciences* 954, no. 1 (January 25, 2006): 140–74, https://doi.org/10.1111/j.1749-6632.2001.tb02751.x.

38. Anna S. Lau, William Tsai, Josephine Shih, Lisa L. Liu, Wei-Chin Hwang, and David T. Takeuchi, "The Immigrant Paradox among Asian American Women: Are Disparities in the Burden of Depression and Anxiety Paradoxical or Explicable?," *Journal of Consulting and Clinical Psychology* 81, no. 5 (October 2013), https://doi.org/10.1037/a0032105; Sheng-Shiung Huang and Hao-Jan Yang, "Is There a Healthy Immigrant Effect Among Women Through Transnational Marriage? Results from Immigrant Women from Southeast Asian Countries in Taiwan," *Journal of Immigrant and Minority Health* 20, no. 1 (February 1, 2018): 178–87, https://doi.org/10.1007/s10903-016-0513-0; W. Parker Frisbie, Youngtae Cho, and Robert A. Hummer, "Immigration and the Health of Asian and Pacific Islander Adults in the United States," *American Journal of Epidemiology* 153, no. 4 (2001): 372–80.

39. Abuelezam et al., "Relevance of the 'Immigrant Health Paradox.'"

40. Mara Loveman, Jeronimo O. Muniz, and Stanley R. Bailey, "Brazil in Black and White? Race Categories, the Census, and the Study of Inequality," *Ethnic and Racial Studies* 35, no. 8 (2012): 1466–83.

41. Hephzibah V. Strmic-Pawl, Brandon A. Jackson, and Steve Garner, "Race Counts: Racial and Ethnic Data on the US Census and the Implications for Tracking Inequality," *Sociology of Race and Ethnicity* 4, no. 1 (2018): 1–13.

42. Nadia N. Abuelezam, Abdulrahman M. El-Sayed, and Sandro Galea, "The Health of Arab Americans in the United States: An Updated Comprehensive Literature Review," *Frontiers in Public Health* 6 (September 11, 2018), https://doi.org/10.3389/fpubh.2018.00262.

43. Sarah Abboud, Perla Chebli, and Em Rabelais, "The Contested Whiteness of Arab Identity in the United States: Implications for Health Disparities Research," *American Journal of Public Health* 109, no. 11 (2019): 1580–83.

44. Abboud, Chebli, and Rabelais, "The Contested Whiteness of Arab Identity in the United States."

45. Florence J. Dallo and Tiffany B. Kindratt, "Disparities in Vaccinations and Cancer Screening Among US- and Foreign-Born Arab and European American Non-Hispanic White Women," *Women's Health Issues* 25, no. 1 (January 1, 2015): 56–62, https://doi.org/10.1016/j.whi.2014.10.002; Florence J. Dallo, Julie J. Ruterbusch, Joseph David Kirma, Kendra Schwartz, and Monty Fakhouri, "A Health Profile of Arab Americans in Michigan: A Novel Approach to Using a Hospital Administrative Database," *Journal of Immigrant and Minority Health* 18, no. 6 (December 1, 2016): 1449–54, https://doi.org/10.1007/s10903-015-0296-8; Nadia N. Abuelezam, Abdulrahman M. El-Sayed, and Sandro Galea, "Differences in Health Behaviors and Health Outcomes among Non-Hispanic Whites and Arab Americans in a Population-Based Survey in California," *BMC Public Health* 19, no. 1 (July 8, 2019): 892, https://doi.org/10.1186/s12889-019-7233-z; Nadia N. Abuelezam, Adolfo G. Cuevas, Sandro Galea, and Summer Sherburne Hawkins, "Maternal Health Behaviors and Infant Health Outcomes Among Arab American and Non-Hispanic White Mothers in Massachusetts, 2012–2016," *Public Health Reports* 135, no. 5 (2020), accessed October 28, 2020, https://journals-sagepub-com.proxy.bc.edu /doi/abs/10.1177/0033354920941146.

46. Nicholas A Jones and Michael Bentley, "Overview of 2015 National Content Test Analysis Report on Race & Ethnicity," 2017.

47. US Census Bureau, "Using Two Separate Questions for Race and Ethnicity in 2018 End-to-End Census," US Department of Commerce, Economics, and Statistics Administration, 2018.

48. Nadia N. Abuelezam, "Health Equity During COVID-19: The Case of Arab Americans," *American Journal of Preventive Medicine* 59, no. 3 (2020): 455–57; Nadia N. Abuelezam, Abdulrahman M. El-Sayed, and Sandro Galea, "Arab American Health in a Racially Charged US," *American Journal of Preventive Medicine* 52, no. 6 (June 1, 2017): 810–12, https://doi.org/10.1016/j.amepre.2017.02.021.

49. Zinzi D. Bailey, Nancy Krieger, Madina Agénor, Jasmine Graves, Natalia Linos, and Mary T. Bassett, "Structural Racism and Health Inequities in the USA: Evidence and Interventions," *Lancet* 389, no. 10077 (2017): 1453–63; Sze Yan Liu, Christina Fiorentini, Zinzi Bailey, Mary Huynh, Katharine McVeigh, and Deborah Kaplan, "Structural Racism and Severe Maternal Morbidity in New York State," *Clinical Medicine Insights: Women's Health* 12 (2019): 1179562X19854778; Whitney R. Robinson and Zinzi D. Bailey, "Invited Commentary: What Social Epidemiology Brings to the Table—Reconciling Social Epidemiology and Causal Inference," *American Journal of Epidemiology* 189, no. 3 (March 2, 2020): 171–74, https://doi.org/10.1093/aje/kwz197.

Chapter 27

1. Ana Teresa Fernández, *Foreign Bodies*, exhibition at Gallery Wendi Norris (April 3 to May 31, 2014), https://anateresafernandez.com/foreign-bodies-paintings/.

See also Gallery Wendi Norris, "Ana Teresa Fernández—*Foreign Bodies*," press release, https://www.gallerywendinorris.com/exhibitions-collection/2014/5/3/foreign-bodies.

2. Rens Bod and Julia Kursell, "Introduction: The Humanities and the Sciences," *Isis* 106, no. 2 (2015): 337–40.

3. Therese Jones, Delese Wear, Lester D. Friedman, and Kathleen Pachucki, eds. *Health Humanities Reader* (New Brunswick: Rutgers University Press, 2014).

4. Robert McRuer, *Crip Theory: Cultural Signs of Queerness and Disability* (New York: New York University Press, 2006).

5. Ibrahim Sirkeci and M. Murat Yücesahin, "Coronavirus and Migration: Analysis of Human Mobility and the Spread of COVID-19," *Migration Letters* 17, no. 2 (2020): 379–98, https://doi.org/10.33182/ml.v17i2.935.

6. Gabriella Sanchez and Luigi Achilli, "Stranded: The Impacts of COVID-19 on Irregular Migration and Migrant Smuggling," *Migration Policy Center: Policy Brief* (2020): 1–12, https://doi.org/10.2870/42411.

7. President Trump's references to Covid-19 as the "Chinese virus" have historical roots in the Chinese Exclusion Act of 1882, which was justified by an outbreak of smallpox in San Francisco. Li Zhou, "How the Coronavirus Is Surfacing America's Deep-seated Anti-Asian Biases," *Vox* (2020), https://www.vox.com/identities/2020/4/21/21221007/anti-asian-racism-coronavirus.

8. Chantal Da Silva, "Donald Trump Says Migrants Bring 'Large Scale Crime and Disease' to America," *Newsweek*, December 11, 2018, https://www.newsweek.com/donald-trump-says-migrants-bring-large-scale-crime-and-disease-america-1253268.

9. "Control of Communicable Diseases; Foreign Quarantine: Suspension of Introduction of Persons into United States from Designated Foreign Countries or Places for Public Health Purposes," *Federal Register: The Daily Journal of the United States Government*, March 24, 2020, https://www.federalregister.gov/documents/2020/03/24/2020-06238/control-of-communicable-diseases-foreign-quarantine-suspension-of-introduction-of-persons-into.

10. Caitlin Dickerson, "US Expels Migrant Children From Other Countries to Mexico," *New York Times*, October 30, 2020, https://www.nytimes.com/2020/10/30/us/migrant-children-expulsions-mexico.html?campaign_id=2&emc=edit_th_2020 1031&instance_id=23683&nl=todaysheadlines&regi_id=39002302&segment_id=42984&user_id=018b165cf69f8632a89636c4c27204cc.

11. "Nationwide Enforcement Encounters: Title 8 Enforcement Actions and Title 42 Expulsions," US Customs and Border Protection, updated October 14, 2020, https://www.cbp.gov/newsroom/stats/cbp-enforcement-statistics/title-8-and-title-42-statistics; Caitlin Dickerson, "Inside the Refugee Camp on America's Doorstep," *New York Times*, October 23, 2020, https://www.nytimes.com/2020/10/23/us/mexico-migrant-camp-asylum.html?action=click&module=RelatedLinks&pgtype=Article.

12. Foundational works include Giorgio Agamben, "We Refugees," *Symposium*

49, no. 2 (1995): 114–19; David Farrier, *Postcolonial Asylum: Seeking Sanctuary before the Law* (Liverpool: Liverpool University Press, 2001); and José David Saldívar, *Border Matters: Remapping American Cultural Studies* (Berkeley: University of California Press, 1997).

13. *Oxford English Dictionary Online*, s.v. "Migration," accessed January 17, 2022, https://www-oed-com.ezproxy.bu.edu.

14. Lin-Manuel Miranda and Jeremy McCarter, *Hamilton: The Revolution* (New York: Grand Central, 2016), 121. Leslie M. Harris, "The Greatest City in the World? Slavery in New York in the Age of Hamilton," in *Historians on Hamilton: How a Blockbuster Musical Is Restaging America's Past* (New Brunswick: Rutgers University Press, 2018): 71–93, 71.

15. Trump later said that he was referring only to MS-13 gang members as "animals." See Linda Qiu, "The Context Behind Trump's 'Animals' Comment," *New York Times*, May 18, 2018, https://www.nytimes.com/2018/05/18/us/politics/fact-check-trump-animals-immigration-ms13-sanctuary-cities.html.

16. Rachel St. John, *Line in the Sand: A History of the Western US-Mexico Border* (Princeton: Princeton University Press, 2012).

17. *USA Today*'s "The Wall" provides an interactive map of the shifting Mexico-US border in Ron Dungan, "A Moving Border, and the History of a Difficult Boundary," *USA Today*, 2017, https://www.usatoday.com/border-wall/story/us-mexico-border-history/510833001/.

18. The foundational reading is Benedict Anderson's *Imagined Communities: Reflections on the Origins and Spread of Nationalism* (London: Verso, [1983] 2006).

19. Ana Teresa Fernández, "Erasing the Border," *Ecotone* 14, no. 2.27 (2019): 37–48, 38.

20. Fernández, "Erasing," 45.

21. Fernández, *Foreign Bodies*; Gallery Wendi Norris, "Ana Teresa Fernández."

22. Fernández, "Erasing," 38.

23. Brooke Binkowski, "Border Report: Artist Aims to 'Make the Border Disappear,'" *Voice of San Diego*, April 11, 2016, https://www.voiceofsandiego.org/topics/news/artist-aims-to-make-the-border-disappear/.

24. Brooke Binkowski, "Border Report: Watch the Border Wall Disappear (Again)," *Voice of San Diego*, December 19, 2016, https://www.voiceofsandiego.org/topics/news/border-report-watch-border-wall-disappear/.

Chapter 28

1. Yang, Jia Lynn. *One Mighty and Irresistible Tide: The Epic Struggle over American Immigration, 1924–1965*. New York: Norton, 2020.

2. Yang, *One Mighty and Irresistible Tide*.

3. UNHCR. "Convention and Protocol Related to the Status of Refugees." https://www.unhcr.org/en-us/3b66c2aa10.

4. UNHCR. "Figures at a Glance." https://www.unhcr.org/en-us/figures-at-a-glance .html.

5. Weiwei, Ai. *Human Flow: Stories from the Global Refugee Crisis*. Princeton: Princeton University Press, 2020, 18–19.

6. Weiwei, *Human Flow*, 19.

7. Yang, *One Mighty and Irresistible Tide*.

8. Trump v. Hawaii, 138 S. Ct. 2392 (2018).

9. Weiwei, *Human Flow*.

10. Hirschfeld Davis, Julie, and Michael D. Shear. *Border Wars: Inside Trump's Assault on Immigration*. New York: Simon & Shuster, 2019.

11. Stillman, Sarah. "The Race to Dismantle Trump's Immigration Policies." *New Yorker* (February 8, 2021): 32–51. https://www.newyorker.com/magazine/2021/02/08 /the-race-to-dismantle-trumps-immigration-policies.

12. Trump v, Hawaii, 138 S. Ct. 2392 (2018).

13. ACLU Research Report. "Justice-Free Zones: US Immigration Detention under the Trump Administration." *Human Rights Watch*. https://www.hrw.org/sites /default/files/supporting_resources/justice_free_zones_immigrant_detention.pdf.

14. Toomey, Russell B., Adriana J. Umaña-Taylor, David R. Williams, Elizabeth Harvey-Mendoza, Laudan B. Jahromi, and Kimberly A. Updegraff. "Impact of Arizona's SB 1070 Immigration Law on Utilization of Health Care and Public Assistance Among Mexican-Origin Adolescent Mothers and Their Mother Figures" *Am J Public Health* 104, no. 1 (February 2014): S28–S34. https://doi.org/10.2105 /AJPH.2013.301655.

15. Novak, Nicole L., Arline T. Geronimus, and Aresha M. Martinez-Cardoso. "Change in Birth Outcomes among Infants Born to Latina Mothers after a Major Immigration Raid." *International Journal of Epidemiology* 46, no. 3 (June 2017): 839–49. https://doi.org/10.1093/ije/dyw346.

16. Hacker, Karen, Jocelyn Chu, Lisa Arsenault, and Robert P. Marlin. "Provider's Perspectives on the Impact of Immigration and Customs Enforcement (ICE) Activity on Immigrant Health." *Journal of Health Care for the Poor and Underserved* 23, no. 2 (2012): 651–65. https://doi.org/10.1353/hpu.2012.0052.

17. Sacchetti, Maria. "ICE Chief Tells Lawmakers Agency Needs Much More Money for Immigration Arrests." *Washington Post*, June 13, 2017. https://www.wash ingtonpost.com/local/social-issues/ice-chief-tells-lawmakers-agency-needs-much -more-money-for-immigration-arrests/2017/06/13/86651e86-5054-11e7-b064-828 ba60fbb98_story.html?utm_term=.4c22b37ee45a.

18. Pew Research Center. "Key Facts about U.S. Immigration Policies and Biden's Proposed Changes," January 11, 2022. https://www.pewresearch.org/fact-tank/2022 /01/11/key-facts-about-u-s-immigration-policies-and-bidens-proposed-changes/.

19. Human Rights First. "Publicly Reported MPP Attacks," February 19, 2021. https://www.humanrightsfirst.org/sites/default/files/PubliclyReportedMPPAttacks 2.19.2021.pdf.

20. Public Health Service Act, 42 U.S.C. §§ 264–272 (2012).

21. Public Health Service Act, 42 U.S.C. §§ 264–272 (2012).

22. Ulrich, Michael R., and Sondra S. Crosby. "Title 42, Asylum, and Politicising Public Health." *Lancet Regional Health–Americas*, March 2022. https://doi.org /10.1016/j.lana.2021.100124.

23. Human Rights First. "A Shameful Record: Biden Administration's Use of Trump Policies Endangers People Seeking Asylum." January 13, 2022. https://www .humanrightsfirst.org/resource/shameful-record-biden-administration-s-use-trump -policies-endangers-people-seeking-asylum.

24. Health Affairs. "Biden's Shot at a Better Public Health Rule." https://www .healthaffairs.org/do/10.1377/forefront.20210924.126765/full/.

25. Wang, R.Y., M. C. Rojo, S. S. Crosby et al. "Examining the Impact of Restrictive Federal Immigration Policies on Healthcare Access: Perspectives from Immigrant Patients across an Urban Safety-Net Hospital." *J Immigrant Minority Health* 24, 178–87 (2022). https://doi.org/10.1007/s10903-021-01177-9.

26. Children's Hospital of Philadelphia PolicyLab. "Thawing the Chill from Public Charge Will Take Time and Investment." https://policylab.chop.edu/blog/thawing -chill-public-charge-will-take-time-and-investment.

27. Artiga, S, R. Garfield, and A. Damico. "Estimated Impacts of Final Public Charge Inadmissibility Rule on Immigrants and Medicaid Coverage: Key Findings." 2019. https://www.kff.org/report-section/estimated-impacts-of-final-public-charge -inadmissibility-rule-on-immigrants-and-medicaid-coverage-key-findings.

28. White House Briefing, February 2, 2021. https://www.whitehouse.gov/brief ing-room/speeches-remarks/2021/02/02/remarks-by-president-biden-at-signing-of -executive-orders-advancing-his-priority-to-modernize-our-immigration-system/.

29. Nguyen, Viet Thanh. "I Can't Forget the Lessons from Vietnam: Neither Should You." *New York Times*, August 8, 2021. https://www.nytimes.com/2021/08/19 /opinion/afghanistan-vietnam-war-refugees.html.

Chapter 29

1. Ingleby, David. "Ethnicity, Migration and the 'Social Determinants of Health' Agenda." *Psychosocial Intervention* 21, no. 3 (2012): 331–41.

2. Labonté, Ronald, and Arne Ruckert. *Health Equity in a Globalizing Era: Past Challenges, Future Prospects*. Oxford: Oxford University Press, 2019.

3. Thomas, Felicity, ed. *Handbook of Migration and Health*. Cheltenham: Edward Elgar, 2016.

4. Arnold, Christine, Jason Theede, and Anita Gagnon. "A Qualitative Exploration of Access to Urban Migrant Healthcare in Nairobi, Kenya." *Social Science and Medicine* 110 (2014): 1–9.

5. Spahl, Wanda, and August Österle. "Stratified Membership: Health Care Access for Urban Refugees in Turkey." *Comparative Migration Studies* 7, no. 42 (2019).

6. Abubakar, Ibrahim, Robert W. Aldridge, Delan Devakumar, Miriam Orcutt, Rachel Burns, Mauricio L. Barreto, Poonam Dhavan et al. "The UCL–Lancet Commission on Migration and Health: The Health of a World on the Move." *Lancet* 392, no. 10164 (2018): 2606–54.

7. United Nations General Assembly. "Transforming Our World: The 2030 Agenda for Sustainable Development," New York, 2015.

8. United Nations General Assembly. "New York Declaration for Refugees and Migrants," New York, 2016.

9. United Nations General Assembly. "New York Declaration for Refugees and Migrants," October 3, 2016, Resolution adopted by the General Assembly on September 19, 2016. https://www.un.org/en/development/desa/population/migration/gen eralassembly/docs/globalcompact/A_RES_71_1.pdf.

10. Wickramage, Kolitha, Jo Vearey, Anthony B. Zwi, Courtland Robinson, and Michael Knipper. "Migration and Health: A Global Public Health Research Priority." *BMC Public Health* 18, no. 1 (2018): 1–9.

11. Kontunen, Kaisa, Barbara Rijks, Nenette Motus, Jenna Iodice, Caroline Schultz, and Davide Mosca. "Ensuring Health Equity of Marginalized Populations: Experiences from Mainstreaming the Health of Migrants." *Health Promotion International* 29, no. 1 (2014): i121–29.

12. Labonté and Ruckert, *Health Equity in a Globalizing Era.*

13. Schierup, Carl-Ulrik, Aleksandra Ålund, and Branka Likić-Brborić. "Migration, Precarization and the Democratic Deficit in Global Governance." *International Migration* 53, no. 3 (2015): 50–63.

14. Lougarre, Claire. "Using the Right to Health to Promote Universal Health Coverage: A Better Tool for Protecting Non-Nationals' Access to Affordable Health Care?" *Health and Human Rights* 18, no. 2 (2016): 35.

15. Abubakar et al., "The UCL–Lancet Commission on Migration and Health."

16. Mladovsky, Philipa, David Ingleby, and Bernd Rechel. "Good Practices in Migrant Health: The European Experience." *Clinical Medicine* 12, no. 3 (2012): 248.

17. Salami, Bukola, Stella Iwuagwu, Oluwakemi Amodu, Mia Tulli, Chizoma Ndikom, Hayat Gommaa, Tina Lavin, and Michael Kariwo. "The Health of Internally Displaced Children in Sub-Saharan Africa: A Scoping Review." *BMJ Global Health* 5, no. 8 (2020): e002584.

18. Whelan, Isabelle. "The Effect of United Kingdom Immigration Policies on Migrant Access to Sexual and Reproductive Healthcare." *BMJ Sexual and Reproductive Health* 45, no. 1 (2019): 74–77.

19. Ingleby, David, Roumyana Petrova-Benedict, Thomas Huddleston, and Elena Sanchez. "The MIPEX Health Strand: A Longitudinal, Mixed-Methods Survey of Policies on Migrant Health in 38 Countries." *European Journal of Public Health* 29, no. 3 (2019): 458–62.

20. Lu, Yao, and Alice Tianbo Zhang. "The Link between Migration and Health." In Thomas, *Handbook of Migration and Health.*

21. Hasan-ul-Bari, S. M., and Tarek Ahmed. "Ensuring Sexual and Reproductive Health and Rights of Rohingya Women and Girls." *Lancet* 392, no. 10163 (2018): 2439–40.

22. Turner, Lewis. "Are Syrian Men Vulnerable Too? Gendering the Syria Refugee Response." *Middle East Institute*, November 29, 2016.

23. Abubakar et al., "The UCL–Lancet Commission on Migration and Health."

24. Chase, Elaine, and Jenny Allsopp. *Youth Migration and the Politics of Wellbeing: Stories of Life in Transition*. Bristol, UK: Bristol University Press, 2020.

25. El-Lahib, Yahya, and Samantha Wehbi. "Immigration and Disability: Ableism In the Policies of the Canadian State." *International Social Work* 55, no. 1 (2012): 95–108.

26. Hargreaves, Sally, Bernadette N. Kumar, Martin McKee, Lucy Jones, and Apostolos Veizis. "Europe's Migrant Containment Policies Threaten the Response to Covid-19." *BMJ* 368 (2020): m1213.

27. Kluge, Hans Henri P., Zsuzsanna Jakab, Jozef Bartovic, Veronika D'Anna, and Santino Severoni. "Refugee and Migrant Health in the COVID-19 Response." *Lancet* 395, no. 10232 (2020): 1237–39.

28. Hargreaves et al., "Europe's Migrant Containment Policies."

29. World Health Organization (WHO). "Coronavirus Disease 2019 (COVID-19): Situation Report 35," 2020.

30. Guadagno, Lorenzo. "Migrants and the COVID-19 Pandemic: An Initial Analysis." *International Organization for Migration, Migration Research Series* 60 (2020).

31. Guadagno, "Migrants and the COVID-19 Pandemic."

32. Phillimore, Jenny. "Migrant Maternity in an Era of Superdiversity: New Migrants' Access to, and Experience of, Antenatal Care in the West Midlands, UK." *Social Science and Medicine* 148 (2016): 152–59.

33. Klein, Jens, and Olaf von dem Knesebeck. "Inequalities in Health Care Utilization among migrants and non-Migrants in Germany: A Systematic Review." *International Journal for Equity in Health* 17, no. 1 (2018): 160.

34. Ingleby, "Ethnicity, Migration and the 'Social Determinants of Health' Agenda."

35. WHO. "Migration and Health: Enhancing Intercultural Competence and Diversity Sensitivity," 2020.

36. Tervalon, Melanie, and Jann Murray-Garcia. "Cultural Humility versus Cultural Competence: A Critical Distinction in Defining Physician Training Outcomes in Multicultural Education." *Journal of Health Care for the Poor and Underserved* 9, no. 2 (1998): 117–25.

37. WHO, "Migration and Health."

38. Bischoff, Alexander, Antonio Chiarenza, and Louis Loutan. "'Migrant-Friendly Hospitals': A European Initiative in an Age of Increasing Mobility." *World Hospitals and Health Services* 45, no. 3 (2009): 7.

39. Owiti, J. Ajaz, A. Ajaz, M. Ascoli, B. De Jongh, A. Palinski, and K. S. Bhui. "Cultural Consultation as a Model for Training Multidisciplinary Mental Healthcare Professionals in Cultural Competence Skills: Preliminary Results." *Journal of Psychiatric and Mental Health Nursing* 21, no. 9 (2014): 814–26.

40. Knipper, Michael. "Joining Ethnography and History in Cultural Competence Training." *Culture, Medicine, and Psychiatry* 37, no. 2 (2013): 373–84.

41. van den Muijsenbergh, Maria, Evelyn van Weel-Baumgarten, Nicola Burns, Catherine O'Donnell, Frances Mair, Wolfgang Spiegel, Christos Lionis et al. "Communication in Cross-Cultural Consultations in Primary Care in Europe: The Case for Improvement. The Rationale for the RESTORE FP 7 Project." *Primary Health Care Research and Development* 15, no. 2 (2014): 122–33.

42. Gray, Ben, Jo Hilder, and Maria Stubbe. "How to Use Interpreters in General Practice: The Development of a New Zealand Toolkit." *Journal of Primary Health Care* 4, no. 1 (2012): 52–61.

43. van den Muijsenbergh et al., "Communication in Cross-Cultural Consultations in Primary Care in Europe."

44. MacFarlane, Anne, Mary O'Reilly-de Brún, Tomas De Brún, Christopher Dowrick, Catherine O'Donnell, Frances Mair, Wolfgang Spiegel et al. "Healthcare for Migrants, Participatory Health Research and Implementation Science—Better Health Policy and Practice through Inclusion. The RESTORE Project." *European Journal of General Practice* 20, no. 2 (2014): 148–52.

45. Gray et al., "How to Use Interpreters in General Practice."

46. Dauvrin, Marie. "Cultural Competence in Health Care: Challenging Inequalities, Involving Institutions." *Université catholique de Louvain* 390 (2013).

47. TIME Project Partnership. "Description of 10 Good Practices in Intercultural Mediation for Immigrants throughout Europe and Suggestions for Transfer," 2015, 39; WHO. "Health Workforce," 2020. https://www.who.int/health-topics/health-workforce#tab=tab_1.

48. WHO, "Health Workforce."

49. Masanjala, Winford H. "Brain Drain in Africa: The Case of Tackling Capacity Issues in Malawi's Medical Migration," 2018.

50. Buchan, James, Barbara McPake, Kwadwo Mensah, and George Rae. "Does a Code Make a Difference—Assessing the English Code of Practice on International Recruitment." *Human Resources for Health* 7, no. 1 (2009): 1–8.

51. Shah, Rebecca. "International Health Worker Migration: Global Inequality and the Right to Health." In *Migration, Health and Inequality*, edited by Felicity Thomas and Jasmine Gideon. London: Zed Books, 2013.

52. Mansuri, Ghazala. *Migration, Sex Bias, and Child Growth in Rural Pakistan.* The World Bank, 2006.

53. Nguyen, Cuong Viet. "Does Parental Migration Really Benefit Left-Behind Children? Comparative Evidence from Ethiopia, India, Peru and Vietnam." *Social Science and Medicine* 153 (2016): 230–39.

54. Fellmeth, Gracia, Kelly Rose-Clarke, Chenyue Zhao, Laura K. Busert, Yun-ting Zheng, Alessandro Massazza, Hacer Sonmez et al. "Health Impacts of Parental Migration on Left-Behind Children and Adolescents: A Systematic Review and Meta-Analysis." *Lancet* 392, no. 10164 (2018): 2567–82.

Chapter 30

1. Abby Budiman. "Key Findings about US Immigrants," FactTank News in the Numbers. Pew Research Center, August 20, 2020. Accessed September 7, 2020. https://www.pewresearch.org/fact-tank/2020/08/20/key-findings-about-u-s-immigrants/.

2. Fernando Riosmena, Randall Kuhn, and Warren C. Jochem. "Explaining the Immigrant Health Advantage: Self-Selection and Protection in Health-Related Factors among Five National-Origin Immigrant Groups in the United States." *Demography* 54, no. 1 (February 2017): 175–200. https:// doi.org/10.1007/s13524-016-0542-2.

3. Howard Markel and Alexandra Minna Stern. "The Foreignness of Germs: The Persistent Association of Immigrants and Disease in American Society." *Milbank Quarterly* 80, no. 4 (December 2002): 757–88. https://doi.org/10.1111/1468-0009.00030.

4. Edna A. Viruell-Fuentes, Patria Y. Miranda, and Sawsan Abdulrahim. "More Than Culture: Structural Racism, Intersectionality Theory, and Immigrant Health." *Social Science and Medicine* 75, no. 12 (December 2012): 2099–106. https://doi.org/10.1016/j.socscimed.2011.12.037.

5. Shazeen Suleman, Kent D. Garber, and Lainie Rutkow. "Xenophobia as a Determinant of Health: An Integrative Review." *Journal of Public Health Policy* 39, no. 4 (November 2018): 407–23. https://doi.org/ 10.1057/s41271-018-0140-1.

6. Heather Antecol and Kelly Bedard. "Unhealthy Assimilation: Why Do Immigrants Converge to American Health Status Levels?" *Demography* 43 (2006): 337–60.

7. Edward D. Vargas, Gabriel R. Sanchez, and Melina Juárez. "Fear by Association: Perceptions of Anti-Immigrant Policy and Health Outcomes." *Journal of Health Politics, Policy and Law* 42, no. 3 (June 2017): 459–83. https://doi.org/10.1215/03616878-3802940.

8. Kaiser Family Foundation. "Health Coverage of Immigrants," March 18, 2020. Accessed September 7, 2020. https://www.kff.org/disparities-policy/fact-sheet/health-coverage-of-immigrants/.

9. Thomas C. Buchmueller, Anthony T. Lo Sasso, Ithai Lurie, and Sarah Dolfin. "Immigrants and Employer-Sponsored Health Insurance." *Health Services Research* 42, no. 1 (2007): 286–310. https:// doi.org/10.1111/j.1475-6773.2006.00600.x.

10. Arloc Sherman et al. "Immigrants Contribute Greatly to US Economy, Despite Administration's 'Public Charge' Rule Rationale." Washington, DC: Center on Budget and Policy Priorities, August 15, 2019. Accessed October 22, 2020. https://

www.cbpp.org/research/poverty-and-inequality/immigrants-contribute-greatly-to
-us-economy-despite-administrations.

11. Daniel Costa, David Cooper, and Heidi Shierholz. "Facts about Immigration and the US Economy: Answers to Frequently Asked Questions." Washington,
DC: Economic Policy Institute, August 12, 2014. Accessed October 22, 2020. https://
www.epi.org/publication/immigration-facts/.

12. Dan Kosten. "Immigrants as Economic Contributors: Immigrant Tax Contributions and Spending Power," National Immigration Forum, September 6, 2018.
Accessed October 22, 2020. https://immigrationforum.org/article/immigrants-as
-economic-contributors-immigrant-tax-contributions-and-spending-power/.

13. 8 U.S.C.A. § 1396.

14. 8 U.S.C.A. § 1396b(v)(1).

15. Pub. L. No. 104-193, 110 Stat. 2105 (August 22, 1996).

16. 8 U.S.C.A § 1395dd.

17. 42 U.S.C.A. § 1395dd(e)(1).

18. Lauren A. Dame. "The Emergency Medical Treatment and Active Labor
Act: The Anomalous Right to Health Care," *Health Care Matrix* 8, no. 1 (1998): 3–
28. https://scholarlycommons.law.case.edu/healthmatrix/vol8/iss1/20.

19. 42 U.S.C.A. § 1395dd(e)(1).

20. Alexia Elejalde-Ruiz. "Fear, Anxiety, Apprehension: Immigrants Fear Doctor Visits Could Leave Them Vulnerable to Deportation," *Chicago Tribune*, June 22,
2018. Accessed November 4, 2020. https://www.chicagotribune.com/business/ct-biz
-immigration-fears-hurt-health-care-access-0225-story.html.

21. Kaiser Family Foundation, "Health Coverage of Immigrants."

22. Scott D. Rhodes, Lilli Mann, Florence H. Simán, Eunyoung Song, Jorge
Alonzo, Mario Downs, Emma Lawlor, Omar Martinez, Christina J. Sun, Mary Claire
O'Brien, Beth A. Reboussin, and Mark A. Hall. "The Impact of Local Immigration
Enforcement Policies on the Health of Immigrant Hispanics/Latinos in the United
States." *American Journal of Public Health* 105, no. 2 (February 2015): 329–37.
https://doi.org/10.2105/AJPH.2014.302218.

23. Cindy Mann. Letter to State Official and Medicaid Director, August 28, 2012,
Center for Medicaid and CHIP Services, "Re: Individuals with Deferred Action
for Childhood Arrivals," SHO# 12-002. Accessed September 7, 2019. https://www
.medicaid.gov/Federal-Policy-Guidance/downloads/SHO-12-002.pdf.

24. Tricia Brooks, Lauren Roygardner, and Samantha Artiga. *Medicaid and CHIP
Eligibility, Enrollment, and Cost Sharing Policies as of January 2019: Findings from a
50-State Survey*. Washington, DC: Kaiser Family Foundation, March 27, 2019. Accessed September 7, 2020. https://www.kff.org/medicaid/report/medicaid-and-chip
-eligibility-enrollment-and-cost-sharing-policies-as-of-january-2019-findings-from
-a-50-state-survey/.

25. Alameda County Public Health Department. *Immigration and Public Health:
An Issue Brief*, July 2017. Accessed November 4, 2020. https://acphd-web-media

.s3-us-west-2.amazonaws.com/media/data-reports/fact-sheets-presentations/docs/immigration.pdf.

26. Rhodes et al., "Impact of Local Immigration Enforcement Policies."

27. Tiffany D. Joseph. "What Health Care Reform Means for Immigrants: Comparing the Affordable Care Act and Massachusetts Health Reforms." *Journal of Health Politics, Policy and Law* 41, no. 1 (2016): 101–16. https://doi.org/10.1215/03616878-3445632.

28. Jennifer Tolbert, Kendal Orgera, Natalie Singer, and Anthony Damico. "Key Facts about the Uninsured Population," Kaiser Family Foundation, December 20, 2019. Accessed September 7, 2020. https://www.kff.org/uninsured/issue-brief/key-facts-about-the-uninsured-population/.

29. Kaiser Family Foundation, "Health Coverage of Immigrants."

30. Arturo Vargas Bustamante, Jie Chen, Ryan M. McKenna, and Alexander N. Ortega. "Health Care Access and Utilization among US Immigrants Before and After the Affordable Care Act." *Journal of Immigrant and Minority Health* 21 (April 2019): 211–18. https://doi.org/10.1007/s10903-018-0741-6.

31. Stephen Zuckerman, Timothy A. Waidman, and Emily Lawson. "Undocumented Immigrants, Left Out of Health Reform, Likely to Continue to Grow as Share of the Uninsured." *Health Affairs* 30, no. 10 (2011): 1997–2004. https://doi.org/10.1377/hlthaff.2011.0604.

32. INA § 212(a)(4), 8 U.S.C. § 1182(a)(4).

33. United States Citizenship and Immigration Services. "Public Charge." Accessed September 7, 2020. https://www.uscis.gov/greencard/public-charge.

34. Immigrant Legal Resource Center. "U Visa/T Visa/VAWA." Accessed October 19, 2020. https://www.ilrc.org/u-visa-t-visa-vawa.

35. National Immigrant Women's Advocacy Project. "VAWA Public Benefits Eligibility Process: VAWA Self-Petitioners, VAWA Cancellation of Removal, and VAWA Suspension of Deportation." Accessed October 18, 2020. https://niwaplibrary.wcl.american.edu/pubs/vawa-eligibility-process.

36. Kaiser Family Foundation, "Health Coverage of Immigrants."

37. Mariana Chilton, Maureen M. Black, Carol Berkowitz, Patrick H. Casey, John Cook, Diana Cutts, Ruth Rose Jacobs, Timothy Heeren, Stephanie Ettinger de Cuba, Sharon Coleman, Alan Meyers, and Deborah A. Frank. "Food Insecurity and Risk of Poor Health Among US-Born Children of Immigrants." *American Journal of Public Health* 99, no. 3 (March 2009): 556–62. https://doi.org/10.2105/AJPH.2008.144394.

38. Department of Homeland Security. "2019 Public Charge Rule Vacated and Removed; DHS Withdraws Proposed Rule Regarding the Affidavit of Support." March 11, 2021. Accessed August 27, 2021. https://www.dhs.gov/news/2021/03/11/2019-public-charge-rule-vacated-and-removed-dhs-withdraws-proposed-rule-regarding.

39. Pub. L. No. 104–208, 110 Stat. 3009-546 (September 30, 1996).

40. 8 U.S.C.A. § 1183a.

41. National Immigrant Law Center. "Sponsored Immigrants & Benefits," August 2009. Accessed October 18, 2020. https://www.nilc.org/wp-content/uploads/2016/05/sponsoredimmsbens-na-2009-08.pdf.

42. Arturo Vargas Bustamante, Jie Chen, John A. Rizzo, and Alexander N. Ortega. "Identifying Health Insurance Predictors and the Main Reported Reasons for Being Uninsured among US Immigrants by Legal Authorization Status." *International Journal of Health Planning and Management* 29 (2014): e83–e96. https://doi.org.10.1002/hpm.2214.

43. Donald W. Light. "Categorical Inequality, Institutional Ambivalence, and Permanently Failing Institutions: The Case of Immigrants and Barriers to Health Care in America." *Ethnic and Racial Studies* 35, no. 1 (2012): 23–39. https://doi.org/10.1080/01419870.2011.594172.

44. Alejandro Portes, Patricia Fernandez-Kelly, and Donald W. Light. "Life on the Edge: Immigrants Confront the American Health System." *Ethnic and Racial Studies* 35, no. 1(2012): 3–22. https://doi.org/10.1080/01419870.2011.594173.

45. Leo R. Chavez. "Undocumented Immigrants and Their Use of Medical Services in Orange County, California." *Social Science and Medicine* 74, no. 6 (March 2012): 887–93. https://doi.org/10.1016/j.socscimed.2011.05.023.

46. Peter Shin, Jessica Sharac, Sara Rosenbaum, and Julia Paradise. "Community Health Centers: A 2013 Profile and Prospects as ACA Implementation Proceeds," Kaiser Family Foundation, March 17, 2015. Accessed September 7, 2020. https://www.kff.org/medicaid/issue-brief/community-health-centers-a-2013-profile-and-prospects-as-aca-implementation-proceeds/.

47. Kaiser Commission on Medicaid and the Uninsured. "Community Health Centers in an Era of Health Reform: An Overview and Key Challenges to Health Center Growth Executive Summary 2013," March 2013. Accessed September 7, 2020. https://www.kff.org/wp-content/uploads/2013/03/8098-03_es.pdf.

48. Jie Chen and Arturo Vargas-Bustamante. "Estimating the Effects of Immigration Status on Mental Health Care Utilizations in the United States." *Journal of Immigrant and Minority Health* 13, no. 4 (February 2011): 671–80. https://doi.org/10.1007/s10903-011-9445-x.

49. Amelia Seraphia Derr. "Mental Health Service Use among Immigrants in the United States: A Systematic Review." *Psychiatric Services* 67, no. 3 (2016): 265–74. https://doi.org/10.1176/appi.ps.201500004.

50. Project on Government Oversight. "Isolated: ICE Confines Some Detainees with Mental Illness in Solitary for Months," August 14, 2019. Accessed September 29, 2020. https://www.pogo.org/investigation/2019/08/isolated-ice-confines-some-detainees-with-mental-illness-in-solitary-for-months/.

51. Veronica Venture and Dana Salvano-Dunn. Office for Civil Rights and Civil Liberties, US Department of Homeland Security, Memorandum to Matthew Albence, Executive Associate Director, Enforcement and Removal Operation, April 25,

2018. Accessed October 18, 2020. https://www.dhs.gov/sites/default/files/publications/adelanto-expert-memo-04-25-18.pdf.

52. Megan Finno-Velasquez, Jodi Berger Cardoso, Alan J. Dettlaff, and Michael S. Hurlburt. "Effects of Parent Immigration Status on Mental Health Service Use among Latino Children Referred to Child Welfare." *Psychiatric Services* 67, no. 2 (February 2016): 192–98. https://doi.org/10.1176/appi.ps.201400444.

53. Lisa R. Fortuna, Michelle V. Porche, and Margarita Alegria. "Political Violence, Psychosocial Trauma, and the Context of Mental Health Services Use among Immigrant Latinos in the United States." *Ethnicity and Health* 13, no. 5 (2008): 435–63. https://doi.org/10.1080/13557850701837286.

54. Rhodes et al., "Impact of Local Immigration Enforcement Policies."

55. Grace Kim, Renee Lahey, Marcus Silva, and Sean Tan. "Public Charge and the Threat to Immigrant Families in California: Reducing the Chilling Effect on Medi-Cal Participation." Los Angeles: UCLA Luskin School of Public Affairs, California Immigrant Policy Center, 2019. Accessed October 11, 2020. https://luskin.ucla.edu/wp-content/uploads/2019/06/4PublicCharge.FINAL_.MP_.pdf.

56. INA § 212(a)(1)(A), 8 U.S.C. § 1182(a)(1)(A).

57. INA § 212(a)(6)(C), 8 U.S.C. § 1182(a)(6)(C).

58. Pub. L. No. 106-386 (October 28, 2000).

59. INA § 214(o)(2), 8 U.S.C. § 1184(o)(2).

60. Kathryn M. Doan. "The T Visa Protection for Young Victims of Narco Human Trafficking." Accessed 2013. https://caircoalition.org/2013/11/04/the-t-visa-protection-for-young-victims-of-narco-human-trafficking.

61. Gosia Wozniacka. "Little Known Visas Free Immigrants from Abuse," *Oregonian*, March 26, 2019 [July 18, 2009]. Accessed August 27, 2021. https://www.oregonlive.com/news/2009/07/littleknown_visas_free_immigra.html.

62. Yael Schacher. "Abused Blamed, and Refused: Protection Denied to Women and Children Trafficked Over the US Southern Border," Field Report. *Refugees International* (May 2019). Accessed August 27, 2021. https://reliefweb.int/sites/reliefweb.int/files/resources/Trafficking%2BReport%2B-%2BMay%2B2019%2B-%2BFinal.pdf.

63. United States Center for Medicare and Medicaid Services. "Immigration Status and the Marketplace." Accessed September 2, 2021. https://www.healthcare.gov/immigrants/immigration-status/.

64. INA § 212(a)(4)(E)(iii), 8 U.S.C. § 1182(a)(4)(E)(iii).

65. INA § 245(l), 8 U.S.C. § 1255(l).

66. 8 C.F.R. § 214.14.

67. INA § 212(a)(4)(E)(ii), 8 U.S.C. § 1182(a)(4)(E)(ii).

68. Pub. L. No. 103-322.

69. INA § 212(a), 8 U.S.C. § 1182(a).

70. United States Center for Medicare and Medicaid Services. "Coverage for Lawfully Present Immigrants." Accessed September 2, 2021. https://www.healthcare.gov/immigrants/lawfully-present-immigrants/.

71. INA § 208, 8 U.S.C. § 1158.

72. Matter of A-R-C-G-, 26 I & N Dec. 388 (BIA 2014).

73. Matter of Kasinga, 21 I & N Dec. 357 (BIA 1996).

74. Bah v. Mukasey, 529 F.3d 99 (2d Cir. 2008).

75. Avendano-Hernandez v. Lynch, 800 F.3d 1072 (9th Cir. 2015).

76. Matter of Toboso-Alfonso, 20 I & N Dec. 819 (BIA 1990).

77. Matter of W-G-R-, 26 I & N Dec. 208 (BIA 2014).

78. Joel Rose. "The Justice Department Overturns Policy That Limited Asylum for Survivors of Violence," NPR. Accessed September 2, 2021. https://www .npr.org/2021/06/16/1007277888/the-justice-department-overturns-rules-that-limited -asylum-for-survivors-of-viol.

79. Katherin Wikholm, Ranit Mishori, Deborah Ottenheimer, Valeriy Korostyshevskiy, Rebecca Reingold, Colin Wikholm, and Kathryn Hampton. "Female Genital Mutilation/Cutting as Grounds for Asylum Requests in the US: An Analysis of More Than 100 Cases." *Journal of Immigrant and Minority Health* 22, no. 4 (2020): 675–81. https://doi.org/10.1007/s10903-020-00994-8.

80. Mary Dutton, Leslye Orloff, and Giselle Aguilar Hass. "Characteristics of Help-Seeking Behaviors, Resources, and Services Needs of Battered Immigrant Latinas: Legal and Policy Implications." *Georgetown Journal on Poverty Law and Policy* 7, no. 2 (2000): 1–53.

81. Leslye Orloff and Janice V. Kaguyutan. "Offering a Helping Hand: Legal Protections for Battered Immigrant Women: A History of Legislative Responses." *American University Journal of Gender, Social Policy, and Law* 10, no. 1 (2002): 95–170.

82. New York City Department of Health and Mental Hygiene. "Femicide in New York City," October 2004. Accessed September 2, 2021. http://www.ncdsv.org /images/NYCDH_femicide-in-nyc-1995-2002.pdf.

Chapter 31

1. Mixed Migration Centre, "Mixed Migration Review 2020." Accessed January 14, 2021. http://www.mixedmigration.org/wp-content/uploads/2020/11/Mixed -Migration-Review-2020.pdf.

2. Russell King, "Migration and Development in the Mediterranean Region," *Geography* 81, no. 1 (1996): 3–14.

3. Corrado Bonifazi and Marija Mamolo, "Past and Current Trends of Balkan Migrations," *Espace Populations Sociétés*, no. 2004/3 (December 1, 2004): 519–31. https://doi.org/10.4000/eps.356.

4. IOM, "Mixed Migration Flows in the Mediterranean and Beyond." Accessed January 19, 2021. https://www.iom.int/sites/default/files/situation_reports/file/Mixed -Flows-Mediterranean-and-Beyond-Compilation-Overview-2015.pdf.

5. UNdata, "Net Migration Rate (per 1,000 Population)." Accessed January 19, 2021. http://data.un.org/Data.aspx?q=MIGRATION&d=PopDiv&f=variableID%3A85.

6. Heaven Crawley et al., "Understanding the Dynamics and Drivers of Mediterranean Migration in 2015," November 2016, 84.

7. IOM, "Flows Compilation Report July 2018." Accessed January 14, 2021. https://migration.iom.int/docs/Flows_Compilation_Report_July_2018.pdf.

8. UNHCR, "Global Trends; Forced Displacement in 2019." Accessed January 19, 2021. https://www.unhcr.org/5ee200e37.pdf.

9. Rebecca Kilberg, "Turkey's Evolving Migration Identity," Migration Policy Institute, July 24, 2014. https://www.migrationpolicy.org/article/turkeys-evolving-migration-identity.

10. Diana Rayes, "Amid an Unfolding Humanitarian Crisis in Syria, the European Union Faces the Perils of Devolving Migration Management to Turkey," Migration Policy Institute, March 20, 2020. https://www.migrationpolicy.org/article/amid-humanitarian-crisis-syria-eu-faces-perils-devolving-migration-third-countries.

11. UNHCR, "Mediterranean Situation." Accessed January 19, 2021. https://data2.unhcr.org/ar/situations/mediterranean/location/5179.

12. European Court of Auditors, "Asylum, Relocation and Return of Migrants: Time to Step up Action to Address Disparities between Objectives and Results," 2019, 86.

13. InfoMigrants, "Over 1,000 Migrants Relocated from Greece in 2020," October 2, 2020. https://www.infomigrants.net/en/post/27697/over-1-000-migrants-relocated-from-greece-in-2020.

14. Martin Altemeyer-Bartscher et al., "On the Distribution of Refugees in the EU," *Intereconomics* 2016, no. 4 (2016): 220–28.

15. World Bank Group, "An Uncertain Recovery: Western Balkans Regular Economic Report, Fall 2020." Accessed January 21, 2021. https://openknowledge.worldbank.org/bitstream/handle/10986/34644/153774.pdf.

16. UNODC, "UNODC New Research: How COVID-19 Restrictions and the Economic Consequences Are Likely to Impact Migrant Smuggling and Cross-Border Trafficking in Persons to Europe and North America." Accessed January 21, 2021. https://www.unodc.org/islamicrepublicofiran/en/unodc-new-research_-how-covid-19-restrictions-and-the-economic-consequences-are-likely-to-impact-migrant-smuggling-and-cross-border-trafficking-in-persons-to-europe-and-north-america.html.

17. IOM, "Turkey—Migrant Presence Monitoring—Situation Report," November 2019. Accessed January 21, 2021. https://dtm.iom.int/reports/turkey-migrant-presence-monitoring-situation-report-november-2019.

18. European Commission, "EU—Turkey Statement: Two Years On," 2018. Accessed January 21, 2021. https://brussels.fes.de/e/the-eu-turkey-statement-two-years-on-lessons-learned.

19. UNHCR Operational Data Portal (ODP), "UNHCR Greece Factsheet October 2020." Accessed January 21, 2021. https://data2.unhcr.org/en/documents/details/83459.

20. IOM, "Flows Compilation Report July 2018."

21. IOM, "Europe— Flow Monitoring." Accessed January 22, 2021. https://relief web.int/report/world/flow-monitoring-europe.

22. Save the Children, "Balkans Migration and Displacement Hub Data and Trend Analysis: Regional Overview (January–March 2019)." Accessed January 22, 2021. https://resourcecentre.savethechildren.net/node/15379/pdf/refugees_and_mi grants_balkans_regional_overview_q1_2019_sc_bmdh_data.pdf.

23. Mixed Migration Centre, "Mixed Migration Review 2020."

24. Jovana Arsenijević et al., "A Crisis of Protection and Safe Passage: Violence Experienced by Migrants/Refugees Travelling along the Western Balkan Corridor to Northern Europe," *Conflict and Health* 11, no. 1 (April 16, 2017): 6. https://doi .org/10.1186/s13031-017-0107-z.

25. REACH, "Migration to Europe through the Western Balkans." Accessed January 22, 2021. https://reliefweb.int/sites/reliefweb.int/files/resources/reach_report _consolidated_report_on_migration_to_europe_through_the_western_balkans_2015 -2016_july_2016.pdf.

26. IOM, "Migrants' Presence Monitoring Quarterly Report Q4 Oct-Nov-Dec-20." Accessed January 22, 2021. https://displacement.iom.int/system/tdf/reports/Q4_quar terly-Oct-Nov-Dec-20.pdf?file=1&type=node&id=10597.

27. UNHCR, "UNHCR Greece Factsheet October 2020."

28. IOM, "DTM Mediterranean—Western Balkans Overview 2019." Accessed January 22, 2021. http://reports/dtm-mediterranean-%E2%80%93-western-balkans -overview-2019.

29. Asylum Information Database, "Identification." Accessed January 22, 2021. https://asylumineurope.org/reports/country/greece/asylum-procedure/guarantees -vulnerable-groups/identification/.

30. Thomas Papadimos et al., "Health Security and the Refugee Crisis in Greece: The Refugee Perspective," *Contemporary Developments and Perspectives in International Health Security* 1 (April 29, 2020). https://doi.org/10.5772/intechopen .91210.

31. Ameer Kakaje et al., "Mental Disorder and PTSD in Syria during Wartime: A Nationwide Crisis," *BMC Psychiatry* 21, no. 1 (January 2, 2021): 2. https://doi .org/10.1186/s12888-020-03002-3.

32. Md Mahbub Hossain et al., "Prevalence of Mental Disorders in South Asia: An Umbrella Review of Systematic Reviews and Meta-Analyses," *Asian Journal of Psychiatry* 51 (June 2020): 102041. https://doi.org/10.1016/j.ajp.2020.102041.

33. Jaimee Stuart and Jemima Nowosad, "The Influence of Premigration Trauma Exposure and Early Postmigration Stressors on Changes in Mental Health Over Time Among Refugees in Australia," *Journal of Traumatic Stress* 33, no. 6 (December 2020): 917–27. https://doi.org/10.1002/jts.22586.

34. Rasheed M. Fakri et al., "Reconstruction of Nonunion Tibial Fractures in War-Wounded Iraqi Civilians, 2006–2008: Better Late than Never," *Journal of*

Orthopaedic Trauma 26, no. 7 (July 2012): e76–82. https://doi.org/10.1097/BOT.0b 013e318225e8d0.

35. WHO, "Annual Report 2016." Accessed January 14, 2021. https://www.who .int/hac/crises/syr/whosyriaannualreport2016.pdf?ua=1.

36. Kaan Sözmen et al., "Cardiovascular Risk Factor Trends in the Eastern Mediterranean Region: Evidence from Four Countries Is Alarming," *International Journal of Public Health* 60, no. 1 (January 2015): S3–11, https://doi.org/10.1007 /s00038-014-0610-6.

37. Shailja Shah et al., "Delivering Non-Communicable Disease Interventions to Women and Children in Conflict Settings: A Systematic Review," *BMJ Global Health* 5, no. 1 (April 2020). https://doi.org/10.1136/bmjgh-2019-002047.

38. Debora Alvarez-Del Arco et al., "High Levels of Postmigration HIV Acquisition within Nine European Countries," *AIDS* 31, no. 14 (September 10, 2017): 1979–88. https://doi.org/10.1097/QAD.0000000000001571.

39. Johann Cailhol and Nichola Khan, "Chronic Hepatitis and HIV Risks amongst Pakistani Migrant Men in a French Suburb and Insights into Health Promotion Interventions: The ANRS Musafir Qualitative Study," *BMC Public Health* 20, no. 1 (September 12, 2020): 1393. https://doi.org/10.1186/s12889-020-09459-x.

40. Lia D'Ambrosio et al., "European Policies in the Management of Tuberculosis among Migrants," *International Journal of Infectious Diseases* 56 (March 2017): 85–89. https://doi.org/10.1016/j.ijid.2016.11.002.

41. Mary Malebranche et al., "Addressing Vulnerability of Pregnant Refugees," *Bulletin of the World Health Organization* 95, no. 9 (September 1, 2017): 611–611A. https://doi.org/10.2471/BLT.17.193664.

42. Brian D. Gushulak and Douglas W. MacPherson, "Population Mobility and Health: An Overview of the Relationships between Movement and Population Health," *Journal of Travel Medicine* 11, no. 3 (June 2004): 171–74. https://doi.org /10.2310/7060.2004.18490.

43. European Council on Refugees and Exiles, "Country Report: Turkey," 2018. Accessed January 22, 2021. https://asylumineurope.org/wp-content/uploads/2019/04 /report-download_aida_tr_2018update.pdf.

44. European Council on Refugees and Exiles, "Country Report: Turkey."

45. InfoMigrants, "Snowstorm Kills 13 Migrants Crossing from Iran to Turkey," February 10, 2020. https://www.infomigrants.net/en/post/22650/snowstorm-kills-13 -migrants-crossing-from-iran-to-turkey.

46. UNHCR, "Mediterranean Situation." Accessed January 22, 2021.

47. RSA, "Greece: Investigate Pushbacks, Violence at Borders," October 6, 2020. https://rsaegean.org/en/greece-investigate-pushbacks-violence-at-borders/.

48. Jovana Arsenijević et al., "A Crisis of Protection and Safe Passage: Violence Experienced by Migrants/Refugees Travelling along the Western Balkan Corridor to Northern Europe," *Conflict and Health* 11 (2017): 6. https://doi.org/10.1186 /s13031-017-0107-z.

49. Jovana Arsenijević et al., "'I Feel like I Am Less than Other People': Health-Related Vulnerabilities of Male Migrants Travelling Alone on Their Journey to Europe," *Social Science and Medicine (1982)* 209 (July 2018): 86–94. https://doi.org/10.1016/j.socscimed.2018.05.038.

50. Ayşen Üstübici and Sibel Karadağ, "Refugee Protection in Turkey during the First Phase of the COVID-19 Pandemic," 2020, 39.

51. "Greek Roads Prove Deadly for Migrants on Busy Land Route to Europe," *The New Humanitarian*, January 17, 2019. https://www.thenewhumanitarian.org/news/2019/01/17/greek-roads-prove-deadly-migrants-busy-land-route-europe.

52. Refugee.info, "Hidden Dangers at the Greece-Turkey Land Border," January 25, 2019. https://blog.refugee.info/major-risks-at-the-greek-land-border/.

53. Jihane Ben Farhat et al., "Syrian Refugees in Greece: Experience with Violence, Mental Health Status, and Access to Information during the Journey and While in Greece," *BMC Medicine* 16, no. 1 (March 13, 2018): 40. https://doi.org/10.1186/s12916-018-1028-4.

54. Roberto Forin and Claire Healy, "Bridging the Gap between Migration Asylum and Anti-trafficking," ICMPD, 2018. Accessed January 22, 2021. https://childhub.org/sites/default/files/webinars/bridging_the_gap_between_migration_asylum_and_anti-trafficking.pdf.

55. Benjamin F. Henwood et al., "Permanent Supportive Housing: Addressing Homelessness and Health Disparities?," *American Journal of Public Health* 103, no. 2 (December 2013): S188–92. https://doi.org/10.2105/AJPH.2013.301490.

56. Vassilis P. Arapoglou and Kostas Gounis, *Contested Landscapes of Poverty and Homelessness In Southern Europe: Reflections from Athens* (Cham: Springer, 2017).

57. Esra S. Kaytaz, "Held at the Gates of Europe: Barriers to Abolishing Immigration Detention in Turkey," *Citizenship Studies* 25, no. 2 (December 22, 2020): 1–21. https://doi.org/10.1080/13621025.2020.1859192.

58. Clare K. Shortall et al., "On the Ferries: The Unmet Health Care Needs of Transiting Refugees in Greece," *International Health* 9, no. 5 (September 1, 2017): 272–80. https://doi.org/10.1093/inthealth/ihx032.

59. E. Kakalou et al., "Demographic and Clinical Characteristics of Refugees Seeking Primary Healthcare Services in Greece in the Period 2015–2016: A Descriptive Study," *International Health* 10, no. 6 (November 1, 2018): 421–29. https://doi.org/10.1093/inthealth/ihy042.

60. Androula Pavli and Helena Maltezou, "Health Problems of Newly Arrived Migrants and Refugees in Europe," *Journal of Travel Medicine* 24, no. 4 (July 1, 2017). https://doi.org/10.1093/jtm/tax016.

61. Assimoula Eonomopoulou et al., "Migrant Screening: Lessons Learned from the Migrant Holding Level at the Greek-Turkish Borders," *Journal of Infection and Public Health* 10, no. 2 (April 2017): 177–84. https://doi.org/10.1016/j.jiph.2016.04.012.

62. Ö. Ergönül et al., "Profiling Infectious Diseases in Turkey after the Influx of 3.5 Million Syrian Refugees," *Clinical Microbiology and Infection* 26, no. 3 (March 2020): 307–12. https://doi.org/10.1016/j.cmi.2019.06.022.

63. Kassiani Mellou et al., "Hepatitis A among Refugees, Asylum Seekers and Migrants Living in Hosting Facilities, Greece, April to December 2016," *Euro Surveillance: Bulletin Europeen Sur Les Maladies Transmissibles = European Communicable Disease Bulletin* 22, no. 4 (January 26, 2017). https://doi.org/10.2807/1560 -7917.ES.2017.22.4.30448.

64. Daniele Mipatrini et al., "Vaccinations in Migrants and Refugees: A Challenge for European Health Systems. A Systematic Review of Current Scientific Evidence," *Pathogens and Global Health* 111, no. 2 (March 2017): 59–68. https:// doi.org/10.1080/20477724.2017.1281374.

65. Üstübici and Karadağ, "Refugee Protection in Turkey."

66. Elias Kondilis et al., "Covid-19 and Refugees, Asylum Seekers, and Migrants in Greece," *BMJ (Clinical Research ed.)* 369 (June 1, 2020): m2168. https://doi .org/10.1136/bmj.m2168.

67. Jane Freedman, "Sexual and Gender-Based Violence against Refugee Women: A Hidden Aspect of the Refugee 'Crisis,'" *Reproductive Health Matters* 24, no. 47 (May 2016): 18–26. https://doi.org/10.1016/j.rhm.2016.05.003.

68. Global Initiative, "Human Trafficking, Sexual Exploitation Growing Risk for Syrian Refugees." Accessed January 22, 2021. https://globalinitiative.net/anal ysis/human-trafficking-sexual-exploitation-growing-risk-for-syrian-refugees/.

69. Perihan Elif Ekmekci, "Syrian Refugees, Health and Migration Legislation in Turkey," *Journal of Immigrant and Minority Health* 19, no. 6 (December 2017): 1434–41. https://doi.org/10.1007/s10903-016-0405-3.

70. Ahmet Içduygu and Evin Millet, "Syrian Refugees in Turkey: Insecure Lives in an Environment of Pseudo-Integration," 2016, 7.

71. Maaike P. J. Hermans et al., "Healthcare and Disease Burden among Refugees in Long-Stay Refugee Camps at Lesbos, Greece," *European Journal of Epidemiology* 32, no. 9 (September 2017): 851–54. https://doi.org/10.1007/s10654-017 -0269-4.

72. Danielle N. Poole et al., "Major Depressive Disorder Prevalence and Risk Factors among Syrian Asylum Seekers in Greece," *BMC Public Health* 18, no. 1 (July 24, 2018): 908. https://doi.org/10.1186/s12889-018-5822-x.

73. Pia Juul Bjertrup et al., "A Life in Waiting: Refugees' Mental Health and Narratives of Social Suffering after European Union Border Closures in March 2016," *Social Science and Medicine* 215 (October 2018): 53–60. https://doi.org/10 .1016/j.socscimed.2018.08.040.

74. European Council on Refugees and Exiles, "Country Report: Turkey."

75. Elena Riza et al., "Determinants of Refugee and Migrant Health Status in 10 European Countries: The Mig-HealthCare Project," *International Journal of Environmental Research and Public Health* 17, no. 17 (August 31, 2020). https://doi .org/10.3390/ijerph17176353.

76. Rojjin Mamuk and Nevin Hotun Şahin, "Reproductive Health Issues of Undocumented Migrant Women Living in Istanbul," *European Journal of Contraception and Reproductive Health Care* (November 16, 2020): 1–7. https://doi.org/10.1080/13625187.2020.1843618.

77. Qais Alemi et al., "Determinants of Health Care Services Utilization among First Generation Afghan Migrants in Istanbul," *International Journal of Environmental Research and Public Health* 14, no. 2 (February 17, 2017). https://doi.org/10.3390/ijerph14020201.

78. Liz Joseph et al., "A Qualitative Research Study Which Explores Humanitarian Stakeholders' Views on Healthcare Access for Refugees in Greece," *International Journal of Environmental Research and Public Health* 17, no. 19 (September 23, 2020). https://doi.org/10.3390/ijerph17196972.

79. Antonis A. Kousoulis, Myrsini Ioakeim-Ioannidou, and Konstantinos P. Economopoulos, "Access to Health for Refugees in Greece: Lessons in Inequalities," *International Journal for Equity in Health* 15, no. 1 (August 2, 2016): 122. https://doi.org/10.1186/s12939-016-0409-6.

80. Caryn Bredenkamp, Mariapia Mendola, and Michele Gragnolati, "Catastrophic and Impoverishing Effects of Health Expenditure: New Evidence from the Western Balkans," *Health Policy and Planning* 26, no. 4 (July 2011): 349–56. https://doi.org/10.1093/heapol/czq070.

81. Milena Santric-Milicevic et al., "Uptake of Health Care Services by Refugees: Modelling a Country Response to a Western Balkan Refugee Crisis," *Healthcare* 8, no. 4 (December 14, 2020). https://doi.org/10.3390/healthcare8040560.

82. Noor C. Gieles et al., "Maternal and Perinatal Outcomes of Asylum Seekers and Undocumented Migrants in Europe: A Systematic Review," *European Journal of Public Health* 29, no. 4 (August 1, 2019): 714–23. https://doi.org/10.1093/eurpub/ckz042.

83. Erik Teunissen et al., "Reporting Mental Health Problems of Undocumented Migrants in Greece: A Qualitative Exploration," *European Journal of General Practice* 22, no. 2 (June 2016): 119–25. https://doi.org/10.3109/13814788.2015.1136283.

84. Miriam Orcutt et al., "EU Migration Policies Drive Health Crisis on Greek Islands," *Lancet* 395, no. 10225 (February 29, 2020): 668–70. https://doi.org/10.1016/S0140-6736(19)33175-7.

85. UN General Assembly, "New York Declaration for Refugees and Migrants," September 19, 2016, 24.

86. MSF, "International Activity Report 2019." Accessed January 24, 2021. https://www.msf.org/sites/msf.org/files/2020-08/international-activity-report-2019.pdf.

87. UN, "The Electronic—Personal Health Record (e-PHR) to Foster Access to Health and Integration of Migrants. Contribution to SDGs 3, 8, 10 and 17— United Nations Partnerships for SDGs Platform." Accessed January 24, 2021. https://sustainabledevelopment.un.org/partnership/?p=30034.

88. Karl Puchner et al., "Time to Rethink Refugee and Migrant Health in Europe: Moving from Emergency Response to Integrated and Individualized Health

Care Provision for Migrants and Refugees," *International Journal of Environmental Research and Public Health* 15, no. 6 (May 28, 2018). https://doi.org/10.3390/ijerph15061100.

89. Puchner et al., "Time to Rethink Refugee and Migrant Health in Europe."

90. Sara Delilovic et al., "What Value for Whom? Provider Perspectives on Health Examinations for Asylum Seekers in Stockholm, Sweden," *BMC Health Services Research* 18, no. 1 (August 3, 2018): 601. https://doi.org/10.1186/s12913-018-3422-1.

91. Kayvan Bozorgmehr and Oliver Razum, "Effect of Restricting Access to Health Care on Health Expenditures among Asylum-Seekers and Refugees: A Quasi-Experimental Study in Germany, 1994–2013," *PloS One* 10, no. 7 (2015): e0131483. https://doi.org/10.1371/journal.pone.0131483.

92. Helena Legido-Quigley et al., "Healthcare Is Not Universal If Undocumented Migrants Are Excluded," *BMJ (Clinical Research ed.)* 366 (September 16, 2019): l4160. https://doi.org/10.1136/bmj.l4160.

93. Elisabetta De Vito et al., *A Review of Evidence on Equitable Delivery, Access and Utilization of Immunization Services for Migrants and Refugees in the WHO European Region*, WHO Health Evidence Network Synthesis Reports (Copenhagen: WHO Regional Office for Europe, 2017). http://www.ncbi.nlm.nih.gov/books/NBK475647/.

94. WHO, "Health Promotion for Improved Refugee and Migrant Health." Accessed January 22, 2021. https://www.euro.who.int/__data/assets/pdf_file/0004/3883 63/tc-health-promotion-eng.pdf.

95. Stephen A. Matlin et al., "Migrants' and Refugees' Health: Towards an Agenda of Solutions," *Public Health Reviews* 39, no. 1 (September 24, 2018): 27. https://doi.org/10.1186/s40985-018-0104-9.

96. Tessa van Loenen et al., "Primary Care for Refugees and Newly Arrived Migrants in Europe: A Qualitative Study on Health Needs, Barriers and Wishes," *European Journal of Public Health* 28, no. 1 (February 1, 2018): 82–87. https://doi.org/10.1093/eurpub/ckx210.

Chapter 32

1. Sanjay Sharma et al., "State of Migration in Nepal," *Centre for the Study of Labour and Mobility*, Research Paper VI, 2014.

2. Kamal Raj Singh Rathaur, "British Gurkha Recruitment: A Historical Perspective," *Voice of History* 16, no. 2 (2001): 19–24; Harka B. Gurung, "Internal and International Migration in Nepal [in Nepali]," Main Report (Kathmandu: HMG Population Commission, 1983).

3. M. Kollmair et al., "New Figures for Old Stories: Migration and Remittances in Nepal.," in *Migration and Remittances in Developing Countries*, ed. N. Kumar

and V. V. Ramani (Hyderabad, Pakistan: Icfai University Press, 2006), 77–85; Susan Thieme and Simone Wyss, "Migration Patterns and Remittance Transfer in Nepal: A Case Study of Sainik Basti in Western Nepal," *International Migration* 43, no. 5 (2005): 59–98; Bandita Sijapati and Amrita Limbu, *Governing Labour Migration in Nepal: An Analysis of Existing Policies and Institutional Mechanisms*, 2017.

4. Government of Nepal, Ministry of Labour and Employment, "Labour Migration for Employment—A Status Report for Nepal: 2014/2015" (Kathmandu, Nepal: Government of Nepal, Ministry of Labour and Employment, 2016).

5. Government of Nepal, Ministry of Labour and Employment, "Labour Migration for Employment"; Patricia Cortes, "The Feminization of International Migration and Its Effects on the Children Left Behind: Evidence from the Philippines," *Migration and Development* 65 (January 1, 2015): 62–78, https://doi.org/10.1016/j.worlddev.2013.10.021; Sharma et al., "State of Migration in Nepal"; Andrew Gardner et al., "A Portrait of Low-Income Migrants in Contemporary Qatar," *Journal of Arabian Studies* 3, no. 1 (June 1, 2013): 1–17, https://doi.org/10.1080/21534764.2013.806076.

6. Raja Ram Dhungana et al., "Psychological Morbidity in Nepali Cross-Border Migrants in India: A Community Based Cross-Sectional Study," *BMC Public Health* 19, no. 1 (November 15, 2019): 1534, https://doi.org/10.1186/s12889-019-7881-z.

7. Government of Nepal, Ministry of Labour, Employment and Social Security, "Nepal Labour Migration Report 2020" (Kathmandu, Nepal: Government of Nepal, Ministry of Labour, Employment and Social Security, 2020), https://moless.gov.np/wp-content/uploads/2020/03/Migration-Report-2020-English.pdf.

8. David Seddon, Jagannath Adhikari, and Ganesh Gurung, "Foreign Labor Migration and the Remittance Economy of Nepal," *Critical Asian Studies* 34, no. 1 (2002): 19–40; Elvira Graner and Ganesh Gurung, "Arab Ko Lahure: Looking at Nepali Labour Migrants to Arabian Countries," *Contributions to Nepalese Studies* 30, no. 2 (2003): 295–325; Thieme and Wyss, "Migration Patterns and Remittance Transfer in Nepal."

9. Gardner et al., "A Portrait of Low-Income Migrants in Contemporary Qatar."

10. Gardner et al., "A Portrait of Low-Income Migrants in Contemporary Qatar."

11. Gardner et al., "A Portrait of Low-Income Migrants in Contemporary Qatar."

12. Vartika Sharma et al., "Life across the Border: Migrants in South Asia" (New Delhi: Population Council, 2015), https://assets.publishing.service.gov.uk/media/57a0897f40f0b649740000e8/61263_Final-Migrant-Report_Life-across-the-border.pdf.

13. Dhungana et al., "Psychological Morbidity in Nepali Cross-Border Migrants in India."

14. Sharma et al., "Life across the Border"; Dhungana et al., "Psychological Morbidity in Nepali Cross-Border Migrants in India"; Maheshwor Shrestha, "Push and Pull: A Study of International Migration from Nepal," *Social Protection and Labor Global Practice Group, World Bank Group*, Policy Research Working Papers, February 8, 2017, https://doi.org/10.1596/1813-9450-7965.

15. Joshi et al., "Health Problems of Nepalese Migrants"; Gardner et al., "A Portrait of Low-Income Migrants in Contemporary Qatar"; Lynn Bennett, "Sex and Motherhood among the Brahmins and Chhetris of East-Central Nepal," *Contribution to Nepalese Studies* 3, no. Special Issue (June 1976): 1–52; Yao Lu, "Test of the 'Healthy Migrant Hypothesis': A Longitudinal Analysis of Health Selectivity of Internal Migration in Indonesia," *Social Science and Medicine* 67, no. 8 (October 1, 2008): 1331–39, https://doi.org/10.1016/j.socscimed.2008.06.017; Diana Hull, "Migration, Adaptation, and Illness: A Review," *Social Science and Medicine. Part A: Medical Psychology and Medical Sociology* 13 (January 1, 1979): 25–36, https://doi.org/10.1016/0271-7123(79)90005-1; Pratik Adhikary, Steven Keen, and Edwin van Teijlingen, "Health Issues among Nepalese Migrant Workers in the Middle East," *Health Science Journal* 5, no. 3 (2011): 169–75; Pratik Adhikary, Steve Keen, and Edwin van Teijlingen, "Workplace Accidents among Nepali Male Workers in the Middle East and Malaysia: A Qualitative Study," *Journal of Immigrant and Minority Health* 21, no. 5 (October 1, 2019): 1115–22, https://doi.org/10.1007/s10903-018-0801-y.

16. Joshi et al., "Health Problems of Nepalese Migrants"; Gardner et al., "A Portrait of Low-Income Migrants in Contemporary Qatar."

17. Gardner et al., "A Portrait of Low-Income Migrants in Contemporary Qatar"; Andrew M Gardner, "Labor Camps in the Gulf States," in *Viewpoints: Migration and the Gulf* (Washington, DC: The Middle East Institute, 2010), 55–57.

18. Joshi et al., "Health Problems of Nepalese Migrants"; Nepal Ministry of Health, New Era, and ICF, *Nepal Demographic and Health Survey 2016* (Kathmandu: Nepal Ministry of Health, 2017); Chandni Singh and Ritwika Basu, "Moving in and out of Vulnerability: Interrogating Migration as an Adaptation Strategy along a Rural–Urban Continuum in India," *The Geographical Journal* 186, no. 1 (2020): 87–102, https://doi.org/10.1111/geoj.12328; Scott T. Yabiku, Victor Agadjanian, and Boaventura Cau, "Labor Migration and Child Mortality in Mozambique," *Social Science and Medicine*, special issue: Place, *Migration and Health*, 75, no. 12 (December 1, 2012): 2530–38, https://doi.org/10.1016/j.socscimed.2012.10.001.

19. Sharma et al., "State of Migration in Nepal."

20. Sharma et al., "State of Migration in Nepal."

21. Bennett, "Sex and Motherhood among the Brahmins and Chhetris of East-Central Nepal."

22. Lu, "Test of the 'Healthy Migrant Hypothesis' "; Hull, "Migration, Adaptation, and Illness."

23. Joshi et al., "Health Problems of Nepalese Migrants"; Adhikary et al., "Health Issues among Nepalese Migrant Workers in the Middle East"; Adhikary et al., "Workplace Accidents among Nepali Male Workers in the Middle East and Malaysia."

24. Gardner et al., "A Portrait of Low-Income Migrants in Contemporary Qatar."

25. Gardner et al., "A Portrait of Low-Income Migrants in Contemporary Qatar"; Andrés A. Agudelo-Suárez et al., "A Metasynthesis of Qualitative Studies Regarding Opinions and Perceptions about Barriers and Determinants of Health

Services' Accessibility in Economic Migrants," *BMC Health Services Research* 12, no. 1 (December 17, 2012): 461, https://doi.org/10.1186/1472-6963-12-461.

26. Shreejana Shrestha, "Mental Cost of Migration," *Nepali Times*, July 15, 2016, sec. Nation.

27. Dhungana et al., "Psychological Morbidity in Nepali Cross-Border Migrants in India."

28. Shrestha, "Mental Cost of Migration."

29. Nathalie E. Williams et al., "A Micro-Level Event-Centered Approach to Investigating Armed Conflict and Population Responses," *Demography* 49, no. 4 (2012): 1521–46.

30. Dhungana et al., "Psychological Morbidity in Nepali Cross-Border Migrants in India."

31. Dhungana et al., "Psychological Morbidity in Nepali Cross-Border Migrants in India."

32. Shrestha, "Mental Cost of Migration"; "वैदेशिक रोजगार बोर्डको सचिवालय."

33. Sharma et al., "State of Migration in Nepal."

34. Sharma et al., "State of Migration in Nepal."

35. Sharma et al., "State of Migration in Nepal."

36. Sharma et al., "State of Migration in Nepal."

37. Sharma et al., "State of Migration in Nepal."

38. Mahesh Puri and John Cleland, "Assessing the Factors Associated with Sexual Harassment among Young Female Migrant Workers in Nepal," *Journal of Interpersonal Violence* 22, no. 11 (November 1, 2007): 1363–81, https://doi.org/10.1177/0886260507305524.

39. Mahesh Puri and John Cleland, "Sexual Behavior and Perceived Risk of HIV/AIDS among Young Migrant Factory Workers in Nepal," *Journal of Adolescent Health* 38, no. 3 (March 1, 2006): 237–46, https://doi.org/10.1016/j.jadohealth.2004.10.001.

40. Williams et al., "A Micro-Level Event-Centered Approach"; Gardner et al., "A Portrait of Low-Income Migrants in Contemporary Qatar."

41. Nepal Ministry of Health, New Era, and ICF, *Nepal Demographic and Health Survey 2011*.

42. Singh and Basu, "Moving in and out of Vulnerability"; Yabiku, Agadjanian, and Cau, "Labor Migration and Child Mortality in Mozambique."

43. Sharma et al., "State of Migration in Nepal"; Vidhya Bir Singh Kansakar, "International Migration and Citizenship in Nepal," in *Population Monograph of Nepal* (Kathmandu: Central Bureau of Statistics, n.d.), 85–119.

44. Sharma et al., "State of Migration in Nepal"; Kansakar, "International Migration and Citizenship in Nepal."

45. "Bhutan Refugees Rally for Help to Go Back Home," *Kathmandu Post*, December 11, 2018, Reliefweb.int, https://reliefweb.int/report/nepal/bhutan-refugees-rally-help-go-back-home; "Nepal," Global Focus UNHCR Operations Worldwide. Accessed October 20, 2020, https://reporting.unhcr.org/node/10316.

46. Mark Van Ommeren et al., "Psychiatric Disorders among Tortured Bhutanese Refugees in Nepal," *Archives of General Psychiatry* 58, no. 5 (2001): 475–82; Edward J. Mills et al., "Prevalence of Mental Disorders and Torture among Tibetan Refugees: A Systematic Review," *BMC International Health and Human Rights* 5, no. 1 (November 9, 2005): 7, https://doi.org/10.1186/1472-698X-5-7.

Chapter 33

1. McAuliffe, Marie, Binod Khadria, and Céline Bauloz. *World Migration Report 2020.* Geneva: IOM, 2019.

2. International Organization for Migration. "International Migration, Health and Human Rights," 2013. https://publications.iom.int/books/international-migration-health-and-human-rights.

3. Kristiansen, Maria, and Aziz Sheikh. "The Health of Low-Income Migrant Workers in Gulf Cooperation Council Countries." *Health and Human Rights Journal: An International Journal* (July 2014).

4. Gardner, Andrew M. "Gulf Migration and the Family." *Journal of Arabian Studies* 1, no. 1 (June 2011): 3–25.

5. Naithani, Pranav, and A. N. Jha. "Challenges Faced by Expatriate Workers in Gulf Cooperation Council Countries." *International Journal of Business and Management* 5, no. 1 (December 2009): 98–104.

6. International Organization for Migration. "Global Migration Data Portal." Migration Data Portal, 2020. https://migrationdataportal.org/.

7. International Organization for Migration, "Global Migration Data Portal."

8. Kristiansen and Sheikh, "The Health of Low-Income Migrant Workers."

9. Alahmad, Barrak, Hussam Kurdi, Kyle Colonna, Janvier Gasana, Jacqueline Agnew, and Mary A Fox. "COVID-19 Stressors on Migrant Workers in Kuwait: Cumulative Risk Considerations." *BMJ Global Health* 5, no. 7 (July 2020): e002995.

10. Amnesty International. "The Dark Side of Migration. Spotlight on Qatar's Construction Sector Ahead of the World Cup," 2013.

11. The European Centre for Democracy and Human Rights (ECDHR). "GCC Countries and Migrant Workers: Background Facts," May 2020. https://www.ecdhr.org/?p=902.

12. Gardner, "Gulf Migration and the Family."

13. Human Rights Watch. "'As If I Am Not Human': Abuses against Asian Domestic Workers in Saudi Arabia," 2008. https://www.hrw.org/reports/2008/saudiarabia0708/.

14. Naithani, "Challenges Faced by Expatriate Workers in Gulf Cooperation Council Countries."

15. Rashad, Hoda. "Health Equity in the Arab World: The Future We Want." *Lancet* 383, no. 9914 (January 2014): 286–87.

16. Fargues, Philippe, and Nasra M. Shah. "Socio-Economic Impacts of GCC Migration." Cambridge: Gulf Research Centre, 2012.

17. Sönmez, Sevil, Yorghos Apostolopoulos, Diane Tran, and Shantyana Rentrope. "Human Rights and Health Disparities for Migrant Workers in the UAE." *Health and Human Rights* 13, no. 2 (December 2011): 17–35.

18. Sönmez et al. "Human Rights and Health Disparities for Migrant Workers in the UAE."

19. Diop, Abdoulaye, Kien Trung Le, and Micheal C. Ewers. "Working and Living Conditions of Migrant Workers in the GCC." In *India Migration Report 2016: Gulf Migration*, edited by S. Irudaya Rajan, 75–89. London: Routledge India, 2017.

20. Diop et al., "Working and Living Conditions of Migrant Workers in the GCC."

21. Sönmez et al., "Human Rights and Health Disparities for Migrant Workers in the UAE."

22. Alahmad et al., "COVID-19 Stressors on Migrant Workers in Kuwait."

23. Diop et al., "Working and Living Conditions of Migrant Workers in the GCC."

24. Human Rights Watch. "Building Towers, Cheating Workers. Exploitation of Migrant Construction Workers in the United Arab Emirates," November 2006. https://www.hrw.org/report/2006/11/11/building-towers-cheating-workers/exploitation-migrant-construction-workers-united.

25. Joffres, Christine, Edward Mills, Michel Joffres, Tinku Khanna, Harleen Walia, and Darrin Grund. "Sexual Slavery without Borders: Trafficking for Commercial Sexual Exploitation in India." *International Journal for Equity in Health* 7 (September 2008): 22.

26. Joshi, Suresh, Padam Simkhada, and Gordon J. Prescott. "Health Problems of Nepalese Migrants Working in Three Gulf Countries." *BMC International Health and Human Rights* 11 (March 2011): 3.

27. Satyanarayana, V. A., P. S. Chandra, K. Vaddiparti. "Mental Health Consequences of Violence against Women and Girls." *Current Opinion in Psychiatry* 5 (September 28, 2015): 350–56.

28. Simkhada, Padam, Edwin van Teijlingen, Manju Gurung, and Sharada P. Wasti. "A Survey of Health Problems of Nepalese Female Migrants Workers in the Middle-East and Malaysia." *BMC International Health and Human Rights* 18, no. 1 (January 2018): 4.

29. McAuliffe et al., *World Migration Report 2020.*

30. GBD 2019 Diseases and Injuries Collaborators. "Global Burden of 369 Diseases and Injuries in 204 Countries and Territories, 1990–2019: A Systematic Analysis for the Global Burden of Disease Study 2019." *Lancet* 396, no. 10258 (October 2020): 1204–22.

31. Spallek, Jacob, Hajo Zeeb, and Oliver Razum. "What Do We Have to Know from Migrants' Past Exposures to Understand Their Health Status? A Life Course Approach." *Emerging Themes in Epidemiology* 8, no. 1 (August 2011): 6.

32. Kronfol, Ziad, Marwa Saleh, and Maha Al-Ghafry. "Mental Health Issues

among Migrant Workers in Gulf Cooperation Council Countries: Literature Review and Case Illustrations." *Asian Journal of Psychiatry* 10 (August 2014): 109–13.

33. Khaled, Salma M., and Richard Gray. "Depression in Migrant Workers and Nationals of Qatar: An Exploratory Cross-Cultural Study." *The International Journal of Social Psychiatry* 65, no. 5 (August 2019): 354–67.

34. Pratik, Adhikary, Steven Keen, and Edwin van Teijlingen. "Health Issues among Nepalese Migrant Workers in the Middle East." *Health Science Journal* 5, no. 3 (2011): 169–75.

35. Zahid, Muhammad Ajmal, and Mohammad Alsuwaidan. "The Mental Health Needs of Immigrant Workers in Gulf Countries." *International Psychiatry: Bulletin of the Board of International Affairs of the Royal College of Psychiatrists* 11, no. 4 (November 2014): 79–81.

36. Alahmad et al., "COVID-19 Stressors on Migrant Workers in Kuwait."

37. Khoja, Tawfiq, Salman Rawaf, Waris Qidwai, David Rawaf, Kashmira Nanji, and Aisha Hamad. "Health Care in Gulf Cooperation Council Countries: A Review of Challenges and Opportunities." *Cureus* 9, no. 8 (August 2017): e1586.

38. Kristiansen and Sheikh, "The Health of Low-Income Migrant Workers."

39. Kristiansen and Sheikh, "The Health of Low-Income Migrant Workers."

40. Human Rights Watch, "Building Towers, Cheating Workers."

41. Modarres, Ali. "Migration and the Persian Gulf: Demography, Identity and the Road to Equitable Policies." *Anthropology of the Middle East* 5, no. 1 (2010): 1–17.

42. Diop et al., "Working and Living Conditions of Migrant Workers in the GCC."

43. Batniji, Rajaie, Lina Khatib, Melani Cammett, Jeffrey Sweet, Sanjay Basu, Amaney Jamal, Paul Wise, and Rita Giacaman. "Governance and Health in the Arab World." *Lancet* 383, no. 9914 (January 2014): 343–55.

44. International Organization for Migration, "International Migration, Health and Human Rights"

45. Kristiansen and Sheikh, "The Health of Low-Income Migrant Workers."

Chapter 34

1. Statistics South Africa, "Census in Brief. Report No. 03-01-41." Pretoria: Statistics South Africa, 2012.

2. UNDESA, "International Migrant Stock 2019: Country Profile—South Africa," United Nations Department of Economic and Social Affairs, 2019.

3. Jo Vearey, Charles Hui, and Kolitha Wickramage, "Migration and Health: Current Issues, Governance and Knowledge Gaps," *World Migration Report*, 2020, 38.

4. J. Vearey, M. Modisenyane, and J. Hunter-Adams, "Towards a Migration-Aware Health System in South Africa: A Strategic Opportunity to Address Health Inequity South African," *South African Health Review*, 2017; Jo Vearey, "Moving

Forward: Why Responding to Migration, Mobility and HIV in South(ern) Africa Is a Public Health Priority," *Journal of the International AIDS Society* 21, no. S4 (2018): e25137, https://doi.org/10.1002/jia2.25137; J. Vearey, "Healthy Migration: A Public Health and Development Imperative for South(ern) Africa," *South African Medical Journal* 104, no. 10 (July 3, 2014): 663, https://doi.org/10.7196/samj.8569.

5. J. Vearey et al., "Exploring the Migration Profiles of Primary Healthcare Users in South Africa," *Journal of Immigrant and Minority Health* (2016), https://doi.org/10.1007/s10903-016-0535-7.

6. Thea de Gruchy and Jo Vearey, "'Left Behind': Why Implementing Migration-Aware Responses to HIV for Migrant Farm Workers Is a Priority for South Africa," *African Journal of AIDS Research* 19, no. 1 (January 2, 2020): 57–68, https://doi.org/10.2989/16085906.2019.1698624; Vearey, "Moving Forward"; MSF, "Providing Antiretroviral Therapy for Mobile Populations: Lesson Learned from a Cross Border ARV Programme in Musina, South Africa," 2012; MSF, "No Refuge, Access Denied: Medical and Humanitarian Needs of Zimbabweans in South Africa," 2009; Thea de Gruchy and Anuj Kapilashrami, "After the Handover: Exploring MSF's Role in the Provision of Health Care to Migrant Farm Workers in Musina, South Africa," *Global Public Health* 14, no. 10 (March 5, 2019): 1–13, https://doi.org/10.1080/17441692.2019.1586976; SADC, "SADC HIV and AIDS Cross Border Initiative—A Global Fund Project." Gaboronne: SADC, 2012, https://www.k4health.org/sites/default/files/SADC_Cross_Border_Initiative_2012.pdf; SADC Directorate for Social and Human Development and Special Programs, "SADC Declaration on Tuberculosis in the Mining Sector," 2012; Jo Vearey, Brittany Wheeler, and S. Jurgens-Bleeker, "Migration and Health in SADC. A Review of the Literature." Pretoria: IOM, 2011; Jo Vearey et al., "A Review of Migrant and Mobile Populations within Border Areas of SADC: Implications for HIV Prevention Programming," *African Centre for Migration and Society (ACMS), University of the Witwatersrand*, 2011, http://www.soulcity.org.za/research/research-reports/regional-alliance/ACMS-Soul%20City%20FINAL.pdf; Matthew Wilhelm-Solomon and Jens Pedersen, "Crossing the Borders of Humanitarianism: Médecins Sans Frontières (MSF) in Inner-City Johannesburg," *Urban Forum*, June 23, 2016, https://doi.org/10.1007/s12132-016-9285-9.

7. IOM, "Forum Responds to Cross Border Migration Challenges between South Africa and Zimbabwe | International Organization for Migration," 2013, https://southafrica.iom.int/news/forum-responds-cross-border-migration-challenges-between-south-africa-and-zimbabwe; IOM, "IOM Hosts a Two-Day Summit on Migration and Health in Ehlanzeni District Municipality," 2014, https://southafrica.iom.int/news/iom-hosts-two-day-summit-migration-and-health-ehlanzeni-district-municipality.

8. Jo Vearey et al., "Analysing Local-Level Responses to Migration and Urban Health in Hillbrow: The Johannesburg Migrant Health Forum," *BMC Public Health* 17, no. 3 (July 4, 2017): 427, https://doi.org/10.1186/s12889-017-4352-2.

9. SADC Directorate for Social and Human Development and Special Programs,

"SADC Policy Framework for Population Mobility and Communicable Diseases in the SADC Region: Final Draft April 2009," 2009, http://www.Arasa.Info/Files /Pub_SADC%20Policy_Framework_FINAL.Pdf.

10. ILO, "Promoting a Rights-Based Approach to Migration, Health, and HIV and AIDS: A Framework for Action." Geneva: ILO, 2017; IOM, "Health of Migrants: Resetting the Agenda. Report of the 2nd Global Consultation. Colombo, Sri Lanka, 21–23 February 2017." Geneva, Switzerland: IOM, 2017, https://www .iom.int/sites/default/files/our_work/DMM/Migration-Health/GC2_SriLanka_Report _2017_FINAL_22.09.2017_Internet.pdf; WHO, "Promoting the Health of Refugees and Migrants. Draft Global Action Plan, 2019–2023." Geneva: WHO, 2019; *Lancet*, "No Public Health without Migrant Health," *Lancet* 3, no. 6 (May 24, 2018), https://doi.org/10.1016/S2468-2667(18)30101-4; Ibrahim Abubakar et al., "The UCL–Lancet Commission on Migration and Health: The Health of a World on the Move," *Lancet* 392, no. 10164 (December 2018): 2606–54, https://doi.org/10.1016 /S0140-6736(18)32114-7; Vearey et al., "Migration and Health: Current Issues."

11. Sasha Frade, Jo Vearey, and Stephen Tollman, "South Africa's Healthcare System Can't Afford to Ignore Migration," 2019, http://theconversation.com/south -africas-healthcare-system-cant-afford-to-ignore-migration-120797.

12. Kolitha Wickramage et al., "Missing. Where Are the Migrants in Pandemic Influenza Preparedness Plans?," *Health and Human Rights* 20, no. 1 (June 2018): 251–58; J. Vearey, "Securing Borders: The Danger of Blurring Global Migration Governance and Health Security Agendas in Southern Africa," *Occasional Paper: South Africa Institute of International Affairs*, 2018.

13. N. Maple et al., "Covid-19 and Migration Governance in Africa," report commissioned by the Open Society Foundation, 2020.

14. Christo Vosloo, "Extreme Apartheid: The South African System of Migrant Labour and Its Hostels," *Image and Text*, no. 34 (2020): 1–33, https://doi.org/10 .17159/2617-3255/2020/n34a1.

15. Vosloo. "Extreme Apartheid."

16. Statistics South Africa, "Census in Brief."

17. Statistics South Africa, "Census in Brief."

18. UNDESA, "International Migrant Stock 2019."

19. Sarah Helen Chiumbu and Dumisani Moyo, "'South Africa Belongs to All Who Live in It': Deconstructing Media Discourses of Migrants during Times of Xenophobic Attacks, from 2008 to 2017," *Communicare* 37, no. 1 (July 2018): 136–52; I. Freemantle and J. P. Misago, "The Social Construction of (Non) Crises and Its Effects: Government Discourse on Xenophobia, Immigration and Social Cohesion in South Africa." In *Crisis and Migration: Critical Perspectives*, edited by A. Lindley, 212. New York: Routledge, 2014, http://www.routledge.com/books /details/9780415645027/.

20. Vearey et al., "Towards a Migration-Aware Health System in South Africa."

21. Janine A. White, Duane Blaauw, and Laetitia C. Rispel, "Social Exclusion

and the Perspectives of Health Care Providers on Migrants in Gauteng Public Health Facilities, South Africa," *PLOS One* 15, no. 12 (December 28, 2020): e0244080, https://doi.org/10.1371/journal.pone.0244080.

22. Johannesburg Migrant Health Forum, "Fact Sheet on Migration and Health in the South African Context," 2015, http://goo.gl/7N4yYM; Vearey, "Healthy Migration"; Vearey et al., "Towards a Migration-Aware Health System in South Africa."

23. H. Coovadia et al., "The Health and Health System of South Africa: Historical Roots of Current Public Health Challenges," *Lancet* 374 (2009): 817–34; Bongani M. Mayosi et al., "Health in South Africa: Changes and Challenges since 2009," *Lancet* 380, no. 9858 (December 14, 2012): 2029–43, https://doi.org/10.1016/S0140 -6736(12)61814-5; Mickey Chopra et al., "Achieving the Health Millennium Development Goals for South Africa: Challenges and Priorities," *Lancet* 374, no. 9694 (September 19, 2009): 1023–31, https://doi.org/10.1016/S0140-6736(09)61122-3.

24. John E. Ataguba, Candy Day, and Di McIntyre, "Monitoring and Evaluating Progress towards Universal Health Coverage in South Africa," *PLOS Medicine* 11, no. 9 (September 22, 2014): e1001686, https://doi.org/10.1371/journal.pmed .1001686; Diane McIntyre, Jane Doherty, and John Ataguba, "Universal Health Coverage Assessment South Africa," Global Network for Health Equity, December 2014, 16.

25. Janet Michel et al., "Universal Health Coverage Financing in South Africa: Wishes vs Reality," *Journal of Global Health Reports* (July 21, 2020), https://doi .org/10.29392/001c.13509.

26. Jean Pierre Misago, "Political Mobilisation as the Trigger of Xenophobic Violence in Post-Apartheid South Africa," *International Journal of Conflict and Violence* 13 (March 6, 2019): 646, https://doi.org/10.4119/UNIBI/ijcv.646; Jean Pierre Misago, "Politics by Other Means? The Political Economy of Xenophobic Violence in Post-Apartheid South Africa," *The Black Scholar* 47, no. 2 (April 3, 2017): 40–53, https://doi.org/10.1080/00064246.2017.1295352.

27. Loren B. Landau, "No Borders: The Politics of Immigration Control and Resistance," *South African Journal of International Affairs* 24, no. 2 (April 3, 2017): 264– 66, https://doi.org/10.1080/10220461.2017.1305286.

28. Sasha Frade and Jo Vearey, "Migrants Must Be Part of South Africa's Universal Health Plan. Here's Why," The Conversation, 2019, http://theconversation.com /migrants-must-be-part-of-south-africas-universal-health-plan-heres-why-120925.

29. Davide T. Mosca et al., "Universal Health Coverage: Ensuring Migrants and Migration Are Included," *Global Social Policy* (June 24, 2020), https://doi.org /10.1177/1468018120922228.

30. J. Vearey, S. Gandar, and Rebecca Walker, "Drones, Dinghies and an Army Helicopter—Why the State's New Toys Won't Help South Africa's Response to Covid-19," *Daily Maverick*, January 8, 2021, https://www.dailymaverick.co.za/article /2021-01-08-drones-dinghies-and-an-army-helicopter-why-the-states-new-toys-wont -help-south-africas-response-to-covid-19/.

31. Maple et al., "Covid-19 and Migration Governance in Africa."

32. Mosca et al., "Universal Health Coverage"; Vearey et al., "Migration and Health."

Chapter 35

1. Diallo, Khassoum. "Data on the Migration of Health-Care Workers: Sources, Uses, and Challenges." *Bulletin of the World Health Organization* 82 (2004): 601–7.

2. Cebotari, Victor, Melissa Siegel, and Valentina Mazzucato. 2018. "Migration and Child Health in Moldova and Georgia." *Comparative Migration Studies* 6, no 1. (2018): 3.

3. Hu, Xiaojiang, Sarah Cook, and Miguel A Salazar. "Internal Migration and Health in China." *Lancet* 372, no. 9651 (2008): 1717–19.

4. Chen, Juan. "Internal Migration And Health: Re-examining the Healthy Migrant Phenomenon in China." *Social Science and Medicine* 72, no. 8 (2011): 1294–301.

5. Tong, Yuying, and Martin Piotrowski. "Migration and Health Selectivity in the Context of Internal Migration in China, 1997–2009." *Population Research and Policy Review* 31, no. 4 (2012): 497–543.

6. Gong, Peng, Song Liang, Elizabeth J. Carlton, Qingwu Jiang, Jianyong Wu, Lei Wang, and Justin V. Remais. "Urbanisation and Health in China." *Lancet* 379, no. 9818 (2012): 843–52.

7. Xiang, B. "Migration and Health in China: Problems, Obstacles and Solutions." Asian Metacenter for Population and Sustainable Development Analysis Research Papers 17 (2004).

8. Chen, Shiyi, Gary H. Jefferson, and Jun Zhang. "Structural Change, Productivity Growth and Industrial Transformation in China." *China Economic Review* 22, no. 1 (2011): 133–50.

9. Huang, Dongya, and Chuanmin Chen. "Revolving out of the Party-State: The Xiahai Entrepreneurs and Circumscribing Government Power in China." *Journal of Contemporary China* 25, no. 97 (2016): 41–58.

10. Li, Bingqin, Chunlai Chen, and Biliang Hu. "Governing Urbanization and the New Urbanization Plan in China." *Environment and Urbanization* 28, no. 2 (2016): 515–34.

11. Li, Bingqin. "Governing Urban Climate Change Adaptation in China." *Environment and Urbanization* 25, no. 2 (2013): 413–27.

12. Wei, Xuan, and Honggen Zhu. "Return Migrants' Entrepreneurial Decisions in Rural China." *Asian Population Studies* 16, no. 1 (2020): 61–81.

13. Li et al., "Governing Urbanization."

14. Ma, Libang, Meimei Chen, Xinglong Che, and Fang. "Farmers' Rural-To-Urban Migration, Influencing Factors and Development Framework: A Case Study of Sihe Village of Gansu, China." *International Journal of Environmental Research and Public Health* 16, no. 5 (2019): 877.

15. Shen, Yang, and Bingqin Li. "Policy Coordination in the Talent War to Achieve Economic Upgrading: The Case of Four Chinese Cities." *Policy Studies* (2020). https://doi.org/10.1080/01442872.2020.1738368.

16. Li, Bingqin, and Yongmei Zhang. "Housing Provision for Rural–Urban Migrant Workers in Chinese Cities: The Roles of the State, Employers and the Market." *Social Policy and Administration* 45, no. 6 (2011): 694–713.

17. Bonnin, Michel. "The 'Lost Generation': Its Definition and Its Role in Today's Chinese Elite Politics." *Social Research* 73, no. 1 (2006): 245–74.

18. Zhao, Qi, Asli Kulane, Yi Gao, and Biao Xu. "Knowledge and Attitude on Maternal Health Care among Rural-to-Urban Migrant Women in Shanghai, China." *BMC Women's Health* 9, no. 1 (2009): 5. https://doi.org/10.1186/1472-6874-9-5.

19. Hu, Feng, Zhaoyuan Xu, and Yuyu Chen. "Circular Migration, or Permanent Stay? Evidence from China's Rural–Urban Migration." *China Economic Review* 22, no. 1 (2011): 64–74.

20. Lin, Qianhan. "Lost in Transformation? The Employment Trajectories of China's Cultural Revolution Cohort." *Annals of the American Academy of Political and Social Science* 646, no. 1 (2013): 172–93.

21. Wang, Shun, and Weina Zhou. "The Unintended Long-Term Consequences of Mao's Mass Send-Down Movement: Marriage, Social Network, and Happiness." *World Development* 90 (2017): 344–59.

22. Zhong, Bao-Liang, Tie-Bang Liu, Jian-Xing Huang, Helene H. Fung, Sandra S. M. Chan, Yeates Conwell, and Helen F. K. Chiu. "Acculturative Stress of Chinese Rural-to-Urban Migrant Workers: A Qualitative Study." *PLoS One* 11, no. 6 (2016): e0157530.

23. Wen, Ming, Zhenzhen Zheng, and Jianlin Niu. "Psychological Distress of Rural-to-Urban Migrants in Two Chinese Cities: Shenzhen and Shanghai." *Asian Population Studies* 13, no. 1 (2017): 5–24.

24. Wang, Bo, Xiaoming Li, Bonita Stanton, and Xiaoyi Fang. "The Influence of Social Stigma and Discriminatory Experience on Psychological Distress and Quality of Life among Rural-to-Urban Migrants in China." *Social Science and Medicine* 71, no. 1 (2010): 84–92.

25. Yang, Min, Martin Dijst, and Marco Helbich. "Mental Health among Migrants in Shenzhen, China: Does It Matter whether the Migrant Population Is Identified by Hukou or Birthplace?" *International Journal of Environmental Research and Public Health* 15, no. 12 (2018): 2671.

26. Wang, Senhu, and Yang Hu. "Migration and Health in China: Linking Sending and Host Societies." *Population, Space and Place* 25, no. 6 (2019): e2231.

27. Lommel, L., X. Hu, M. Sun, and J-L. Chen. "Frequency of Depressive Symptoms among Female Migrant Workers in China: Associations with Acculturation, Discrimination, and Reproductive Health." *Public Health* 181 (2020): 151–57.

28. Deng, Zihong, and Bingqin Li. "Parents' Experiences of Discrimination and Children's Depressive Symptoms: Evidence from China." *Journal of Child and Family Studies* (2021): 1–16.

29. Göbel, Christian. "The Political Logic of Protest Repression in China." *Journal of Contemporary China* (2020): 1–17. https://doi.org/10.1080/10670564.2020.17 90897.

30. Pils, Eva. "Peasants' Struggle for Land in China." In *Marginalized Communities and Access to Justice*, edited by Yash Ghai and Jill Cottrell, 136–60. Oxfordshire: Routledge, 2009.

31. Sargeson, Sally. "Violence as Development: Land Expropriation and China's Urbanization." *Journal of Peasant Studies* 40, no. 6 (2013): 1063–85.

32. Sun, Meiping, Rui Ma, Yang Zeng, Fengji Luo, Jing Zhang, and Wenjun Hou. 2010. "Immunization Status and Risk Factors of Migrant Children in Densely Populated Areas of Beijing, China." *Vaccine* 28, no 5 (2010): 1264–74.

33. Li, Bingqin, Bo Hu, Tao Liu, and Lijie Fang, 249–66.

34. Zhuang, Lihui, Jizhi Guo, and Yang Wang. 2006. "Research on the Mental Health of Three Gorges Migrants." *Chinese Journal of Social Medicine* 4 (2006): 10.

35. Yang, Hui, Hua Hu, and Hua-qing Meng. "Study on Mental Health, Life Events and Personality Character of Migration in Three Gorges Reservoir Area." *Chongqing Medicine* 7 (2009).

36. Jiang, Yanpeng, Paul Waley, and Sara Gonzalez. "'Nice Apartments, No Jobs': How Former Villagers Experienced Displacement and Resettlement in the Western Suburbs of Shanghai." *Urban Studies* 55, no. 14 (2018): 3202–17.

37. Tang, Wanjie, Gang Wang, Tao Hu, Qian Dai, Jiajun Xu, Yanchun Yang, and Jiuping Xu. "Mental Health and Psychosocial Problems among Chinese Left-Behind Children: A Cross-Sectional Comparative Study." *Journal of Affective Disorders* 241 (2018): 133–41.

38. Ge, Ying, Jun Se, and Jingfu Zhang. "Research on Relationship among Internet-Addiction, Personality Traits and Mental Health of Urban Left-Behind Children." *Global Journal of Health Science* 7, no. 4 (2015): 60–69.

39. Sun, Meng, Zhimin Xue, Wen Zhang, Rui Guo, Aimin Hu, Yihui Li, Tumbwene Elieza Mwansisya et al. "Psychotic-Like Experiences, Trauma and Related Risk Factors among 'Left-Behind' Children in China." *Schizophrenia Research* 181 (2017): 43–48.

40. Wang, F., X. Zhou, and T. Hesketh. "Psychological Adjustment and Behaviours in Children of Migrant Workers in China." *Child Care, Health and Development* 43, no. 6 (2017): 884–90.

41. Wu, Z. "A Total of 975,000 Cases of Occupational Diseases Have Been Reported in China, and the Actual Number of Cases Is Even Higher" (Zhōngguó lěijì bàogào zhíyèbìng 97.5 Wàn lì shíjì fābìng rénshù gèng gāo). *China News*, July 30, 2019. http://www.chinanews.com/gn/2019/07-30/8911495.shtml.

42. Tang, X. Z., Q. Zeng, and D. S. Liu. "A Cost-Benefit Analysis of Occupational Disease Reporting in China." *Chinese Journal of Industrial Hygiene and Occupational Diseases* 35, no. 3 (2017): 226–29.

43. Ning, Huacheng, Yao Zhou, Ziwen Zhou, Sixiang Cheng, and Ruixue Huang.

"Challenges to Improving Occupational Health in China." *Occupational and Environmental Medicine* 74, no. 12 (2017): 924–25.

44. Fitzgerald, Simon, Xin Chen, Hui Qu, and Mira Grice Sheff. "Occupational Injury among Migrant Workers in China: A Systematic Review." *Injury Prevention* 19, no. 5 (2013): 348–54.

45. Mo, Jingfu, Lu Wang, William Au, and Min Su. "Prevalence of Coal Workers' Pneumoconiosis in China: A Systematic Analysis of 2001–2011 Studies." *International Journal of Hygiene and Environmental Health* 217, no. 1 (2014): 46–51.

46. Wang, Di, Caie Yang, Tieji Kuang, Hong Lei, Xianghong Meng, Aihua Tong, Jufang He, Ying Jiang, Fengjie Guo, and Mei Dong. "Prevalence of Multidrug and Extensively Drug-Resistant Tuberculosis in Beijing, China: A Hospital-Based Retrospective Study." *Japanese Journal of Infectious Diseases* 63, no. 5 (2010): 368–71.

47. He, T. J., Z. Lan, and T. Yumeng. "Analysis of the Prevalence of Major Chronic Diseases among the Floating Population in Hubei Province." *Chronic Diseases Prevention and Control of China* 24, no. 3 (2016): 175–78.

48. Shen, Xin, Kathryn DeRiemer, Z-An Yuan, M. Shen, Z. Xia, X. Gui, L. Wang, Qian Gao, and Jian Mei. "Drug-Resistant Tuberculosis in Shanghai, China, 2000–2006: Prevalence, Trends and Risk Factors." *The International Journal of Tuberculosis and Lung Disease* 13, no. 2 (2009): 253–59.

49. Wang, W., J. Wang, Q. Zhao, N. D. Darling, M. Yu, B. Zhou, and B. Xu. "Contribution of Rural-to-Urban Migration in the Prevalence of Drug Resistant Tuberculosis in China." *European Journal of Clinical Microbiology and Infectious Diseases* 30, no. 4 (2011): 581–86.

50. Jiang, Qi, Qingyun Liu, Lecai Ji, Jinli Li, Yaling Zeng, Liangguang Meng, Geyang Luo et al. "Citywide Transmission of Multidrug-resistant Tuberculosis Under China's Rapid Urbanization: A Retrospective Population-Based Genomic Spatial Epidemiological Study." *Clinical Infectious Diseases* 71, no. 1 (2020): 142–51.

51. Wang, Di, Caie Yang, Tieji Kuang, Hong Lei, Xianghong Meng, Aihua Tong, Jufang He, Ying Jiang, Fengjie Guo, and Mei Dong. "Prevalence of Multidrug and Extensively Drug-Resistant Tuberculosis in Beijing, China: A Hospital-Based Retrospective Study." *Japanese Journal of Infectious Diseases* 63, no. 5 (2010): 368–71.

52. Zhang, Lei, Eric P. F. Chow, Heiko J. Jahn, Alexander Kraemer, and David P. Wilson. "High HIV Prevalence and Risk of Infection among Rural-to-Urban Migrants in Various Migration Stages in China: A Systematic Review and Meta-analysis." *Sexually Transmitted Diseases* 40, no. 2 (2013): 136–47.

53. Zou, Xia, Eric P. F. Chow, Peizhen Zhao, Yong Xu, Li Ling, and Lei Zhang. "Rural-to-Urban Migrants Are at High Risk of Sexually Transmitted and Viral Hepatitis Infections in China: A Systematic Review and Meta-analysis." *BMC Infectious Diseases* 14, no. 1 (2014): 1–8.

54. Wei, Wang, Zhang Wei-Sheng, Alayi Ahan, Yan Ci, Zhang Wei-Wen, and Cao Ming-Qin. "The Characteristics of TB Epidemic and TB/HIV Co-infection Epidemic:

A 2007–2013 Retrospective Study in Urumqi, Xinjiang Province, China." *PloS One* 11, no. 10 (2016): e0164947.

55. Su, Lina, Long Sun, and Lingzhong Xu. "Review on the Prevalence, Risk Factors and Disease Management of Hypertension among Floating Population in China during 1990–2016." *Global Health Research and Policy* 3, no. 1 (2018): 24.

56. Guan, Ming. "Epidemiology of Hypertensive State among Chinese Migrants: Effects of Unaffordable Medical Care." *International Journal of Hypertension* 2018 (2018). https://www.hindawi.com/journals/ijhy/2018/5231048/abs/.

57. Zhao, Qi, Asli Kulane, Yi Gao, and Biao Xu. "Knowledge and Attitude on Maternal Health Care among Rural-to-Urban Migrant Women in Shanghai, China." *BMC Women's Health* 9, no. 1 (2009): 5.

58. Feng, Wang, Ping Ren, Zhan Shaokang, and Shen Anan. "Reproductive Health Status, Knowledge, and Access to Health Care among Female Migrants in Shanghai, China." *Journal of Biosocial Science* 37, no. 5 (2005): 603.

59. Hesketh, Therese, Ye Xue Jun, Li Lu, and Wang Hong Mei. "Health Status and Access to Health Care of Migrant Workers in China." *Public Health Reports* 123, no. 2 (2008): 189–97.

60. Li, Qiang, Gordon Liu, and Wenbin Zang. "The Health of Left-Behind Children in Rural China." *China Economic Review* 36 (2015): 367–76.

61. Ma, Sha, Minmin Jiang, Feng Wang, Jingjing Lu, Lu Li, and Therese Hesketh. "Left-Behind Children and Risk of Unintentional Injury in Rural China—A Cross-Sectional Survey." *International Journal of Environmental Research and Public Health* 16, no. 3 (2019): 403.

62. Hu, Hongwei, Jiamin Gao, Haochen Jiang, and Pingnan Xing. "A Comparative Study of Unintentional Injuries among Schooling Left-Behind, Migrant and Residential Children in China." *International Journal for Equity in Health* 17, no. 1 (2018): 47.

63. Li, Qiang, Gordon Liu, and Wenbin Zang, "The Health of Left-Behind Children in Rural China."

64. Sun, Meiping, Rui Ma, Yang Zeng, Fengji Luo, Jing Zhang, and Wenjun Hou. "Immunization Status and Risk Factors of Migrant Children in Densely Populated Areas of Beijing, China." *Vaccine* 28, no. 5 (2010): 1264–74.

65. Gao, Xiao-Li, Colman McGrath, and Huan-Cai Lin. "Oral Health Status of Rural–Urban Migrant Children in South China." *International Journal of Paediatric Dentistry* 21, no. 1 (2011): 58–67.

66. Li, Ling, and Hongqiao Fu. "China's Health Care System Reform: Progress and Prospects." *The International Journal of Health Planning and Management* 32, no. 3 (2017): 240–53.

67. Lu, Liping, Qi Jiang, Jianjun Hong, Xiaoping Jin, Qian Gao, Heejung Bang, Kathryn DeRiemer, and Chongguang Yang. "Catastrophic Costs of Tuberculosis Care in a Population with Internal Migrants in China." *BMC Health Services Research* 20, no 1. (2020): 1–9.

68. Hong, Yan, Xiaoming Li, Bonita Stanton, Danhua Lin, Xiaoyi Fang, Mao Rong, and Jing Wang. "Too Costly to Be Ill: Health Care Access and Health Seeking Behaviors among Rural-to-Urban Migrants in China." *World Health and Population* 8, no. 2 (2006): 22.

69. Wang, Nan Christine. "Understanding Antibiotic Overprescribing in China: A Conversation Analysis Approach." *Social Science and Medicine* 262 (2020): 113251.

70. Meng, Qingyue, Anne Mills, Longde Wang, and Qide Han. "What Can We Learn from China's Health System Reform?" *BMJ* 365 (2019): l2349.

Chapter 36

We wish to thank Dr. Yan (Ivy) Zhao (The Hong Kong Polytechnic University) for assistance in chapter formatting and reference editing.

1. Statistics New Zealand. "Migration Trends Report 2019." Wellington: Statistics New Zealand, 2020.

2. Ricci, Harris, Donna Cormack, Martin Tobias, Li-Chia Yeh, Natalie Talamaivao, Joanna Minster, and Roimata Timutimu. "Self-Reported Experience of Racial Discrimination and Health Care Use in New Zealand: Results from the 2006/07 New Zealand Health Survey." *American Journal of Public Health* 102, no. 5 (2012): 1012–19; Came, Heather, Claire Doole, and Brian McKenna. "Institutional Racism in Public Health Contracting: Findings of a Nationwide Survey from New Zealand." *Social Science and Medicine* 199 (2018): 132-9.

3. Ricci et al. "Self-Reported Experience of Racial Discrimination."

4. Ameratunga, Shanthi, Sandar Tin, Kumanan Rasanathan, Elizabeth Robinson, and Peter Watson. "Use of Health Care by Young Asian New Zealanders: Findings from a National Youth Health Survey." *Journal of Paediatrics and Child Health* 44, no. 11 (2008): 636–41; Scragg, Robert. "Asian Health in Aotearoa in 2006–2007: Trend since 2002–2003." Edited by Agency ANDHBS. Auckland: Auckland Northern District Health Board Support Agency, 2010; Kudakwashe, Tuwe. "African Communities in New Zealand: An Investigation of Their Employment Experiences and Impact on Their Wellbeing Using African Oral Tradition of Storytelling as a Research Methodology." Auckland: Auckland University of Technology, 2018; Kanengoni, Blessing, Sari Andajani-Sutjahjo, and Eleanor Holroyd. "Setting the Stage: Reviewing Current Knowledge on the Health of New Zealand Immigrants—an Integrative Review." *PeerJ* 6 (2018): e5184.

5. Immigration New Zealand. "Evidence of Good Health," 2020. https://www.immigration.govt.nz/new-zealand-visas/apply-for-a-visa/tools-and-information/medical-info/evidence-you-in-good-health.

6. Kanengoni et al., "Setting the Stage."

7. Kanengoni et al., "Setting the Stage."

8. Came, Heather, Dominic O'Sullivan, Jacquie Kidd, and Timothy McCreanor. "The Waitangi Tribunal's WAI 2575 Report: Implications for Decolonizing Health Systems." *Health and Human Rights* 22, no. 1 (2020): 209; Came, Heather, Dominic O'Sullivan, and T. McCreanor. "Introducing Critical Tiriti Policy Analysis through a Retrospective Review of the New Zealand Primary Health Care Strategy." *Ethnicities* 20, no. 3 (2020): 434–56.

9. Hoare, Karen J., Jane Mills, and Karen Francis. "The Role of Government Policy in Supporting Nurse-Led Care in General Practice in the United Kingdom, New Zealand and Australia: An Adapted Realist Review." *Journal of Advanced Nursing* 68, no. 5 (2012): 963–80.

10. Stats NZ. "National Ethnic Population Projections: 2013 (Base)–2038 (Update)," 2017. http://archive.stats.govt.nz/browse_for_stats/population/estimates_and _projections/NationalEthnicPopulationProjections_HOTP2013-2038.aspx.

11. Stats NZ, "National Ethnic Population Projections."

12. Zhou, Lifeng, Sue Lim, and Janine Pratt. "Asian Health Action Plan for Waitemata Dhb." Waitemata District Health Board, July 2010.

13. Zhou, Lifeng, and Samantha Bennett. "International Benchmarking of Asian Health Outcomes for Waitemata and Auckland Dhbs." Waitemata District Health Board, 2017.

14. Ministry of Health. "Adults Topic: Emergency Department Use," 2019. https:// minhealthnz.shinyapps.io/nz-health-survey-2017-18-annual-data-explorer/_w_0811 ceee/_w_67e825f2/_w_cc2512ca/#!/explore-topics.

15. Montayre, Jed, and Mu-Hsing Ho. "Factors Associated with ED Use Among New Asian Immigrants in New Zealand: A Cross-Sectional Analysis of Secondary Data." *Journal of Emergency Nursing* (2020).

16. Zhou, Lifeng. "Health Needs Assessment for Asian people in Waitemata." Waitemata District Health Board, 2009.

17. Montayre, Jed, Stephen Neville, and Eleanor Holroyd. "Moving Backwards, Moving Forward: The Experiences of Older Filipino Migrants Adjusting to Life in New Zealand." *International Journal of Qualitative Studies on Health and Well-being* 12, no. 1 (2017): 1347011.

18. Your Local Doctor. "An Enrolment Drive for Auckland's New Migrant Communities," 2020. https://www.yourlocaldoctor.co.nz/.

19. Neville, Stephen, and Jeffery Adams. "Views about HIV/STI and Health Promotion among Gay and Bisexual Chinese and South Asian Men Living in Auckland, New Zealand." *International Journal of Qualitative Studies on Health and Well-being* 11, no. 1 (2016): 30764.

20. Neville and Adam, "Views about HIV/STI and Health Promotion."

21. Adams, Jeffery, Rommel Coquilla, Jed Montayre, Eric Julian Manalastas, and Stephen Neville. "Views about HIV and Sexual Health among Gay and Bisexual Filipino Men Living in New Zealand." *International Journal of Health Promotion and Education* (2020): 1–12.

22. Martinez, Omar, Elwin Wu, Theo Sandfort, Brian Dodge, Alex Carballo-Dieguez, Rogeiro Pinto, Scott Rhodes, Eva Moya, and Silvia Chavez-Baray. "Evaluating the Impact of Immigration Policies on Health Status among Undocumented Immigrants: A Systematic Review." *Journal of Immigrant and Minority Health* 17, no. 3 (2015): 947–70.

23. Cheung, Gary. "Characteristics of Chinese Service Users in an Old Age Psychiatry Service in New Zealand." *Australasian Psychiatry* 18, no. 2 (2010): 152–57.

24. Cheung, "Characteristics of Chinese Service Users."

25. Connor, Jennie, Robyn Kydd, Kevin Shield, and Jurgen Rehm. "The Burden of Disease and Injury Attributable to Alcohol in New Zealanders under 80 Years of Age: Marked Disparities by Ethnicity and Sex." *New Zealand Medical Journal* 128, no. 1409 (2015): 15–28.

26. Statistics New Zealand. "Key Facts About Drinking in New Zealand," 2019. https://www.alcohol.org.nz/research-resources/nz-statistics.

27. Rasanathan, Kumanan, Shanthi Ameratunga, Janet Chen, and Elizabeth Robinson. "A Health Profile of Young Asian New Zealanders Who Attend Secondary School." *Adolescent Health* 116 (2006): U380.

28. Montayre, Jed, Jaden De-Arth, Jagamaya Shrestha-Ranjit, Stephen Neville, and Eleanor Holroyd. "Challenges and Adjustments in Maintaining Health and Well-Being of Older Asian Immigrants in New Zealand: An Integrative Review." *Australasian Journal on Ageing* 38, no. 3 (2019): 154–72.

29. Montayre, Jed, Stephen Neville, Valerie Wright-St. Clair, Eleanor Holroyd, and Jeffery Adams. "Older Filipino Immigrants' Reconfiguration of Traditional Filial Expectations: A Focus Ethnographic Study." *Contemporary Nurse* 56, no. 1 (2020): 1–13; Montayre, Jed, Stephen Neville, Valerie Wright-St. Clair, Eleanor Holroyd, and Jeffery Adams. "Late-Life Living and Care Arrangements of Older Filipino New Zealanders." *Journal of Clinical Nursing* 28, no. 3–4 (2019): 480–88.

30. Montayre et al., "Older Filipino Immigrants' Reconfiguration of Traditional Filial Expectations."

31. Montayre et al., "Late-Life Living and Care Arrangements of Older Filipino New Zealanders."

32. United Nations Population Division. "World Population Ageing 2020 Highlights," 2020. https://www.un.org/development/desa/pd/news/world-population-ageing-2020-highlights.

Chapter 37

1. Andrew, N. L., P. Bright, L. de la Rua, S. J. Teoh, and M. Vickers. "Coastal Proximity of Populations in 22 Pacific Island Countries and Territories." *PLoS One* 14, no. 9 (2019): e0223249.

2. Jackson, K. "Islands, Maps, Conflicts: The Recurring Relevance of Physical

Geography in the Asia Pacific." *Asia Pacific Business Review* 2, no. 4 (2019). https://doi.org/10.1080/13602381.2019.1686244.

3. Hau'ofa, E. "Our Sea of Islands." *Contemporary Pacific* 6, no. 1 (1994): 147–61.

4. Hugo, G., and R. Bedford. "Pacific Islands, Migration 18th Century to Present." In *The Encyclopedia of Global Human Migration*, edited by I. Ness. Hoboken, NJ: Wiley-Blackwell, 2013.

5. Hau'ofa, E. "Our Sea of Islands." In *A New Oceania: Rediscovering Our Sea of Islands*, edited by Vijay Naidu, Eric Waddell, and Epeli Hau'ofa. Suva: SSED (USP), 1993.

6. Voigt-Graf, C. "Pacific Islanders and the Rim: Linked By Migration." *Asian and Pacific Migration Journal* 16 (2007): 143–56.

7. ILO. *International Labour Migration Statistics: A Guide for Policymakers and Statistics Organizations in the Pacific*, 2015. http://www.ilo.org/wcmsp5/groups/public/---asia/---ro-bangkok/---ilo-suva/documents/publication/wcms_371837.pdf.

8. IOM. "Migration Data Portal," 2020. Accessed July 1, 2020. https://migrationdataportal.org/?i=stock_abs_&t=2019&m=2&sm49=61.

9. Hugo and Bedford, "Pacific Islands."

10. ILO, *International Labour Migration*.

11. Hugo and Bedford, "Pacific Islands."

12. Naidu, V., and L. Vaike. "Internal Migration in the Pacific Islands: A Regional Overview." *Journal of Pacific Studies* 35, no. 3 (2016): 91–110.

13. Nurse, L. A., R. F. McLean, J. Agard, L. P. Briguglio, V. Duvat-Magnan, N. Pelesikoti et al. "Small Islands." In *Climate Change 2014: Impacts, Adaptation, and Vulnerability*, Part B: Regional Aspects. Contribution of Working Group II to the Fifth Assessment Report of the Intergovernmental Panel on Climate Change, edited by V. R. Barros, C. B. Field, D. J. Dokken, M. D. Mastrandrea, K. J. Mach, T. E. Bilir et al., 1613–54. Cambridge, UK: Cambridge University Press, 2014.

14. ILO, *International Labour Migration*.

15. WHO. "Division of Pacific Technical Support," 2020. https://www.who.int/westernpacific/about/how-we-work/pacific-support/4.

16. Hugo and Bedford, "Pacific Islands."

17. IOM. *IOM in Asia and the Pacific 2017–2020*. Bangkok: International Organisation for Migration, 2017.

18. ILO, *International Labour Migration*.

19. IOM. *World Migration Report 2020*, 2020. https://publications.iom.int/system/files/pdf/wmr_2020.pdf.

20. Abubakar, I., R. Aldridge, D. Devakumar, M. Orcutt, R. Burns et al. "The UCL-Lancet Commission on Migration and Health: The Health of a World on the Move." *Lancet* 392 (2018): 2606–54.

21. Connell, J., and K. Petrou. *Pacific Labour Mobility*. Sydney: University of Sydney, 2019. http://pacificlabour.siteindev.com.au/wordpress-content-dir/uploads/2019/10/Pacific-Labour-Mobility-Towards-a-future-research-agenda.pdf.

22. Gamlen, A., W. Murray, and J. Overton. "Investigating Education, Migration and Development—Moving Triangles in the Pacific." *New Zealand Geographer* 73 (2017): 3–14.

23. World Bank. "Migration and Remittances Data," 2020. Accessed July 1, 2020. https://www.worldbank.org/en/topic/migrationremittancesdiasporaissues/brief/migration-remittances-data.

24. Brown, R. P. C., J. Connell, and E. Jiminez-Soto. "Migrants' Remittances, Poverty and Social Protection in the South Pacific: Fiji and Tonga." *Population, Space and Place* 20 (2014): 434–54.

25. Smith, R. "Changing Standards of Living: The Paradoxes of Building a Good Life in Rural Vanuatu." In *The Quest for the Good Life in Precarious Times: Ethnographic Perspectives on the Domestic Moral Economy*, edited by C. Gregory and J. Altman, 33–55. Canberra: ANU, 2018.

26. UN-Habitat. *Urbanization and Climate Change in Small Island Developing States*. Nairobi: UN-Habitat, 2015.

27. UN-Habitat, *Urbanization and Climate Change*.

28. ILO, *International Labour Migration*.

29. Naidu and Vaike, "Internal Migration in the Pacific Islands."

30. ADB. *The Emergence of Pacific Urban Villages: Urbanization Trends in the Pacific Islands*. Manila: Asian Development Bank, 2016.

31. ADB, *The Emergence of Pacific Urban Villages*.

32. Schrecongost, A., et al. "Delivering Water and Sanitation to Melanesian Informal Settlements: Preliminary Findings of a Review of WASH Services in Informal Settlements of the Melanesian Region." *Journal of the Australian Water Association* 42, no. 3 (2015): 40–43.

33. Getahun, A., A. Batikawai, D. Nand, S. Khan, A. Sahukhan, and D. Faktaufon. "Dengue in Fiji: Epidemiology of the 2014 DENV-3 Outbreak." *Western Pacific Surveillance and Response Journal* 10, no. 2 (2019). https://doi.org/10.5365/wpsar .2018.9.3.001.

34. Gero, A., J. Kohlitz, and J. Willetts. "Informal Settlements in the Pacific and Links to Sustainable Development." *Development Bulletin* 78 (2017): 91–96. https:// opus.lib.uts.edu.au/handle/10453/118057.

35. WHO. *Human Health and Climate Change in Pacific Island Countries*, 2015.

36. Gero et al., Informal Settlements in the Pacific.".

37. UN-Habitat, *Urbanization and Climate Change*.

38. Kuruppu, N. "Turning the Tide on Urbanisation Policy in the Pacific Islands." United Nations University, October 20, 2016. https://unu.edu/publications/articles /urbanisation-in-pacific-islands.html.

39. Naidu and Vaike, "Internal Migration in the Pacific Islands."

40. World Bank. "World Urbanization Prospects: 2018 Revision," 2018. Accessed July 1, 2020. https://data.worldbank.org/indicator/SP.URB.TOTL.IN.ZS?locations=NR.

41. UN-Habitat. "5th Pacific Urban Forum Summary Report," 2019. Accessed July 1, 2020. https://www.fukuoka.unhabitat.org/info/news/pdf/PUF5_Summary_Re port.pdf.

42. Day, S., T. Forster, J. Himmelsbach, L. Korte, P. Mucke et al. *World Risk Report 2019*, 2019. https://reliefweb.int/sites/reliefweb.int/files/resources/WorldRisk Report-2019_Online_english.pdf.

43. IOM, *IOM in Asia and the Pacific*.

44. Shultz, J. M., J. Russell, and Z. Espinel. "Epidemiology of Tropical Cyclones: The Dynamics of Disaster, Disease, and Development." *Epidemiologic Reviews* 27, no. 1 (2005): 21–35; WHO, *Human Health and Climate Change*.

45. WHO. "Outbreak Surveillance and Response Priorities for Mitigating the Health Impact of Disaster." Tenth Pacific health ministers meeting, agenda item 9, 2013. www.wpro.who.int/southpacific/pic_meeting/2013/documents/PHMM_PIC10 _9_Outbreak.

46. IOM, *IOM in Asia and the Pacific*; IOM, *World Migration Report 2020*.

47. Uscher-Pines, L. "Health Effects of Relocation Following Disaster: A Systematic Review of the Literature." *Disasters* 33, no. 1 (2009): 1–22.

48. ILO. *Climate Change and Migration Issues in the Pacific*. Fiji: United Nations Economic and Social Commission for Asia and the Pacific, 2014.

49. McMichael, C., M. Katonivualiku, and T. Powell. "Planned Relocation and Everyday Agency in Low-Lying Coastal Villages in Fiji." *The Geographical Journal* 185, no. 3 (2019), 325–27.

50. Lee, H., and S. T. Francis. *Migration and Transnationalism: Pacific Perspectives*. Canberra: ANU, 2009.

51. WHO. *Universal Health Coverage: Moving Towards Better Health—Action Framework for the Western Pacific Region*. Manila: WHO Regional Office for the Western Pacific, 2016. https://iris.wpro.who.int/handle/10665.1/13371.

52. WHO. *Regional Action Agenda on Achieving the Sustainable Development Goals in the Western Pacific*. Manila: WHO Regional Office for the Western Pacific, 2017.

53. WHO. *Regional Framework for Urban Health in the Western Pacific 2016–2020: Healthy and Resilient Cities*. Manila: WHO Regional Office for the Western Pacific, 2016.

54. WHO, *Human Health and Climate Change*.

55. IOM, *IOM in Asia and the Pacific*.

56. Abubakar et al., "The UCL-Lancet Commission on Migration and Health."

Chapter 38

1. Mattia Mazzolii, Boris Diechtiareff, Antònia Tugores, William Wives, Natalia Adler, Pere Colet, and José J. Ramasco. "Migrant Mobility Flows Characterized

with Digital Data," *PLoS One* 15, no. 3 (2020). https://doi.org/10.1371/journal.pone .0230264.

2. United Nations Department of Economic and Social Affairs, Population Division, "The World Counted 258 Million International Migrants in 2017, Representing 3.4 per Cent of Global Population," *Popfacts*, no. 5 (2017): 1–4.

3. Economic Commission for Latin America and the Caribbean (ECLAC), *Social Panorama of Latin America, United Nations*, 2019.

4. Adela Pellegrino, *La Migración Internacional En América Latina y El Caribe: Tendencias y Perfiles de Los Migrantes, Migración Internacional: Serie Población y Desarrollo*, 2003.

5. Abraham F. Lowenthal and Felix Mostajo, "Estados Unidos de América Latina, 1960-2010: De La Pretensión Hegemonica a las Relaciones Diversas y Complejas," *Foro Internacional* (2010).

6. World Bank, "The New Wave of Globalization and Its Economic Effects," *Globalization, Growth and Poverty: Building an Inclusive World Economy* (2002): 23–52.

7. Pellegrino, *La Migración Internacional*.

8. Gloria Marcela Gómez Builes, Gilberto Mauricio Astaiza Arias, and Maria Cecília de Souza Minayo, "Las migraciones forzadas por la violencia: el caso de Colombia," *Ciência & Saúde Coletiva* 13, no. 5 (October 2008): 1649–60. https://doi .org/10.1590/S1413-81232008000500028.

9. IDMC, "Global Report on Internal Displacement Summary GRID 2019," *Internal Displacement Monitoring Centre*, no. 5 (2019): 16.

10. UNHCR, "Venezuela Situation," accessed December 7, 2020. https://www .unhcr.org/venezuela-emergency.html.

11. UN Refugee Agency, "Situación Venezuela," 2020.

12. Inter-American Development Bank, "Migrants in Latin America: Disparities in Health Status and in Access to Healthcare," accessed July 15, 2021. https:// publications.iadb.org/publications/english/document/Migrants-in-Latin-America -Disparities-in-Health-Status-and-in-Access-to-Healthcare.pdf.

13. UNHCR, "Venezuela Situation."

14. Francisco Javier Sánchez Chacón, "La Frontera Táchira (Venezuela)-Norte de Santander (Colombia) en Las Relaciones Bi-Nacionales y en la Integración Regional," *Revista de Estudios Transfronterizos* 11, no. 1 (2011): 63–84.

15. William Mejía Ochoa, "Colombia y Las Migraciones Internacionales: Evolución Reciente y Panorama Actual a Partir de Las Cifras," *Revista Interdisciplinar Da Mobilidade Humana* 20, no. 39 (2012): 185–210. https://doi.org/10.1590 /s1980-85852012000200010.

16. Pellegrino, *La Migración Internacional*.

17. Pellegrino, *La Migración Internacional*.

18. Tomás Milton Muñoz Bravo, "Políticas Migratorias En México y Venezuela: Análisis de Respuestas Gubernamentales Disímiles Ante Procesos de Inmigración

y Emigración Internacionales," *Desafíos* 28, no. 1 (2016): 333–66. https://doi.org /10.12804/desafios28.2.2016.09; Anitza Freitez, "La Emigración Desde Venezuela Durante La Última Década," *Temas de Coyuntura* 63 (Julio 2011): 11–38.

19. Manuel Felipe García Arias and Jair Eduardo Restrepo Pineda, "Aproximación al Proceso Migratorio Venezolano En El Siglo XXI," *Hallazgos* (2019). https://doi.org/10.15332/2422409x.5000.

20. Julían Fernandez-Niño and Karen Luna-Orozco, "Migración Venezolana En Colombia: Retos En Salud Pública," *Revista de La Universidad Industrial de Santander. Salud* 50, no. 1 (2018): 5–6; Claudia Vargas, "La Migración En Venezuela Como Dimensión de La Crisis," *Pensamiento Propio*, no. 47 (2018): 91–128; Julián Alfredo Fernández-Niño et al., "Necesidades Percibidas de Salud Por Los Migrantes Desde Venezuela En El Asentamiento de Villa Caracas—Barranquilla, 2018: Reporte de Caso En Salud Pública," *Revista de La Universidad Industrial de Santander. Salud* 50, no. 3 (2018): 269–76. https://doi.org/10.18273/revsal.v50n3 -2018002; Tomás Castillo Crasto and Mercedes Reguant Álvarez, "Percepciones Sobre La Migración Venezolana: Causas, España Como Destino, Expectativas de Retorno," *Migraciones* 41, no. 41 (2017): 133–63. https://doi.org/10.14422/mig.i41 .y2017.006.

21. Consejo Nacional De Política Económica y Social, "Estrategia Para La Atención de La Migración Desde Venezuela," 2018.

22. Migración Colombia, "Venezolanos En Colombia: 30 Junio de 2020," 2020.

23. Juan Thomas Ordóñez and Hugo Eduardo Ramírez Arcos, "National Dis-(Order): The Construction of Venezuelan Migration as a Public Health and Security Threat in Colombia," *Revista Ciencias de La Salud* 17, special issue (2019): 48–68. https://doi.org/10.12804/revistas.urosario.edu.co/revsalud/a.8119.

24. Ordóñez and Ramírez Arcos, "National Dis(Order)"; Migración Colombia, "Venezolanos En Colombia."

25. Dan Biswas, Brigit Toebes, Anders Hjern, Henry Ascher, and Marie Norredam. "Access to Health Care for Undocumented Migrants from a Human Rights Perspective: A Comparative Study of Denmark, Sweden, and the Netherlands," *Health and Human Rights* (2012).

26. Esther Pineda and Keymer Avila, "Aproximaciones a La Migración Colombo-Venezolana: Desigualdad, Prejuicio y Vulnerabilidad," *Revista Misión Jurídica* (2019): 59–78.

27. Pineda and Avila, "Aproximaciones a La Migración Colombo-Venezolana."

28. UN Refugee Agency, "Situación Venezuela."

29. Organización Internacional para las Migraciones, "Migración y Migrantes: Características y Novedades Regionales," *Informe Sobre Las Migraciones En El Mundo 2020* (2019): 67–165.

30. Martha Ardila and Diana Rengifo, "Colombia y La Migración Andina: Contexto, Cambios y Necesidades" *Grupo países vecinos* (2006).

31. Organización Internacional para las Migraciones, "Migración y Migrantes."

32. Agencia de las Naciones Unidas para los Refugiados, "Emergencia En

Venezuela: Crisis de Refugiados y Migrantes," 2020; Organización Internacional para las Migraciones, "Migración y Migrantes."

33. Agencia de las Naciones Unidas para los Refugiados, "Situación En Venezuela," 2019.

34. UNHCR and ACNUR, "Aspectos Claves Del Monitoreo de Protección. Situación de Venezuela: Enero–Junio 2019," 2019. https://www.acnur.org/5d321d124.pdf.

35. Stefano Farné and Cristian Sanín, *Panorama Laboral de Los Migrantes Venezolanos En Colombia 2014–2019* (Bogotá: Universidad Externado de Colombia 2020).

36. Farné and Sanín, *Panorama Laboral de Los Migrantes Venezolanos.*

37. Farné and Sanín, *Panorama Laboral de Los Migrantes Venezolanos.*

38. Farné and Sanín, *Panorama Laboral de Los Migrantes Venezolanos.*

39. UNHCR and ACNUR, "Refugiados y Migrantes de Venezuela Durante La Crisis Del COVID-19: Según Aumentan Las Necesidades, Son Esenciales Más Medidas Inclusivas y Ayuda," 2020.

40. Agencia de las Naciones Unidas para los Refugiados, "Situación En Venezuela."

41. Organización Internacional para las Migraciones, "Reflexiones Sobre Las Contribuciones de Los Migrantes En Una Era de Creciente Disrupción y Desinformación," *Informe Sobre Las Migraciones En El Mundo 2020* (2019); Organización Internacional para las Migraciones, "Migración, Inclusión y Cohesion Social: Retos, Novedades Recientes y Oportunidades," *Informe Sobre Las Migraciones En El Mundo 2020* (2019): 211–57.

42. Alfonso J. Rodríguez-Morales, D. Katherine Bonilla-Aldana, Miguel Morales, José A. Suárez, and Ernesto Martínez-Buitrago, "Migration Crisis in Venezuela and its Impact on HIV in Other Countries: The Case of Colombia," *Annals of Clinical Microbiology and Antimicrobials* 18, no. 9 (2019). https://doi.org/10.1186/s12941-019-0310-4.

43. Irina Maljkovic Berry, Wiriya Rutvisuttinunt, Rachel Sippy, Efrain Beltran-Ayala, Katherine Figueroa, Sadie Ryan, Abhinaya Srikanth, Anna M. Stewart-Ibarra, Timothy Endy, and Richard G. Jarman, "The Origins of Dengue and Chikungunya Viruses in Ecuador Following Increased Migration from Venezuela and Colombia," *BMC Evolutionary Biology* 20, no. 31 (2020). https://doi.org/10.1186/s12862-020-1596-8.

44. Rodríguez-Morales et al., "Migration Crisis in Venezuela."

45. Jaime R. Torres and Julio S. Castro, "Venezuela's Migration Crisis: A Growing Health Threat to the Region Requiring Immediate Attention," *Journal of Travel Medicine* 26, no. 2 (2019). https://doi.org/10.1093/jtm/tay141.

46. K. Rebolledo-Ponietsky, C. V. Munayco, and E. Mezones-Holguín, "Migration Crisis in Venezuela: Impact on HIV in Peru," *Journal of Travel Medicine* 26, no. 2 (2019). https://doi.org/10.1093/jtm/tay155; Torres and Castro, "Venezuela's Migration Crisis."

47. Ministerio de Salud y Protección Social, "Población Venezolana En Colombia," 2019, 10–12.

48. Julián Alfredo Fernández-Nino and Ietza Bojorquez-Chapela, "Migration of Venezuelans to Colombia," *Lancet* 392, no. 10152 (2018): 1013–14. https://doi .org/10.1016/S0140-6736(18)31828-2.

49. Rebolledo-Ponietsky et al., "Migration Crisis in Venezuela."

50. Ietza Bojorquez-Chapela et al., "Health Policies for International Migrants: A Comparison between Mexico and Colombia," *Health Policy OPEN* 1 (2020). https://doi.org/10.1016/j.hpopen.2020.100003.

51. Alejandra Carrillo Roa, "O Sistema de Saúde Na Venezuela: Um Paciente Sem Remédio?," *Cadernos de Saude Publica* 34, no. 3 (2018). https://doi.org/10.1590 /0102-311x00058517.

52. Asociación Civil de Planificación Familia, "Informe Sobre Venezuela Asociación Civil de Planificación Familiar," 2016.

53. Roa, "O Sistema de Saúde Na Venezuela."

54. Asociación Civil de Planificación Familia, "Informe Sobre Venezuela Asociación Civil de Planificación Familiar."

55. Asociación Civil de Planificación Familia, "Informe Sobre Venezuela Asociación Civil de Planificación Familiar."

56. Dulce K. Ramírez-López et al., "Vulnerabilidad, Derechos Sexuales y Reproductivos de Mujeres Centroamericanas Residentes En Dos Comunidades de La Zona Rural de Tapachula, Chiapas, México," *Papeles de Poblacion* 18, no. 72 (2012): 113–45.

57. Profamilia and International Planned Parenhood Federation (IPPF), "Evaluación de las necesidades insatisfechas en salud sexual y reproductiva de la población migrante venezolana en cuatro ciudades de la frontera colombo-venezolana: Arauca, Cúcuta, Riohacha y Valledupar," 2019. https://profamilia.org.co/wp-content /uploads/2019/05/LIBRO-Evaluacion-de-las-necesidades-insatisfechas-SSR-y-Mi grantes-Venezolanos-Digital.pdf.

58. Ministerio de Salud y Protección Social, "Plan de Respuesta Del Sector Salud al Fenómeno Migratorio," 2018.

59. Ministerio de Salud y Protección Social, "Plan de Respuesta Del Sector Salud al Fenómeno Migratorio."

60. Ministerio de Salud y Protección Social, "Plan de Respuesta Del Sector Salud al Fenómeno Migratorio."

61. Economic Commission for Latin America and the Caribbean (ECLAC), *Migración y Desarrollo Sostenible: La Centralidad de Los Derechos Humanos. Textos Seleccionados 2008–2019*, 2019.

Chapter 39

1. Worldometer, "Population of Southern Asia," 2020, https://www.worldometers .info/world-population/southern-asia-population/.

2. S. Irudaya Rajan, *South Asia Migration Report 2020 : Exploitation, Entrepreneurship and Engagement* (Oxford: Routledge India, 2020).

3. Vazira Zamindar, "India–Pakistan Partition 1947 and Forced Migration," in *The Encyclopedia of Global Human Migration* (London: Blackwell, 2013).

4. Anchita Borthakur, "Afghan Refugees: The Impact on Pakistan," *Asian Affairs* 48, no. 3 (2017): 488–509.

5. D. A. Kronenfeld, "Afghan Refugees in Pakistan: Not All Refugees, Not Always in Pakistan, Not Necessarily Afghan?," *Journal of Refugee Studies* 21, no. 1 (2008): 43–63.

6. Azeem Ibrahim and Muhammad Yunus, *The Rohingyas: Inside Myanmar's Genocide* (Oxford: C. Hurst and Co., 2018).

7. Ginu Zacharia Oommen, "South Asia–Gulf Migratory Corridor: Emerging Patterns, Prospects and Challenges," *Migration and Development* 5, no. 3 (2015): 394–412.

8. Pierre Centlivres and Micheline Centlivres-Demont, "The Afghan Refugee in Pakistan: An Ambiguous Identity," *Journal of Refugee Studies* 1, no. 2 (1988): 141–52.

9. Sarah Kenyon Lischer, *Dangerous Sanctuaries: Refugee Camps, Civil War, and the Dilemmas of Humanitarian Aid* (Ithaca: Cornell University Press, 2005).

10. Sabyasachi Basu Ray Chaudhury and Ranabir Samaddar, *The Rohingya in South Asia: People Without a State*, 1st ed. (Milton: Routledge, Taylor and Francis, 2018).

11. Muhammad Abbas Khan, "Pakistan's Urban Refugees: Steps towards Self-Reliance," *Forced Migration Review*, no. 63 (2020): 50–52.

12. Lifespan, "Refugee Medical Aid with Immediate, Lifelong Impact," 2020, https://www.lifespan.org/centers-services/infectious-diseases/global-and-local-health -programs/refugee-medical-aid-immediate.

13. M. J. Toole and R. J. Waldman, "Prevention of Excess Mortality in Refugee and Displaced Populations in Developing Countries," *JAMA : Journal of the American Medical Association* 263, no. 24 (1990): 3296–302.

14. Muhammad Suleman Malik, Muhammad Afzal, Alveena Farid, Fati Ullah Khan, Bushra Mirza, and Mohammad Tahir Waheed, "Disease Status of Afghan Refugees and Migrants in Pakistan," *Frontiers in Public Health* 7 (2019).

15. UNAIDSWHO, "UNAIDSWHO Working Group on Global HIV/AIDS and STI Surveillance Myanmar: HIV/AIDS Updates," 2004, https://data.unaids .org/publications/fact-sheets01/myanmar_en.pdf.

16. Md Mahbub Hossain, Abida Sultana, Hoimonty Mazumder, and Munzur-E-Murshid, "Sexually Transmitted Infections among Rohingya Refugees in Bangladesh," *Lancet HIV* 5, no. 7 (2018): E342.

17. K. M. Amran Hossain, Lori M. Walton, S. M. Yasir Arafat, Nidiorin Maybee, Rubel Hossen Sarker, Shahoriar Ahmed, and Feroz Kabir, "Expulsion from the Motherland: Association between Depression & Health-Related Quality of Life for Ethnic Rohingya Living with Refugee Status in Bangladesh," *Clinical Practice and Epidemiology in Mental Health* 16 (2020): 46–52; Save the Children, "Over

80,000 Refugee Children in Cox's Bazar Suffering from Severe Mental Health Issues," August 25, 2019, https://www.savethechildren.org.uk/news/media-centre/press-releases/80000-refugee-children-coxsbazar-mental-health-issues.

18. Bernadette Rosbrook and Robert D. Schweitzer, "The Meaning of Home for Karen and Chin Refugees from Burma: An Interpretative Phenomenological Approach," *European Journal of Psychotherapy and Counselling* 12, no. 2 (2010): 159–72.

19. Marie Jahoda, *Marienthal: The Sociography of an Unemployed Community* (Chicago: Aldine, Atherton, 1971).

20. Andrew Riley, Andrea Varner, Peter Ventevogel, Hasan Taimur, and Courtney Welton-Mitchell, "Daily Stressors, Trauma Exposure, and Mental Health among Stateless Rohingya Refugees in Bangladesh," *Transcultural Psychiatry* 54, no. 3 (2017): 304–31; Silvia Guglielmi, Nicola Jones, Jennifer Muz, Sarah Baird, Khadija Mitu, and Muhammad Ala Uddin, "'How Will My Life Be?': Psychosocial Well-Being among Rohingya and Bangladeshi Adolescents in Cox's Bazar," GAGE, 2020.

21. Jutta Lindert, Mauro Giovanni Carta, Ingo Schäfer, and Richard F. Mollica, "Refugees Mental Health—A Public Mental Health Challenge," *European Journal of Public Health* 26, no. 3 (2016): 374–75.

22. Roselinde Den Boer, "Liminal Space in Protracted Exile: The Meaning of Place in Congolese Refugees' Narratives of Home and Belonging in Kampala," *Journal of Refugee Studies* 28, no. 4 (2015): 486–504.

23. Nicholas Kristof, "I Saw a Genocide in Slow Motion," *New York Times*, March 2, 2018, https://www.nytimes.com/2018/03/02/opinion/i-saw-a-genocide-in-slow-motion.html; Syed S. Mahmood, Emily Wroe, Arlan Fuller, and Jennifer Leaning, "The Rohingya People of Myanmar: Health, Human Rights, and Identity," *Lancet* 389, no. 10081 (2017): 1841–50.

24. Abhishek Bhatia, Ayesha Mahmud, Arlan Fuller, and Rebecca Shin, "The Rohingya in Cox's Bazar," *Health and Human Rights* 20, no. 2 (2018): 105–22.

25. Ronald J. Waldman and William Newbrander, "Afghanistan's Health System: Moving Forward in Challenging Circumstances 2002–2013," *Global Public Health* 9, no. sup1 (2014): S1–5.

26. Willem van de Put, "Addressing Mental Health in Afghanistan," *Lancet* 360 (2002): S41–42.

27. Adnan A. Hyder, Zarin Noor, and Emma Tsui, "Intimate Partner Violence among Afghan Women Living in Refugee Camps in Pakistan," *Social Science and Medicine* 64, no. 7 (2007): 1536–47.

28. Jeanne Ward, "If Not Now, When? Addressing Gender-Based Violence in Refugee, Internally Displaced, and Post-Conflict Settings," Reproductive Health for Refugees Consortium, 2002, https://www.womensrefugeecommission.org/research-resources/if-not-now-when-addressing-gender-based-violence-in-refugee-internally-displaced-and-post/.

29. Farzana Islam, Mohiuddin Hussain Khan, Masako Ueda, N. M. Robiul

Awal Chowdhurry, Salim Mahmud Chowdhury, Mshauri David Delem, and Aminur Rahman, "724 Situation of Sexual and Gender Based Violence among the Rohingya Migrants Residing in Bangladesh," *Injury Prevention* 22 (2016): A260; Mahasti Khakpour and Hassan Vatanparast, "Afghan Refugees in Karachi: Food Insecurity of Protracted Refugee Households," *South Asia@LSE* (blog), November 18, 2019, https://blogs.lse.ac.uk/southasia/2019/11/18/afghan-refugees-in-karachi -food-insecurity-of-protracted-refugee-households/.

30. Islam et al., "724 Situation of Sexual and Gender Based Violence"; Hidayet Siddikoglu, "Pakistan's Inconsistent Refugee Policy: Identity and Cultural Crisis for Afghan Refugees in Pakistan," GPM Migration Policy Institute, January 1, 2016.

31. Linda A. Bartlett, Denise J. Jamieson, Tila Kahn, and Munawar Sultana, "Maternal Mortality among Afghan Refugees in Pakistan, 1999–2000," *Lancet* 359, no. 9307 (2002): 643–49.

32. Khakpour and Vatanparast, "Afghan Refugees in Karachi."

33. Toby Leslie, Harpakash Kaur, Nasir Mohammed, Kate Kolaczinski, Rosalynn L. Ord, and Mark Rowland, "Epidemic of Plasmodium Falciparum Malaria Involving Substandard Antimalarial Drugs, Pakistan, 2003," *Emerging Infectious Diseases* 15, no. 11 (2009): 1753–59.

34. Malik et al., "Disease Status of Afghan Refugees and Migrants in Pakistan."

35. Malik et al., "Disease Status of Afghan Refugees and Migrants in Pakistan."

36. Sohail Jannesari, Stephani Hatch, and Siân Oram, "Seeking Sanctuary: Rethinking Asylum and Mental Health," *Epidemiology and Psychiatric Sciences* 29 (2020): E154.

37. Evan Easton-Calabria, "Warriors of Self-Reliance: The Instrumentalization of Afghan Refugees in Pakistan," *Journal of Refugee Studies* 33, no. 1 (2020): 143–66.

38. Elizabeth A. Rowley, Gilbert M. Burnham, and Rabbin M. Drabe, "Protracted Refugee Situations: Parallel Health Systems and Planning for the Integration of Services," *Journal of Refugee Studies* 19, no. 2 (2006): 158–86.

39. Muhammed Aasim Yusuf, Fahad Hussain, Faisal Sultan, and Farhana Badar, "Cancer Care in Times of Conflict: Cross Border Care in Pakistan of Patients from Afghanistan," *Ecancermedicalscience* 14 (2020): 1018.

40. Brett Moore, "Refugee Settlements and Sustainable Planning," *Forced Migration Review*, no. 55 (2017): 5–6.

41. Patricia Gossman and Saroop Ijaz, "'What Are You Doing Here?' Police Abuses against Afghans in Pakistan," Human Rights Watch, 2015, 37.

42. Bill Frelick, "India Can't Mistreat Refugees By Not Signing Refugee Convention," Human Rights Watch, September 24, 2017, https://www.hrw.org/news/2017 /09/25/india-cant-mistreat-refugees-not-signing-refugee-convention; Hanne Sofie Lindahl, "The Legal Status of Afghan Refugees in Pakistan: Beyond Decades of 'Generosity' and 'Hospitality,'" 2020, http://hdl.handle.net/10852/79188.

43. Issa Ibrahim Berchin, Isabela Blasi Valduga, Jéssica Garcia, and Salgueirinho Osório de Andrade Guerra, "Climate Change and Forced Migrations: An Effort towards Recognizing Climate Refugees," *Geoforum* 84 (2017): 147–50.

Chapter 40

1. Lisa M. Sullivan and Sandro Galea. 2019. *Teaching Public Health*. Baltimore: Johns Hopkins University Press.

2. Sandro Galea, Catherine Ettman, and Muhammad Zaman. 2022. *Migration and Health*. Chicago: University of Chicago Press.

3. Veronica Boix Mansilla. 2020. *The Re-Imagining Migration Guide to Creating Curriculum: A Planning Tool to Support Quality Teaching for a World on the Move*. https://reimaginingmigration.org/guide-to-creating-curriculum/.

4. Boix Mansilla, *The Re-Imagining Migration Guide to Creating Curriculum*.

5. Boix Mansilla, *The Re-Imagining Migration Guide to Creating Curriculum*.

6. Boix Mansilla, *The Re-Imagining Migration Guide to Creating Curriculum*.

7. Boix Mansilla, *The Re-Imagining Migration Guide to Creating Curriculum*.

8. Boix Mansilla, *The Re-Imagining Migration Guide to Creating Curriculum*.

9. James M. Shultz, Lisa M. Sullivan, and Sandro Galea. 2021. *Public Health: An Introduction to the Science and Practice of Population Health*. New York: Springer.

10. Galea et al., *Migration and Health*.

11. Galea et al., *Migration and Health*.

12. Galea et al., *Migration and Health*.

13. Boix Mansilla, *The Re-Imagining Migration Guide to Creating Curriculum*.

14. Boix Mansilla, *The Re-Imagining Migration Guide to Creating Curriculum*.

15. Boix Mansilla, *The Re-Imagining Migration Guide to Creating Curriculum*.

16. Boix Mansilla, *The Re-Imagining Migration Guide to Creating Curriculum*.

17. Boix Mansilla, *The Re-Imagining Migration Guide to Creating Curriculum*.

18. Galea et al., *Migration and Health*.

Chapter 41

1. Maria Nicola, Zaid Alsafi Catrin Sohrabi, Ahmed Kerwan, Ahmed Al-Jabir, Christos Iosifidis, Maliha Agha, and RiazAgha. "The Socio-economic Implications of the Coronavirus Pandemic (COVID-19): A Review," *International Journal of Surgery* 78 (2020): 185–93. https://doi.org/10.1016/j.ijsu.2020.04.018.

2. Rodrik, Dani. "Will COVID 19 Remake the World?," *Project Syndicate*, April 6, 2020. https://www.project-syndicate.org/commentary/will-covid19-remake -the-world-by-dani-rodrik-2020-04?barrier=accesspaylog.

3. Safi, Michael. "Revealed: 46M Displaced People Excluded from Covid Jab Programmes," *Guardian*, May 7, 2021. https://www.theguardian.com/world/2021/may /07/at-least-46m-displaced-people-excluded-from-covid-jabs-who-study-shows.

Index

Page numbers in italics refer to figures and tables.